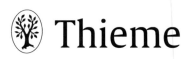

Color Atlas of Dental Hygiene

Periodontology

Herbert F. Wolf
Thomas M. Hassell

Forewords by Gail L. Aamodt
and Susan J. Jenkins

1174 Ilustrations

Thieme
Stuttgart · New York

Color Atlas of Dental Hygiene—Periodontology

Authors—*Periodontology*:

Dr. Herbert F. Wolf
Private Practitioner—Periodontics SSO/SSP
Löwenstrasse 55/57, 8001 Zurich
Switzerland
Email: herbert.wolf@bluewin.ch

Dr. Thomas M. Hassell
Professor, D. D. S., Dr. med. dent., Ph. D.
Associate Vice Chancellor for Research and Dean of
Graduate Studies
North Carolina A&T State University
Greensboro, NC
Email: thomashassell@aol.com

Important note: Medicine is an ever-changing science undergoing continual development. Research and clinical experience are continually expanding our knowledge, in particular our knowledge of proper treatment and drug therapy. Insofar as this book mentions any dosage or application, readers may rest assured that the authors, editors, and publishers have made every effort to ensure that such references are in accordance with **the state of knowledge at the time of production of the book.**

Nevertheless, this does not involve, imply, or express any guarantee or responsibility on the part of the publishers in respect to any dosage instructions and forms of applications stated in the book. **Every user is requested to examine carefully** the manufacturers' leaflets accompanying each drug and to check, if necessary in consultation with a physician or specialist, whether the dosage schedules mentioned therein or the contraindications stated by the manufacturers differ from the statements made in the present book. Such examination is particularly important with drugs that are either rarely used or have been newly released on the market. Every dosage schedule or every form of application used is entirely at the user's own risk and responsibility. The authors and publishers request every user to report to the publishers any discrepancies or inaccuracies noticed. If errors in this work are found after publication, errata will be posted at www.thieme.com on the product description page.

Some of the product names, patents, and registered designs referred to in this book are in fact registered trademarks or proprietary names even though specific reference to this fact is not always made in the text. Therefore, the appearance of a name without designation as proprietary is not to be construed as a representation by the publisher that it is in the public domain.

© 2006 Georg Thieme Verlag,
Rüdigerstraße 14, 70469 Stuttgart,
Germany
http://www.thieme.de
Thieme New York, 333 Seventh Avenue,
New York, NY 10001, USA
http://www.thieme.com

Typesetting by primustype Hurler GmbH,
Notzingen
Printed by Grammlich, Pliezhausen

ISBN-10: 3-13-141761-7 (GTV)
ISBN-13: 978-3-13-141761-9 (GTV)
ISBN-10: 1-58890-440-7 (TNY)
ISBN-13: 978-1-58890-440-9 (TNY)   1 2 3 4 5

Preface

We are pleased to present *Color Atlas of Dental Hygiene—Periodontology,* a new book dedicated exclusively to practicing dental hygienists, dental hygiene educators, and students in dental hygiene education and training programs.

For many decades, periodontics has been the most prominent aspect of the clinical practice of dental hygiene. Calculus removal has been a primary goal of each patient appointment; indeed, the ability to physically remove subgingival calculus remains still today the *sine qua non* of virtually all Dental Hygiene State Board examinations. Many excellent textbooks have been published over the years to teach successful mechanical instrumentation. Manufacturers of dental hand instruments – scalers and curettes – each year introduce innovative and sometimes even fanciful designs touted to improve calculus removal. Manufacturers have also given the dental hygiene profession powerful tools such as sonic and ultrasonic scalers, air scalers and powder-water spray devices; again, to better or more efficiently clean tooth surfaces.

But the turn of the century seemed an appropriate opportunity to freshly analyze the role of periodontics in the profession of dental hygiene, to ascertain new realities, and to define new goals for the profession. Our intent was to integrate new and relevant scientific and clinical knowledge into daily professional practice. We know now that this effort is leading rapidly – world wide – to total paradigm shifts within dental practice generally and dental hygiene in particular. In only the past ten years, progress in periodontology has accelerated exponentially! This has been the result of teamwork, by teams including clinicians, biologists, behavioral scientists, epidemiologists, and specialists from many medical disciplines.

We now know that inflammatory periodontal diseases today represent some of the most widespread health problems in the world. The effects of periodontal diseases upon general systemic health are becoming clearer almost daily. For any dental hygienist to ignore – or be ignorant of – these now obvious medical/dental interrelationships is simply unacceptable.

Therefore, this new book emphasizes a much broader spectrum of new dental and medical knowledge, targeted especially for the dental hygienist. Chapter presentations include:

- Etiology – Dental plaque as a "biofilm", the periodontopathic microorganisms
- Pathogenesis – Host response, risk factors
- Oral pathological changes in gingiva and periodontium
- Oral manifestations of HIV disease. Treatment
- Gingival recession – Prevention!
- New diagnostic tests
- The "systemic pre-phase" of dental hygiene treatment
- Phase I therapy
- "Closed", non-surgical periodontal treatment—Promising new techniques
- FMT – "Full Mouth Therapy"
- Pharmacologic strategies for periodontitis
- Phase II therapy – Summary of surgical treatment
- Phase III therapy – Risk-managed periodontal maintenance – Success and failure
- Periodontal diseases in elderly patients

As Bob Dylan said more than 40 years ago: "The times, they are a'changing." The demands of daily dental practice are leading quickly to the necessity that the dental hygienist assume more and more responsibility, beyond "tooth cleaning", during the routine "recall appointment." Such responsibilities include measures beyond therapy, into clinical and radiographic diagnosis of oral and head-neck pathology, smoking cessation programs, cancer detection, and the performance of tests for genetic risk factors. The trend nationwide, although not yet supported by all participants in the dental community, is toward independent clinical practice for dental hygienists. Indeed, the dental practice laws of five states already permit such practice. And therefore, today's dental hygienist must be prepared to take on a much higher level of clinical responsibility for her/his patients, and this demands a higher level of knowledge as well as a deeper understanding of disease pathogenesis.

The overriding goal of this new textbook is to present and impart the information required in periodontology for the dental hygienist of today, and of tomorrow.

Herbert F. Wolf, Zurich
Thomas M. Hassell, Greensboro

Foreword – I

Gail L. Aamodt, BS, RDH, MS

Department of Dental Hygiene
Northern Arizona University
Flagstaff

The widespread nature of periodontal disease today among the world's population puts the dental hygienist in a key position at the forefront in the diagnosis, treatment, and prevention of oral conditions. Today's dental hygienist must be able to evaluate clinical, radiographic, and historical information, and participate in the team effort of diagnosis, treatment planning, care, and maintenance of the periodontal patient. The long-term success of periodontal therapy depends on a combined effort of the "preventive team," with the dental hygienist occupying a critical role in the prevention, success, and maintenance achieved by periodontal therapeutic measures.

There are many excellent textbooks on periodontology available today, but this *new* book provides a comprehensive, easy-to-read text, extensive diagrams, and exceptionally presented clinical photographs, which make it an ideal medium to capture both theoretical and clinical concepts in an effective, time-efficient manner. The summaries provide clear understanding and easy reference for practicing dental hygienists, dental hygiene educators, and especially students of dental hygiene at all levels. This book provides the knowledge base required of today's dental hygienist, who has a wide scope of responsibilities ranging from comprehensive clinical examinations to the placement of antimicrobials in combination with a wide array of periodontal debridement protocols.

One major requisite for understanding contemporary concepts of periodontology is having an appropriate resource that contains time-proven fundamentals, while also providing new information. For the dental hygienist, this book presents very comprehensive and contemporary information on the microbiology, pathogenesis, cell biology, immunology, host response, disease progression and healing of periodontal diseases. Serious attention is given to the importance of data collection, because without this an accurate diagnosis cannot be made. Of special interest is the section on oral pathological alterations of the periodontium, which must be recognized, thus helping the team coordinate appropriate periodontal and preventive care. A comprehensive classification of the most recent categories of periodontal disease is included as a synthesis of the information covered in the text.

This text is unique in its attention to Phase 3 Therapy (periodontal maintenance therapy), focusing long-term success on rigorous follow up by the dental hygienist as part of the preventive team. The idea of prevention in periodontology or "continuous risk management" is targeted toward recognition of a multilevel assessment of risks. The authors suggest practical periodontal maintenance guidelines in an effort to follow the long-term health status of the periodontal patient.

As the percentage of elderly individuals within a population increases, so does the need to enhance our knowledge and expertise in the treatment/maintenance of this population. This text addresses the structural/biological changes in the periodontal tissues of the elderly individual, leading the clinician to consider modified treatment planning to create a sense of oral well-being for the elderly.

The international appeal of this text is apparent with the extensive array of instruments, devices, products, and medicaments discussed and pictured in the text. This new atlas will serve as an excellent reference in establishing a broader scope of dental hygiene practice, helping to enhance the understanding of periodontology for students, educators, and current practitioners as we strive toward a better future for the health of patients through the most comprehensive dental hygiene care available.

It is with particular pleasure that I offer this foreword to introduce the *Color Atlas of Dental Hygiene—Periodontology*. My thanks go to the Wolf/Hassell team for this masterful contribution.

Foreword – II

Susan J. Jenkins, BS, RDH, MS

Forsyth Dental Hygiene Program
Massachusetts College of Pharmacy & Health Sciences
Boston

It is with great enthusiasm that I write this foreword to the new book *Color Atlas of Dental Hygiene—Periodontology*. The art and science of periodontology are changing rapidly; the practicing dental hygienist and the dental hygiene educator are looking for current information presented in the most up-to-date manner. They will find it here.

For dental hygiene students the *Color Atlas of Dental Hygiene—Periodontology* will be a formidable book that they will utilize throughout their entire education and for years to come. For the novice, the book is presented in clear and concise language. The chapter "Initial Therapy 1" will give the new student a wonderful understanding of his/her future profession. There are few dental hygiene text books that present such an all inclusive approach to the profession. The exquisite color photographs with their fine detail will be a wonderful educational tool not only for the student but for the practicing dental hygienist as well. As I read the book, the old adage "a picture paints a thousand words" kept resonating in my head. In today's age of computer technology our patients are becoming much savvier in their dental knowledge. Many of the questions posed by the patients can be answered clearly and succinctly with the aid of this atlas as a chair-side educator.

This high-tech age in which we live has produced an evolution of power-driven scalers. The new designs of the inserts permit much more effective debridement and lavage in deeper pockets. However, there is still a very prominent place for hand instrumentation. Students must learn the basics of hand instrumentation prior to using the power-driven instruments. The discussion of hand instrumentation in the Therapy sections (pp. 242–243, 257–275) not only contains excellent detailed pictures of the various types of curettes, but also presents proper adaptation of the instruments and correct operator positioning for successful debridement. This book will be a valuable addition in the preclinical phase of the dental hygiene student's education.

It is universally acknowledged that the dental hygienist is the dental team member with whom patients spend the majority of their patient time. Hygienists are called upon to answer questions concerning oral and systemic conditions. As research continues, the connections between the patients's oral cavity and systemic health will continue to evolve. This new book will enable both the student and practicing dental hygienist to educate their patients regarding the contemporary paradigm shift connecting oral and systemic conditions.

One of the largest segments of the US population is the baby boomer. According to the US Census Bureau, in 2006 75 million people, or 29% of the population, fall within this group. We are all aging gracefully and living longer. This will have an impact on our oral health. The chapters "Geriatric Periodontology?" and "Phase 3 Therapy" clearly explain the oral changes that will occur within this population, along with the most innovative recommendations for customizing maintenance care for this group.

For the dental hygiene educator, this atlas will be a versatile text. As the teacher of our periodontology course at MCPHS Forsyth, I often found it difficult to locate high-quality illustrations to use in my lectures. The authors and publisher of the *Color Atlas of Dental Hygiene—Periodontology* have agreed to permit the reproduction of the lovely photographs, crisp diagrams, and artful illustrations in your lectures. This generosity can greatly enhance lectures and enrich the learning experiences of not only the visual learners but of all students.

Congratulations to Dr. Wolf and Dr. Hassell for their foresight in creating this first-class book.

Acknowledgments

First and foremost, we thank our families and our friends for their unflagging encouragement and support, and for their deep understanding and even deeper patience over more than a decade of work as this new book evolved and became a reality.

The creation of this book, which became ever more comprehensive and detailed, was made possible only through the collaboration and assistance of the coworkers in Dr. Wolf's private dental practice (Zurich, Switzerland), our colleague *Edith Rateitschak* in the Center for Dental Medicine (Basle, Switzerland), and the faculty, staff, and students at the College of Health Professions, Northern Arizona University (Flagstaff, AZ). In our work, we were helped greatly by contributions from other universities and many private dental and periodontal practices. Contributions of clinical cases and photographs are acknowledged in detail on page 332.

We also thank especially *Gail Aamodt and Susan Jenkins* for their generous, original, and we believe objective Forewords to this special edition.

Our thanks go to our many colleagues worldwide for their participation as contributors, assistants, photographers, therapists, problem-solvers, and "critics": *Sandra Augustin-Wolf, Zurich; Christine Baca, Flagstaff; Manuel Battegay, Basle—Jean-Pierre Ebner, Basle; Joachim Hermann, Stuttgart; Markus Hürzeler, Munich; Thomas Lambrecht, Basle; Niklaus Lang, Berne; Samuel Low, Gainesville; Carlo Marinello, Basle; Jürg Meyer, Basle; Andrea Mombelli, Geneva; Lucca Ritz, Basle; Hubert Schroeder, Zurich; Ulrich Saxer, Zurich; Peter Schüpbach, Horgen; Nicola Zitzmann, Basle; Edith Rateitschak-Plüss, Basle; Professor Klaus H. Rateitschak, Basle (in memoriam).*

All of the graphic illustrations, schematic diagrams, and tables conceived by Herbert Wolf were realized on the computer with great competence (and understanding for the authors' unending litany of desires!) by *Joachim Hormann*, Graphic Design Co., Stuttgart. He deserves our special thanks. Also *so* worthy of our thanks and praise is Ms. *Censeri Abare* (Gainesville, FL), who prepared the original typescript for this book and then also performed countless corrections and modifications of innumerable drafts, always with precision and with patience.

The enormous costs for all of the color illustrations were born by the authors and by our publisher, and the following commercial entities made significant financial contributions:

Procter & Gamble Co., Trisa Co., Deppeler Co., Gaba Co., Lever Co., and the *Walter-Fuchs Foundation.*

Our text and illustrative materials were prepared for final printing in the *Kaltnermedia* Co. in *Bobingen*, by *Martin Maschke, Markus Christ,* and *Angelika Schönwälder*, who performed brilliantly with understanding, know-how, and enduring patience. Despite the ever-present time pressure, *Grammlich* Co., *Pliezhausen*, carried out the work with precision and persistence.

We are immensely grateful for the excellent guidance and support provided to us by Thieme Medical Publishers, Stuttgart and New York. Special thanks are due to *Dr. Cliff Bergman, Dr. Christian Urbanowicz, Stefanie Langner and Gert Krueger.* These individuals put every ounce of energy, dedication, and personal creativity into this book, and always exhibited understanding (and patience!) for the authors' numerous "impossible" wishes.

Herbert F. Wolf
Thomas M. Hassell

Table of Contents

Therapy

Introduction

"Periodontology" is the study of the tooth-supporting tissues, the "periodontium." The periodontium is made up of those tissues that surround each tooth and which anchor each tooth into the alveolar process (Greek: para = adjacent, odus = tooth).

The following soft and hard tissues constitute the structure of the periodontium:

- Gingiva
- Root Cementum
- Periodontal Ligament
- Alveolar Bone

The structure and function of these periodontal tissues have been extensively researched (Schroeder 1992). Knowledge of the interplay between and among the cellular and molecular components of the periodontium leads to optimum therapy, and also helps to establish the goals for future intensive research.

Periodontal Diseases

Gingivitis – Periodontitis

There are numerous diseases that affect the periodontium. By far the most important of these are plaque-associated gingivitis (gingival inflammation without attachment loss) and periodontitis (inflammation-associated loss of periodontal supporting tissues).

- *Gingivitis* is limited to the marginal, supracrestal soft tissues. It is manifested clinically by bleeding upon probing of the gingival sulcus, and in more severe cases by erythema and swelling, especially of the interdental papillae (Fig. 3).
- *Periodontitis* can develop from a pre-existing gingivitis in patients with compromised immune status, the presence of risk factors and pro-inflammatory mediators, as well as the presence of a predominately periodontopathic microbial flora. The inflammation of the gingiva may then extend into the deeper structures of the tooth-supporting apparatus. The consequences include destruction of collagen and loss of alveolar bone (attachment loss). The junctional epithelium degenerates into a "pocket" epithelium, which proliferates apically and laterally. A true periodontal pocket forms. Such a pocket is a predilection site and a reservoir for opportunistic, pathogenic bacteria; these bacteria sustain periodontitis and enhance the progression of the disease processes (Fig. 4).

Gingival Recession

Gingival recession is not actually a "disease," but rather an anatomic alteration that is elicited by morphology, improper oral hygiene (aggressive scrubbing), and possibly functional overloading.

- Teeth are not lost due to classical gingival recession, but patients may experience cervical hypersensitivity and esthetic complications. If gingival recession extends to the mobile oral mucosa, adequate oral hygiene is often no longer possible. Secondary inflammation is the consequence.

  In addition to classical gingival recession, apical migration of the gingiva is often observed in patients with long-standing, untreated periodontitis, and it may be a consequence of periodontitis *therapy* in elderly patients ("involution"; Fig. 2).

These three periodontal disorders – gingivitis, periodontitis, gingival recession – are observed world-wide; they affect almost the entire population of the earth to greater or lesser degree. In addition to these common forms of oral pathology, there are many less frequently encountered diseases and defects of the periodontal tissues. All of these diseases were comprehensively classified at an international World Workshop in 1999 (see Appendix, p. 327).

1 Healthy Periodontium

The most important characteristic of the periodontium is the special connection between soft and hard tissues:

- In the marginal region, one observes inflammation-free gingiva, which provides the epithelial attachment to the tooth by means of its junctional epithelium (pink collar). This connection protects the deeper-lying components of the periodontium from mechanical and microbiologic insult.
- Subjacent to the junctional epithelium, one observes the supracrestal fibers, which serve to connect the tooth with the gingiva, and also the periodontal ligament fibers in the region of the alveolar bone, which insert into the bone and the cementum of the root surface.

Prevention of disease: Maintaining the health of the periodontium is the highest goal in periodontics, and should also be the patient's goal. It is achieved by optimum, purely mechanical oral hygiene. Disinfectant mouthwashes may enhance mechanical hygiene.

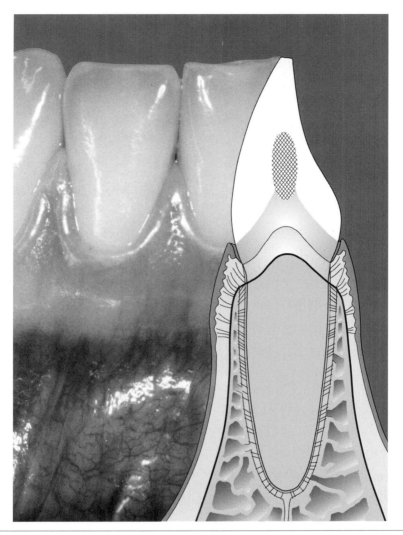

Healthy Periodontium

2 Gingival Recession

The main characteristic of this condition, which is often esthetically objectionable to patients, is an inflammation-free apical migration of the gingival margin. A morphological prerequisite is generally a facial bony lamella that is either extremely thin or entirely lacking. Gingival recession can be initiated and propagated by improper traumatic tooth brushing (horizontal scrubbing), and functional overloading may also play a role (?). Thus gingival recession cannot be classified as a true periodontal *disease*.

The best way for a patient to prevent gingival recession is by using an adequate but gentle oral hygiene technique (vertical-rotatory brushing or use of a sonic toothbrush).

Treatment: Incipient or progressing gingival recession can be halted by altering the patient's oral hygiene techniques; in severe cases, mucogingival surgery may be employed to stop the progression or re-cover the exposed root surfaces.

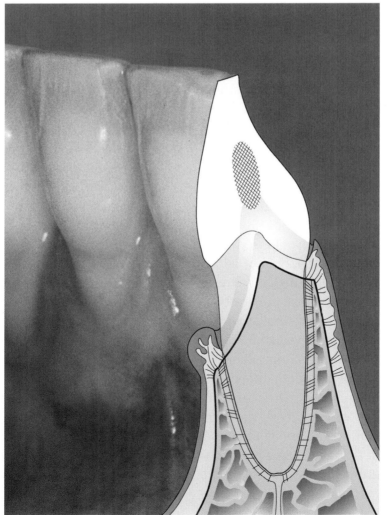

Gingival Recession

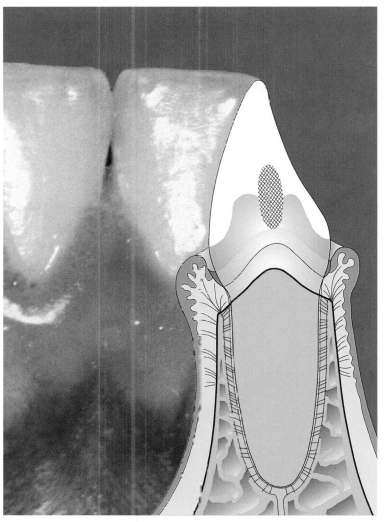

3 Gingivitis

Gingivitis is characterized by plaque-induced inflammation of the papillary and marginal gingivae. Clinical symptoms include bleeding on probing, erythema, and eventual swelling. Gingivitis may be more or less pronounced depending upon the plaque—a biofilm—(quantity/quality) and the host response. Deeper lying structures (alveolar bone, periodontal ligament) are not involved. Gingivitis *may* be a precursor to periodontitis, but this does *not* always occur.

Treatment: Gingivitis can be completely controlled simply through adequate plaque control. Following initiation or improvement of oral hygiene procedures, coupled with professional plaque and calculus removal, complete healing can be expected. Nevertheless, freedom from inflammation, e. g., absence of bleeding on probing, will be impossible to achieve if the patient is not capable of maintaining a high standard of oral hygiene over the long term, or is not willing to do so (compliance!).

Gingivitis

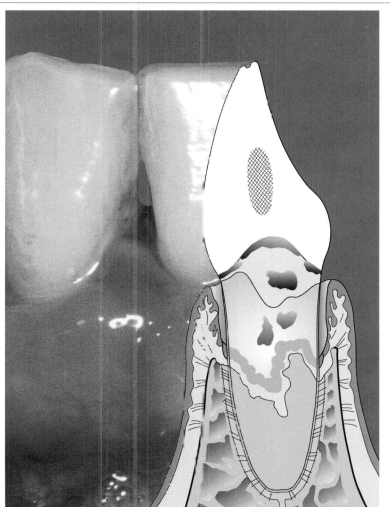

4 Periodontitis

At the gingival margin, the characteristics of periodontitis are similar to those of gingivitis, but the inflammatory processes extend further, into the deeper-lying periodontal structures (alveolar bone and periodontal ligament). True periodontal pockets are formed and connective tissue attachment is lost. Loss of hard and soft tissues is usually localized and not generalized.
Periodontitis may be classified as *chronic* (Type II) or *aggressive* (Type III), with varying degrees of severity. Approximately 90 % of all cases are characterized as "chronic periodontitis" (p. 108, 327).

Treatment: Most cases of periodontitis can be treated successfully. However, the required therapeutic endeavor can vary enormously from case to case. The treatment effort may be relatively small in early stages of periodontitis. Mechanical treatment remains today in the foreground. In special cases, topical and systemic medications may be used as supportive therapy.

Periodontitis

The Clinical Course of Untreated Periodontitis

Periodontitis is usually a very slowly progressing disease (Locker & Leake 1993; Albandar et al. 1997), which in severe cases—particularly when untreated—can lead to tooth loss. Enormous variation in the speed of progression of periodontitis is observed when one differentiates between individual patients. In addition to the quantity and composition of the bacterial plaque, individually varying influences also play important roles: the systemic health of the patient, the patient's genetic constitution, psychically influenced immune response status, ethnic and social factors, as well as risk factors such as smoking and stress (p. 22, Fig. 41). All of these circumstances can influence the onset and the speed at which the disease process accelerates in different patient age groups.

Not all teeth or individual surfaces of teeth are equally susceptible (Manser & Rateitschak 1996):

- Molars are the most endangered
- Premolars and anterior teeth are less susceptible
- Canines are the most resistant.

5 Clinical Course of Untreated Periodontitis
In the aggressive forms of periodontitis (pp. 95, 97), the manifestation of tissue loss on individual teeth occurs in successive acute phases rather than in a gradual, chronic progression. Phases of progression and quiescence alternate. Destructive phases may occur rapidly one after another, or longer quiescent phases may be in evidence.

Red   Acute phase/destruction
Blue Phase of quiescence

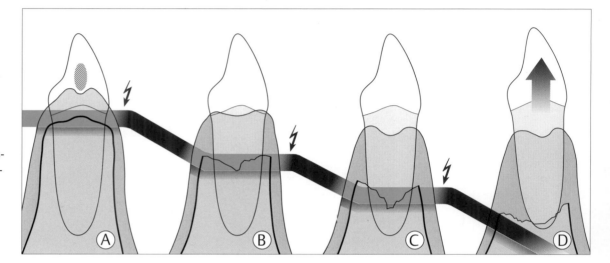

Periodontitis—Concepts of Therapy

The primary goal is *prevention* of periodontal diseases, and the secondary goal is to enhance the healing of existent periodontitis, as far as possible toward complete *Restitutio ad integrum*. Clinical and basic research is targeted today toward realization of these goals in the near future.

At the present time, proven therapeutic concepts are available for the elimination of inflammation and the cessation of the progression of disease. In addition, to a certain degree, it is possible today to regenerate lost periodontal attachment (GTR, p. 301). The following treatment modalities are available to the periodontal therapist:

1 Closed or open root planing ("causal therapy," the "gold standard")
2 Regenerative surgical therapies
3 Resective surgical therapies
4 Alternatives: extraction and dental implants?

1 *Root planing* is the *Conditio sine qua non* in all periodontal therapy. This is pure *causal therapy,* during which the causative "biofilm" (plaque) and subgingival calculus are removed. If the pockets are shallow and the morphological relationships simple (single-rooted teeth), treatment can be performed *closed,* but in advanced cases *open* treatment with direct visual access following reflection of a tissue flap is often preferable (e.g., modified Widman procedure). The result of such treatment is usually healing in the sense of "repair" (p. 206). A long junctional epithelium forms.

2 *Regenerative therapeutic methods* ("guided tissue regeneration" [GTR]; autogenous, alloplastic implants) have taken on increased significance in recent years. These procedures are constantly being further developed, and in the future they may be enhanced by the use of growth and differentiation factors.
Regenerative therapy can lead to the actual re-formation of significant periodontal tissues.

3 *Radical surgery* for the elimination of periodontal pockets has lost some its popularity in recent years, although the results are generally more predictable and the tendency toward recurrence is low.

4 In cases of complex, severely advanced periodontitis, e.g., with severe furcation involvement in the molar region, the dentist may consider tooth extraction and *replacement with a root-form implant* instead of resective or regenerative periodontal surgery. Even in such cases, periodontal treatment of the remaining dentition must be performed, as well as optimum plaque control by the patient and the creation of an adequate amount of bone for the implant.

Initial situation	Clinical treatment	Result

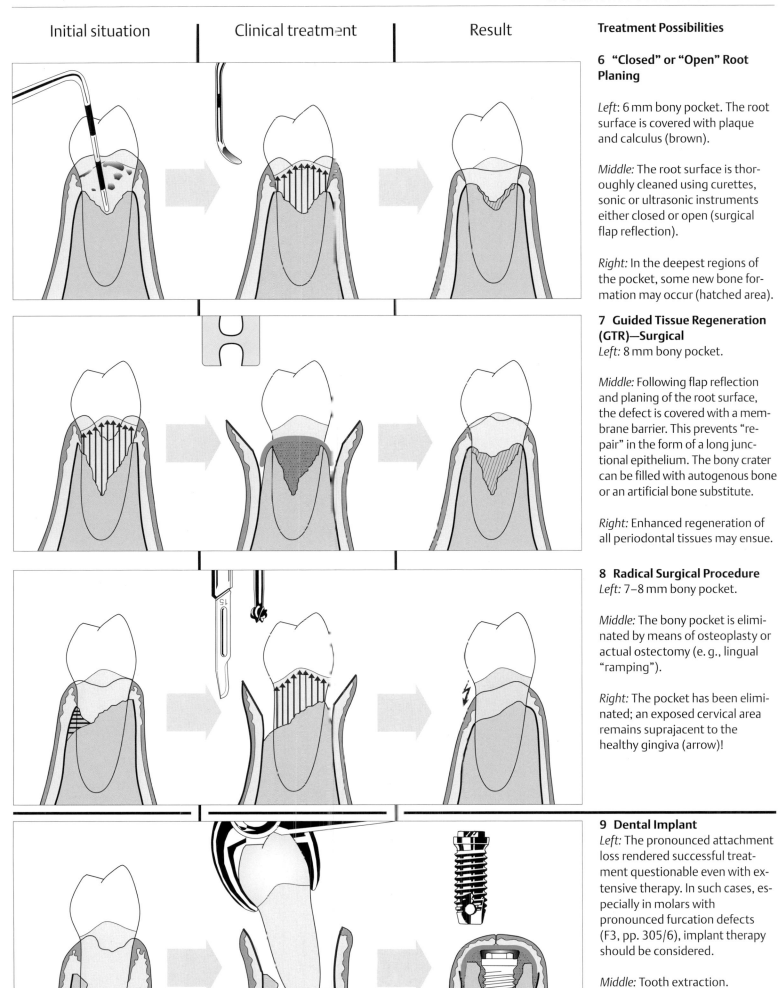

Treatment Possibilities

6 "Closed" or "Open" Root Planing

Left: 6 mm bony pocket. The root surface is covered with plaque and calculus (brown).

Middle: The root surface is thoroughly cleaned using curettes, sonic or ultrasonic instruments either closed or open (surgical flap reflection).

Right: In the deepest regions of the pocket, some new bone formation may occur (hatched area).

7 Guided Tissue Regeneration (GTR)—Surgical
Left: 8 mm bony pocket.

Middle: Following flap reflection and planing of the root surface, the defect is covered with a membrane barrier. This prevents "repair" in the form of a long junctional epithelium. The bony crater can be filled with autogenous bone or an artificial bone substitute.

Right: Enhanced regeneration of all periodontal tissues may ensue.

8 Radical Surgical Procedure
Left: 7–8 mm bony pocket.

Middle: The bony pocket is eliminated by means of osteoplasty or actual ostectomy (e. g., lingual "ramping").

Right: The pocket has been eliminated; an exposed cervical area remains suprajacent to the healthy gingiva (arrow)!

9 Dental Implant
Left: The pronounced attachment loss rendered successful treatment questionable even with extensive therapy. In such cases, especially in molars with pronounced furcation defects (F3, pp. 305/6), implant therapy should be considered.

Middle: Tooth extraction.

Right: The implant is covered by mucosa. Osseous regeneration occurs beneath a membrane.

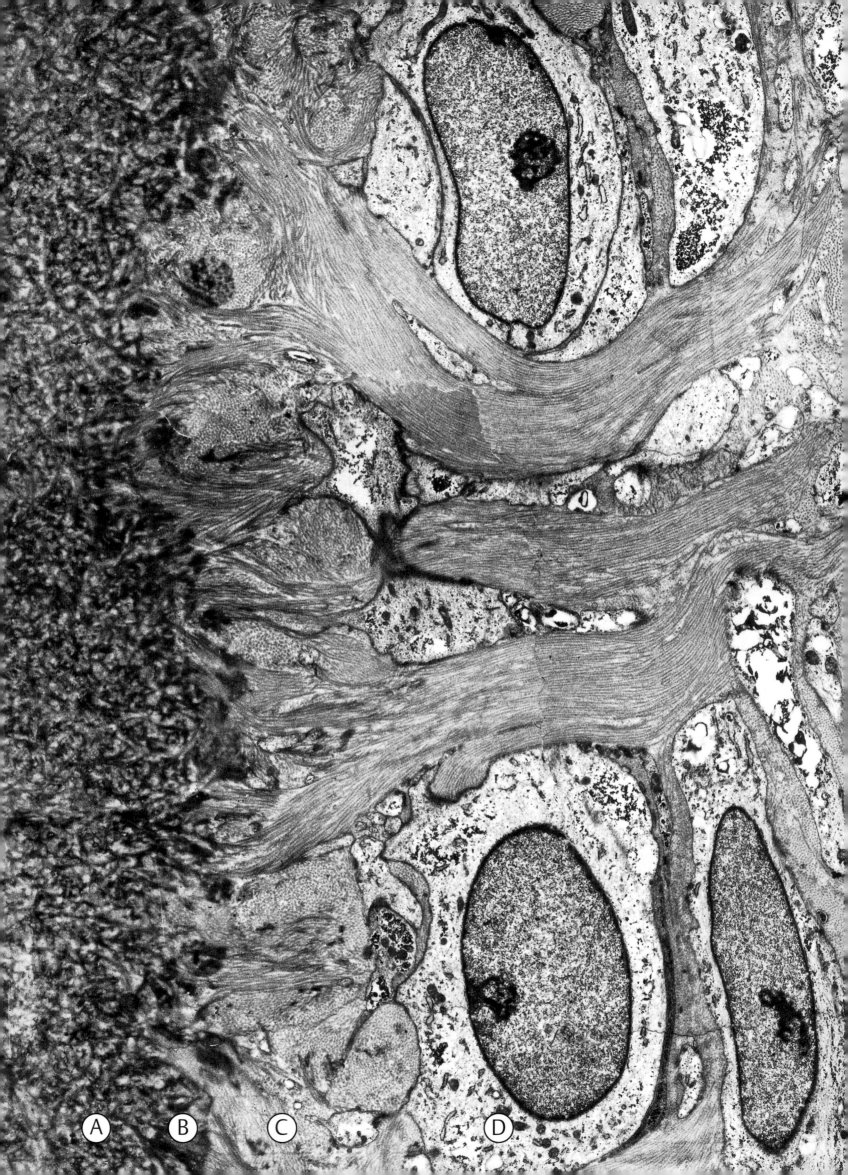

Structural Biology

"Structural biology" is a general term referring to the classical macromorphology and histology of tissues, as well as their function, including the biochemistry of the cells and the intercellular substances.

Basic knowledge of the normal structural biology of periodontal tissues and their dynamics (mediator-guided homeostasis, "turnover") is a prerequisite for full understanding of pathobiological changes in the periodontium, which can involve adaptations of the normal structures or an imbalance of otherwise normal functions (Schroeder 1992).

The term "periodontium" encompasses four different soft and hard tissues: gingiva, root cementum, alveolar bone, and the periodontal ligament, which attaches root cementum to bone. Each of these four tissues can be further differentiated in terms of structure, function and localization.

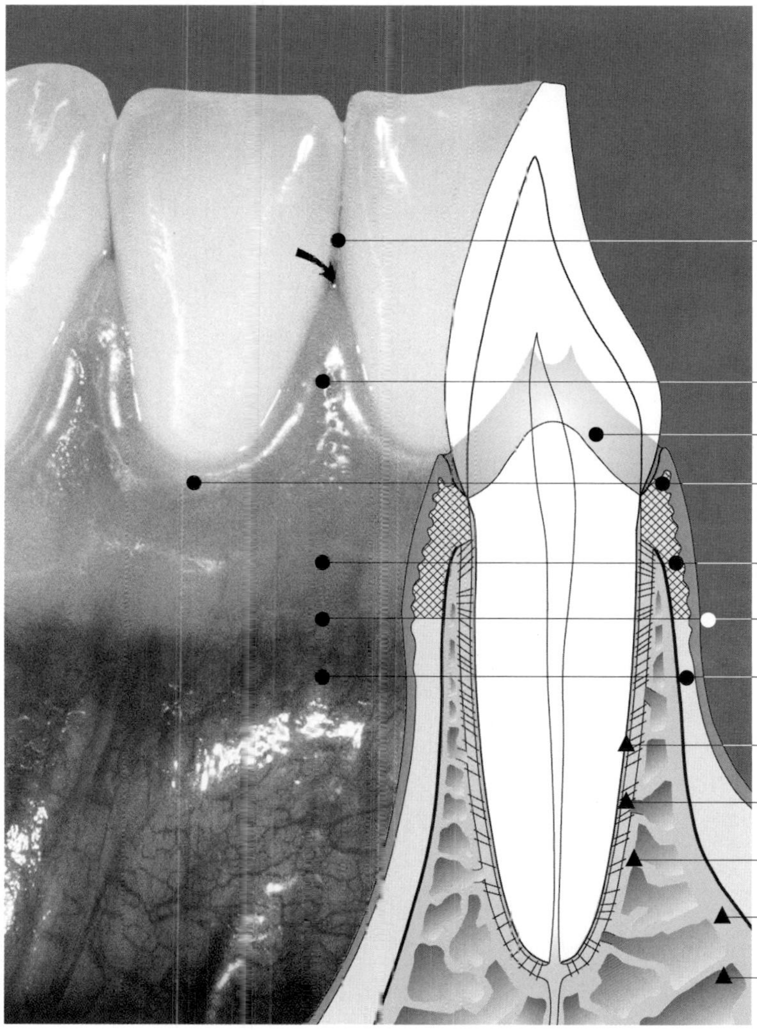

10 Periodontal Structures

Left Side:

Transmission electron photomicrograph (TEM) of root formation in humans (ca. 6-year-old)
This TEM depicts the growing demarcation between dentin, cementum and periodontal ligament during root formation.
Initial mineralization of the "cementoid" directly apposed to the dentin, with penetrating collagen fibers and fibroblast-like cementoblasts, which are involved in the formation of acellular exogenous fiber cementum.

A Dentin
B Cementoid
C Radiating collagen fibers
D Cementoblast (fibroblast-like) building acellular exogenous fiber cement

Courtesy *D. Bosshardt,*
H. Schroeder

Col, interpapillary saddle

Facial papilla

Junctional epithelium

Free gingival margin

Attached gingiva

Mucogingival junction

Alveolar mucosa

Root cementum

Periodontal ligament

Alveolar bone (cribriform plate)

Compact bone

Trabecular bone

Gingiva

The gingiva is one portion of the oral mucosa. It is also the most peripheral component of the periodontium. Gingiva begins at the mucogingival line, and covers the coronal aspect of the alveolar process. On the palatal aspect, the mucogingival line is absent; here, the gingiva is a part of the keratinized, non-mobile palatal mucosa.

The gingiva ends at the cervix of each tooth, surrounds it, and forms there the epithelial attachment by means of a ring of specialized epithelial tissue (junctional epithelium; p. 10). Thus the gingiva provides for the continuity of the epithelial lining of the oral cavity.

The gingiva is demarcated clinically into the *free marginal* gingiva, ca. 1.5 mm wide; the *attached* gingiva, which may be of varying width; and the *interdental* gingiva.

Healthy gingiva is described as "salmon" pink in color; in Blacks (seldom also in Caucasians) the gingiva may exhibit varying degrees of brownish pigmentation. Gingiva exhibits varying consistency and is not mobile upon the underlying bone. The gingival surface is keratinized and may be firm, thick and deeply stippled ("thick phenotype"), or thin and scarcely stippled ("thin phenotype"; Müller & Eger 1996, Müller et al. 2000).

11 Healthy Gingiva
The free gingival margin courses parallel to the cementoenamel junction. The facial interdental papillae extend to the contact area of adjacent teeth. A gingival groove can be observed in some areas, demarcating the free gingival margin from the attached gingiva.

Right: The radiograph depicts normal interdental septa. In the original radiograph, the crest of the alveolar bone was observed ca. 1.5 mm apical to the CEJ.

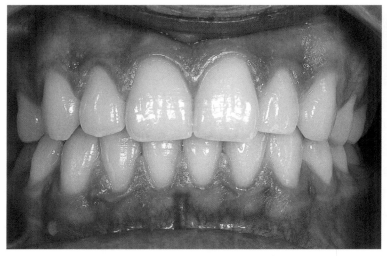
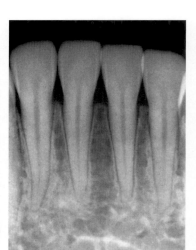

12 Variations in Consistency of Healthy Gingiva
Left: Firm, fibrous gingiva = "thick" phenotype.

Right: Delicate, scarcely stippled gingiva = "thin" phenotype. The subjacent bone covering the roots is clearly visible.

Thicker gingiva provides better conditions for treatment and wound healing (blood flow; stable position of the gingival margin).

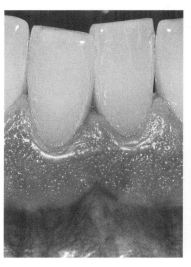
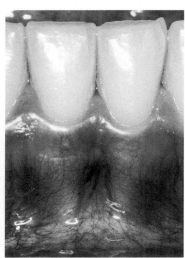

13 Healthy, Pigmented Gingiva
Note the symmetrical pigmentation of the attached gingiva in this 16-year-old African female.

Right: This pigmentation results from the synthesis of melanin by melanocytes located in the basal layer of the epithelium. The melanocytes in this histologic section appear as brown spots.

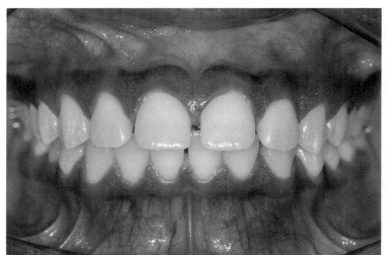
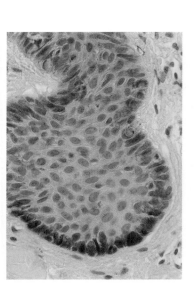

Gingival Width

The attached gingiva becomes wider as a patient ages (Ainamo et al. 1981). The width varies between individuals and among various groups of teeth in the same person. Although it was once believed that a minimum width of attached gingiva (ca. 2 mm) is necessary to maintain the health of the periodontium (Lang & Löe 1972), this concept is not accepted today. However, a wide band of attached gingiva does offer certain advantages in the case of periodontal surgery, both therapeutically and esthetically.

Col—Interpapillary Saddle

Apical to the contact area between two teeth, the interdental gingiva assumes a concave form when viewed in labiolingual section. The concavity, the "col," is thus located between the lingual and facial interdental papillae and is not visible clinically. Depending on the expanse of the contacting tooth surfaces, the col will be of varying depth and breadth. The epithelium covering the col consists of the marginal epithelia of the adjacent teeth (Cohen 1959, 1962; Schroeder 1992). The col is not keratinized. In the absence of contact between adjacent teeth, the keratinized gingiva courses uninterrupted from the facial to the oral aspect.

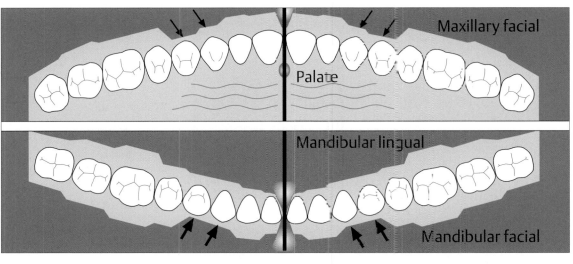

14 Mean Width of Attached Gingiva
- In the *maxilla*, the *facial* gingiva in the area of the incisors is wide, but narrow around the canines and first premolars. On the *palatal* aspect, the marginal gingiva blends without demarcation into the palatal mucosa.
- In the *mandible*, the *lingual* gingiva in the area of the incisors is narrow, but wide on the molars. On the *facial*, the gingiva around the canines and first premolars is narrow (arrow), but wide around the lateral incisors.

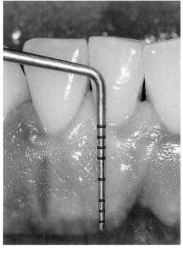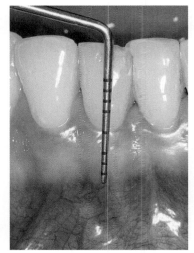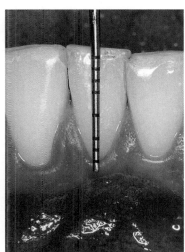

15 Variability of Gingival Width
Width of attached gingiva can vary dramatically. The three patients depicted here, all about the same age, exhibit gingival width varying from 1 to 10 mm in the mandibular anterior area.

Right: After staining the mucosa with iodine (Schiller or Lugol solution) the mucogingival line is easily visible because the non-keratinized alveolar mucosa is *iodine-positive* while the keratinized gingiva is not (cf. p. 161).

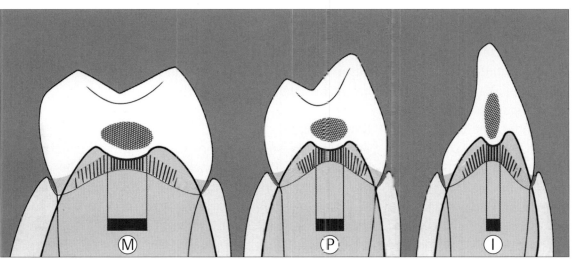

16 Col—Interpapillary Saddle
The col consists essentially of a connection between the junctional epithelia (JE; p. 10) of any two adjacent teeth. Tooth morphology, width of the tooth crowns and relative tooth position will determine the extent of the contact surfaces (hatched), their breadth (2–7 mm, red bar), as well as the depth (1–2 mm) of the interpapillary saddle.

I Incisor
P Premolar
M Molar

Epithelial Attachment

Junctional Epithelium—Epithelial Attachment— Gingival Sulcus

The marginal gingiva attaches to the tooth surface by means of the junctional epithelium, an attachment that is continuously being renewed throughout life (Schroeder 1992).

Junctional Epithelium

The junctional epithelium (JE) is approximately 1–2 mm in coronoapical dimension, and surrounds the neck of each tooth. At its apical extent, it consists of only a few cell layers; more coronally, it consists of 15–30 cell layers. Subjacent to the sulcus bottom, the JE is about 0.15 mm wide.

The junctional epithelium consists of two layers, the basal (mytotically active) and the suprabasal layer (daughter cells). It remains undifferentiated and does not keratinize. The basal cell layer interfaces with the connective tissue via hemidesmosomes and an external basal lamina. Healthy JE exhibits no rete ridges where it contacts the connective tissue. JE turnover rate is very high (4–6 days) compared to oral epithelium (6–12 days, Skougaard 1965; or up to 40 days, Williams et al. 1997).

17 Junctional Epithelium and Gingiva in Orofacial Section
The gingiva consists of three tissues:
- Junctional epithelium
- Oral epithelium
- Lamina propria (connective tissue)

The *junctional epithelium* (JE) assumes a key role in maintenance of periodontal health: It produces the *epithelial attachment* and therefore creates the firm connection of soft tissue to the tooth surface. It is quite permeable, and thus serves as a pathway for diffusion of the metabolic products of plaque bacteria (toxins, chemotactic agents, antigens, etc.). There is also diffusion in the opposite direction, of host defense substances (serum exudates, antibodies, etc.). Even when the gingivae do not appear inflamed clinically, the JE is constantly transmigrated by polymorphoneuclear leukocytes (PMNs) moving towards the sulcus (p. 55, Fig. 109). The red arrows depict the migration of daughter cells from the basal layer toward the gingival sulcus. The circled areas A–C are depicted in detail on page 11.

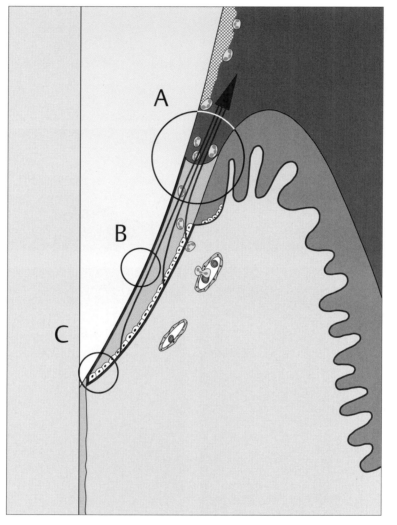

Structure of the Junctional Epithelium (JE)

Height: 1–2 mm
Coronal width: 0.15 mm

A Gingival Sulcus (GS)
Histologic
– Width: 0.15 mm
– Depth: 0–0.5 mm
Clinical
– Depth: 0.5–3 mm
  (dependent upon penetration of the probe into the junctional epithelium; Fig. 378)

B Epithelial Attachment
– Internal basal lamina (IBL)
  Thickness: 35–140 nm
  $(1 \text{ nm} = 10^{-9} \text{ m})$
– Hemidesmosomes

C Apical Extent
of the junctional epithelium

Epithelial Attachment

The epithelial attachment to the tooth is formed by the JE, and consists of an *internal basal lamina* (IBL) and *hemidesmosomes*. It provides the epithelial attachment between gingiva and tooth surface. This can be upon enamel, cementum or dentin in the same manner. The basal lamina and the hemidesmosomes of the epithelial attachment are structural analogs of their counterparts comprising the interface between epithelium and connective tissues.

All cells of the JE are in continual coronal migration, even those cells in immediate contact with the tooth surface. Such cells must continually dissolve and reestablish their hemidesmosomal attachments. Between the basal lamina and the tooth surface, a 0.5–1 µm thick "dental cuticle" is observed; this is possibly a serum precipitate or a secretion product of the junctional epithelial cells.

Gingival Sulcus

The sulcus is a narrow groove surrounding the tooth, about 0.5 mm deep. The bottom of the sulcus is made up of the most coronal cells of the junctional epithelium, which are sloughed (exfoliated) in rapid succession. One lateral wall of the sulcus is made up of the tooth structure, the other wall is the oral sulcular epithelium (OSE; Schroeder 1992).

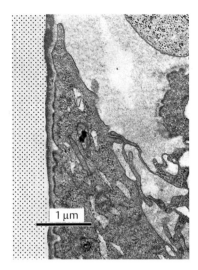

1 μm

1   Junctional Epithelium   JE

2   Oral Sulcular Epithelium OSE

3   Connective Tissue   CT

4   Gingival Sulcus   GS

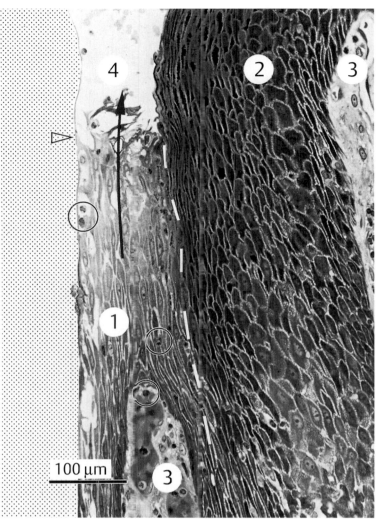

4   2   3

1

100 μm

3

18 Gingival Sulcus and Junctional Epithelium
The junctional epithelial cells (**1**) are oriented parallel to the tooth surface and are sharply demarcated (broken line) from the more deeply staining cells of the oral sulcular epithelium (**2**). All of the daughter cells that emanate from the entire 1–2 mm length of the basal layer of the junctional epithelium must transmigrate the exceptionally narrow (100–150 μm) sulcus bottom (red arrow). Note the polymorphonuclear leukocytes (circled), which emigrate from the venule plexus in the subepithelial connective tissue (**3**) without altering it in any way.

Left: In the enlargement, a portion of the most coronal JE cells (cf. empty black arrow in lower power view) is shown still manifesting hemidesmosomes and an internal basal lamina attached to the enamel surface.

Courtesy *H. Schroeder*

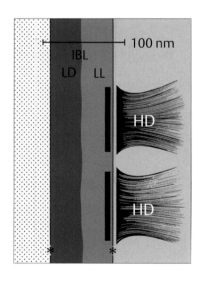

100 nm

IBL

LD   LL

HD

HD

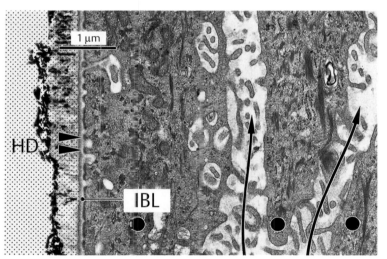

1 μm

HD

HD

IBL

19 Internal Basal Lamina and Hemidesmosomes
Each JE cell adjacent to the tooth forms hemidesmosomes (**HD**) that enable these cells to attach to the internal basal lamina (**IBL**) and ultimately to the surface of the tooth. Remnants of enamel crystals are visible at the left. The long arrows indicate intercellular spaces between three JE cells (●).

Left: The basal lamina is comprised of two layers: the Lamina lucida (**LL**) and the Lamina densa (**LD**).

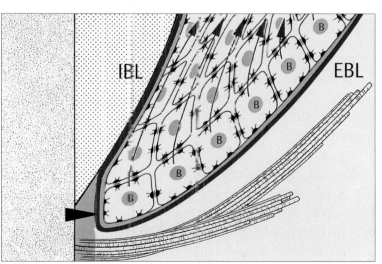

IBL   EBL   B

20 Apicalmost Portion of the Junctional Epithelium
In a young, healthy patient, the JE ends apically at the cementoenamel junction. Daughter cells of the cuboidal basal cells (**B**) migrate toward the sulcus (red arrows). If a JE cell comes into contact with the tooth surface, it establishes the attachment mechanism described above. The internal basal lamina (**IBL**) is continuous with the external basal lamina (**EBL**) around the apical extent of the JE (black arrowhead).

Connective Tissue Attachment

Gingival and Periodontal Fiber Apparatus

The fibrous connective tissue structures provide the attachment between teeth (via cementum) and their osseous alveoli, between teeth and gingiva, as well as between each tooth and its neighbor. These structures include:

- Gingival fiber groups
- Periodontal fiber groups (periodontal ligament)

Gingival Fiber Groups

In the supra-alveolar area, collagen fiber bundles course in various directions. These fibers give the gingiva its resiliency and resistance, and attach it onto the tooth surface subjacent to the epithelial attachment. The fibers also provide resistance to forces and stabilize the individual teeth into a closed segment (Fig. 22). The periosteogingival fibers are also a component of the gingival fiber complex. These connect the attached gingiva to the alveolar process.

21 Localization and Orientation of Gingival and Periodontal Ligament Fiber Bundles
(see also Fig. 22)
In the supra-alveolar region, within the free marginal gingiva and partially also the attached gingiva, the connective tissue compartment is composed primarily of collagen fiber bundles (**A**). These splay from the cementum of the root surface into the gingiva. Other fiber bundles course more or less horizontally within the gingiva and between the teeth, forming a complex architecture (Fig. 22). In addition to collagen fibers, one may also observe a small number of reticular (argyrophilic) fibers.
The periodontal ligament space (**B**) in adults is ca. 0.15–0.2 mm wide. About 60 % of the space is occupied by collagen fiber bundles. These fibers traverse from cementum to alveolar bone (**C**).

Right: Marginal gingiva. Fiber-rich connective tissue (**A**, blue), junctional epithelium and oral epithelium (reddish brown).

Histology courtesy *N. Lang*

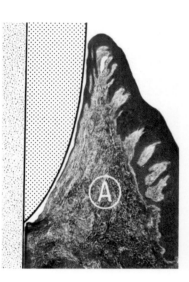

A Gingival Fibers

B Periodontal Ligament Fibers

C Alveolar Bone

X Sulcus and Junctional Epithelium

Y Connective Tissue Attachment

X+Y "Biologic Width" (BW)
(cf. p. 319)

Periodontal Fiber Groups, Periodontal Ligament

The periodontal ligament (PDL) occupies the space between the root surface and the alveolar bone surface. The PDL consists of connective tissue fibers, cells, vasculature, nerves and ground substance. An average of 28,000 fiber bundles insert into each square millimeter of root cementum!

The building block of a fiber bundle is the 40–70 nm thick collagen fibril. Many such fibrils in parallel arrangement make up a collagen fiber. Numerous fibers combine to form collagen fiber bundles. These collagen fiber bundles (Sharpey's fibers) insert into the alveolar bone on one end and into cementum at the other (Feneis 1952). The most ubiquitous cells are fibroblasts, which appear as spindle-shaped cells with oval nuclei and numerous cytoplasmic processes of varying lengths. These cells are responsible for the synthesis and break-down of collagen ("turnover").
Cells responsible for the hard tissues are the cementoblasts and osteoblasts. Osteoclastic cells are only observed during phases of active bone resorption. Near the cementum layer, within the PDL space, one often observes string-like arrangements of epithelial rest cells of Malassez.

The periodontal ligament tissues are highly vascularized (p. 18) and innervated (p. 19).

Course of the Gingival Fiber Bundles (see also Fig. 21)

 1 Dentogingival
   – Coronal
   – Horizontal
   – Apical
 2 Alveologingival
 3 Interpapillary
 4 Transgingival
 5 Circular, semicircular
 6 Dentoperiosteal
 7 Transseptal
 8 Periosteogingival
 9 Intercircular
10 Intergingival

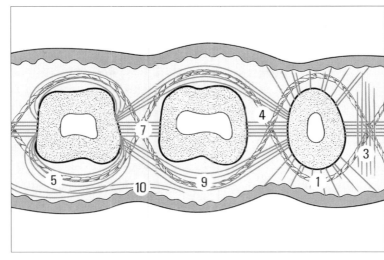

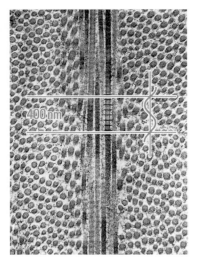

Course of the Periodontal Fiber Bundles

11 Crestal
12 Horizontal
13 Oblique
14 Interradicular
15 Apical

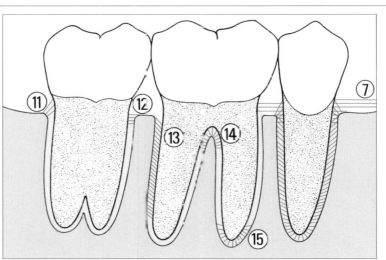

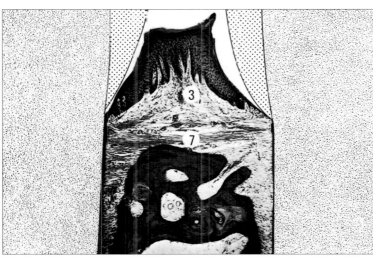

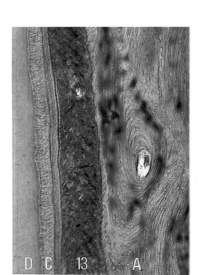

Gingival Fibers

22 Fiber Apparatus in Horizontal Section
The course of the most important supracrestal (gingival) fiber bundles is depicted. The connections between teeth and gingiva as well as between individual teeth are clearly shown.

23 Fiber Bundles Viewed in Mesiodistal Section
In the interdental area, the transseptal fiber bundles (**7**) extend supracrestally from one tooth to its neighbor. The fibers stabilize the arch in its mesiodistal dimension (courtesy N. Lang).

Left: The basic element of the fiber bundle is the collagen fibril; such fibrils are secreted by fibroblasts, and exhibit a regular 64 nm banding pattern (compare the wavelength of blue light, 400 nm).

TEM courtesy *H. Schroeder*

Periodontal Fibers

24 Fiber Apparatus in Mesiodistal Section
The anchoring of a tooth in the alveolar bone is accomplished via the dentoalveolar fibers of the periodontal ligament (PDL). Occlusal forces are absorbed primarily by the oblique fibers, which course from bone to cementum (**13**). The remaining fiber bundles (**11**, **12**, **14**, **15**) counteract tipping and rotating forces.

25 Periodontal Ligament— Details
Collagen fiber bundles (**13**) are intertwined. Osteoblasts (**OB**) line the surface of the bone; cementoblasts (**CB**) line the cementum surface; numerous fibroblasts (**FIB**) occupy the PDL space.

Left: The histologic section (Azan, x50) depicts the fiber-rich periodontal ligament (**13**) and its relationship to cementum (**C**) and bone (**A**). **D** = Dentin.

Histology courtesy *N. Lang*

Root Cementum

Types of Cementum

From a purely anatomic standpoint, root cementum is part of the tooth, but also part of the periodontium. Four types of cementum have been identified (Bosshardt & Schroeder 1991, 1992; Bosshardt & Selvig 1997):

1 Acellular, afibrillar cementum   (AAC)
2 Acellular, extrinsic-fiber cementum   (AEC)
3 Cellular intrinsic-fiber cementum   (CIC)
4 Cellular mixed fiber cementum   (CMC)

AEC and CMC are the most important types of cementum.

Cementum-forming Cells

Fibroblasts and cementoblasts collaborate in the formation of cementum. *Periodontal ligament fibroblasts* secrete acellular extrinsic cementum. *Cementoblasts* secrete cellular intrinsic cementum, and a portion of the cellular mixed fiber cementum, and probably also acellular afibrillar cementum. *Cementocytes* evolve from the cementoblasts, which become entrapped in cementum during cementogenesis. As a result, cementocytes are observed within cellular mixed fiber cementum and frequently in cellular intrinsic cementum (see also Cementum Formation and Healing, p. 206).

26 Types of Cementum—Structure, Localization and Development

1 **Acellular, Afibrillar Cementum** (AAC; red) AAC is formed at the most cervical enamel border following completion of pre-eruptive enamel maturation, and sometimes also during tooth eruption. It is probably secreted by cementoblasts.
2 **Acellular, Extrinsic-fiber Cementum** (AEC; green) AEC forms both pre- and post-eruptively. It is secreted by fibroblasts. On the apical portions of the root, it comprises a portion of the mixed-fiber cementum.
3 **Cellular, Intrinsic-fiber Cementum** (CIC; blue) CIC is formed both pre- and post-eruptively. It is synthesized by cementoblasts, but does not contain extrinsic Sharpey's fibers.
4 **Cellular, Mixed-fiber Cementum** (CMC; orange/green) CMC is formed by both cementoblasts and fibroblasts; it is a combination of cellular intrinsic-fiber cementum and acellular extrinsic-fiber cementum.

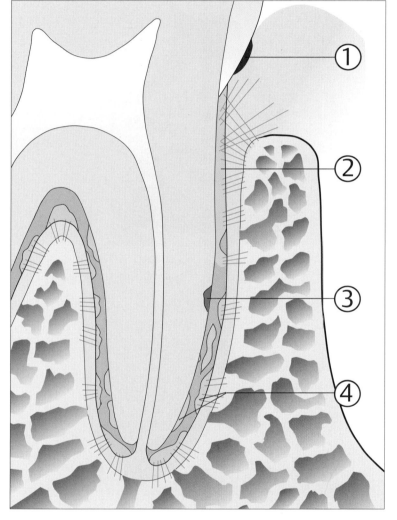

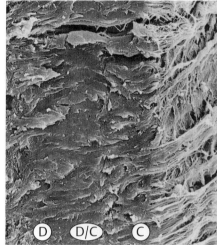

See p. 15, Fig. 29, left

Acellular Extrinsic Cementum (AEC)

The AEC is primarily responsible for the anchorage of the tooth in the alveolus. It is found in the cervical third of all deciduous and permanent teeth. The AEC consists of tightly packed and splaying fiber bundles (Sharpey's fibers), which are embedded in the calcified cementum.

The collagenous structures of cementum and dentin intertwine with each other during root formation and before calcification. This phenomenon explains the tight connection between these two hard tissues.

AEC is the type of cementum that is desired following regenerative periodontal surgical procedures.

Cellular Mixed-fiber Cementum (CMC)

The CMC is also of importance for the anchorage of the tooth in its alveolus. But it is only the acellular extrinsic-fiber cementum portion (AEC) within the mixed cementum, into which the Sharpey's fibers secreted by fibroblasts insert and therefore affix the tooth. CMC is layered vertically but also horizontally to the root surface. The portions secreted by cementoblasts contains high numbers of cementocytes (Fig. 30, left). The CMC is also tightly affixed to the dentin because of the intertwining of the collagen fiber bundles during tooth formation. The CMC "grows" faster than AEC.

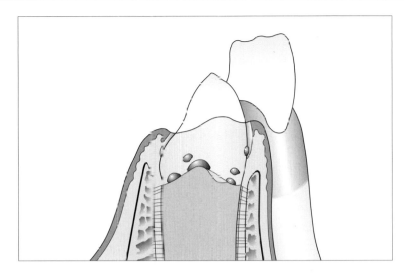

27 Acellular, Afibrillar Cementum (AAC)

AAC is observed only at the cervical region of the tooth, at the cementoenamel junction. It appears as small "islands" upon the enamel and sometimes also on the marginal areas of the root. AAC is formed during tooth eruption, when the reduced enamel epithelium partially dissolves as the enamel surface comes into contact with connective tissue.

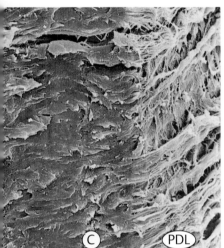

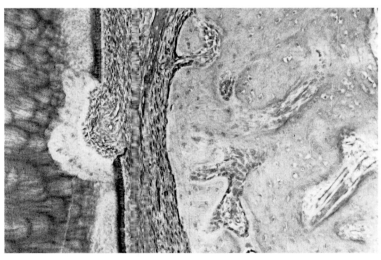

28 Acellular, Extrinsic-Fiber Cementum (AEC)

AEC is localized to the coronal third of the root (**C**), and exhibits a horizontal fiber structure (blue). Variations in the directionality may occur when the tooth encounters positional changes during cementum formation.

Left and p. 14: Note the intense intertwining and connections between dentin (**D**) and cementum (**C**), as well as of cementum and periodontal ligament (**PDL**).

Abbreviations

D   Dentin

D/C   Dentin-Cementum interface

C   Cementum
     C2   AEC
     C4   CMC

PDL   Periodontal ligament

29 Cellular, Intrinsic-Fiber Cementum (CIC)

CIC is usually a component of mixed-fiber cementum. It is localized to the middle, apical and furcal regions of the roots and usually contains embedded cementocytes.

As shown in this figure, CIC is also "reparative" cementum, i. e., it can repair resorption areas and root fractures.

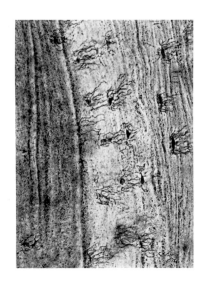

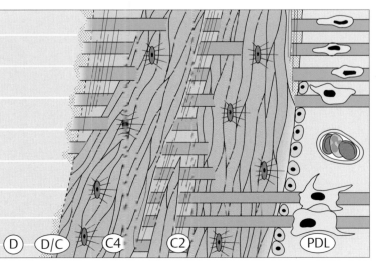

30 Cellular, Mixed-Fiber Cementum (CMC)

CMC is found in the apical portion of the root and in the furcation region. It represents a mixture of acellular extrinsic-fiber cementum (**C2**) and cellular intrinsic-fiber cementum (**C4**).

Left: "Medusa"-like cementocytes in the apical region of a multi-rooted tooth.

Adapted from *D. Bosshardt, H. Schroeder*

Osseous Support Apparatus

Alveolar Process—Alveolar Bone

The *alveolar processes* of the maxilla and the mandible are tooth-dependent structures. They develop with the formation of and during the eruption of the teeth, and they atrophy for the most part after tooth loss. Three structures of the alveolar process may be discriminated:

- Alveolar bone proper
- Trabecular bone
- Compact bone

Compact bone covers and contains the alveolar processes. At the entrance to the alveoli, the alveolar crest, it blends into the cribriform plate, the alveolar bone proper, which forms the alveolar wall and is approximately 0.1–0.4 mm thick. It is perforated with numerous small canals (Volkmann canals) through which vessels as well as nerve fibers enter into and exit the periodontal ligament space. The *trabecular bone* occupies the space between compact bone and alveolar bone proper. The distance between the marginal gingiva and the alveolar crest is referred to as the "biologic width" of 2–3 mm (BW; Gargiulo et al. 1961, see p. 319).

31 Osseous Support Apparatus
The tooth-supporting alveolar process consists of the alveolar bone (**1**), trabecular bone (**2**), and compact bone (**3**). Alveolar bone and compact bone join at the margin to form the alveolar crestal bone (arrow). In this region, the alveolar process is often extremely thin, especially on the facial aspect, and unsupported by trabecular bone (Fig. 36).

Right: Histologic section (HE, x10) through the periodontium (the location is indicated by the rectangle superimposed in the main figure). On the right side of the picture, the alveolar bone with its osteons and a Haversian canal is clearly visible. Bundle bone has been deposited adjacent to the structures on the periodontal aspect.
The periodontal ligament is cell-rich, and exhibits a thin layer of cementum-forming fibroblasts along the acellular, extrinsic-fiber cementum (left).

Histology courtesy *H. Schroeder*

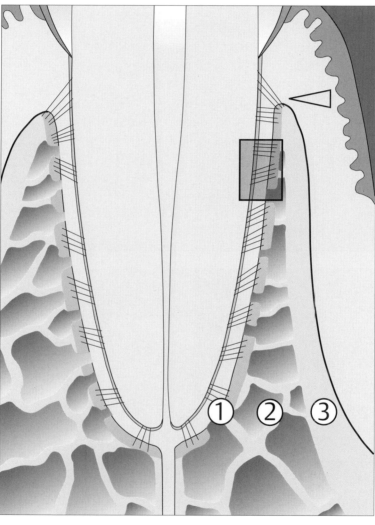

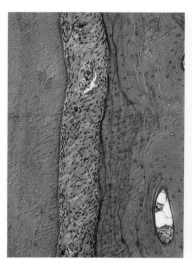

1 **Alveolar Bone**
  Synonyms:

  Anatomically
  – Alveolar Wall
  – Cribriform Plate

  Radiographically
  – Lamina dura

2 **Trabecular Bone**

3 **Compact Bone**

32 Mandibular Alveolar Process in Sagittal Section
In this histologic section (H and E, x1) the elegant structure of the trabecular bone and the more or less large marrow spaces are visible. The *alveolar bone proper* is depicted only as a very thin, often partially broken line.

Right: In this transilluminated bone preparation, it becomes clear that the alveolar bone is perforated by numerous small holes, as in a sieve (cribriform plate).

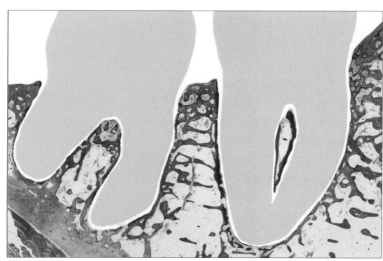

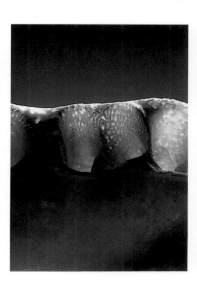

Maxillary Bone

33 Maxillary Alveolar Process in Horizontal Section

The section is through the alveolar process and tooth roots at about the midpoint. With the exception of the molar areas, the bone is thicker on the oral surface than on the facial. The trabecular bone is variably thick. Clearly visible is the varying mass of the bony interdental and interradicular septa, as well as the varying shape of the root cross sections.

Maxilla

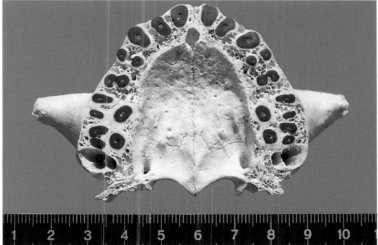

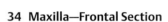

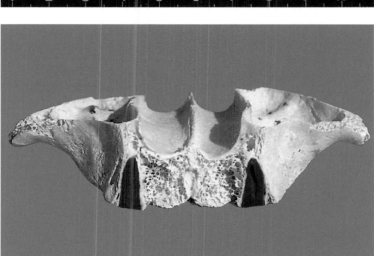

34 Maxilla—Frontal Section

This section was cut through the plane of the canine, and it shows the relationship of the root to the nasal sinus. Clearly visible is the very thin bony layer on the facial surface of the root (Fig. 36).

Left: The sagittal section shows how the root tips of premolars and molars sometimes extend into the maxillary sinus. The alveolar bone may actually border directly on the sinus mucosa.

Mandibular Bone

35 Mandibular Alveolar Process in Horizontal Section

The section represents a cut approximately halfway down the tooth root. In contrast to the maxilla, the orofacial width of the mandibular alveolar process is considerably less. All roots exhibit an "hourglass" profile (proximal concavities).

Mandible

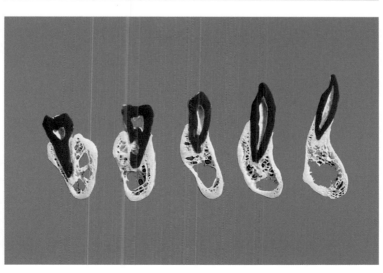

36 Orofacial Sections through the Mandible

From right to left, an incisor, a canine, a premolar and two molars were sectioned. Impressive is the thin, tapered bony lamella on the facial aspect; it is impossible to distinguish between compact bone and alveolar bone proper.

Left: Sagittal section through the alveolar process and alveoli. Especially in the molar area, the alveolar bone is traversed by numerous Volkmann canals.

Blood Supply of the Periodontium

All periodontal tissues, but especially the periodontal ligament, have a copious blood supply even in the healthy state. This is due not only to the high metabolism of this cell- and fiber-rich tissue, but also to the peculiar mechanical/functional demands on the periodontium. Occlusal forces are resisted not only by the periodontal ligament and the alveolar process, but also by means of the tissue fluid and its transfer within the periodontal ligament space (*hydraulic pressure distribution,* dampening).

The most important afferent vessels for the alveolar process and the periodontium are:

- In the *maxilla*, the anterior and posterior alveolar arteries, the infraorbital artery and the palatine artery
- In the *mandible*, the mandibular artery, the sublingual artery, the mental artery, and the buccal and facial arteries.

Lymph vessels follow for the most part the blood vascular tree.

37 Diagram of Periodontal Blood Supply
The periodontal ligament (**1**), the alveolar process (**2**) and the gingiva (**3**) are supplied by three vascular sources. These vessels exhibit frequent anastomoses.
Within the periodontal ligament, the vascular network is especially dense. Adjacent to the junctional epithelium, these vessels splay into a very dense vascular system, the capillary-venule plexus (**A**). This plexus is of great significance for host defense against infection (p. 55).
The oral epithelium contacts the subjacent connective tissue through a series of rete ridges. Each rete ridge of connective tissue contains *capillary loops* (**B**).

Right: In this section beneath the JE, a dense *vascular plexus* (**X**) is observed even in health. Above the white arrows, one observes the most marginal vascular loops in the area of the adjacent, non-keratinized oral sulcular epithelium (**OSE**).

Courtesy J. Egelberg

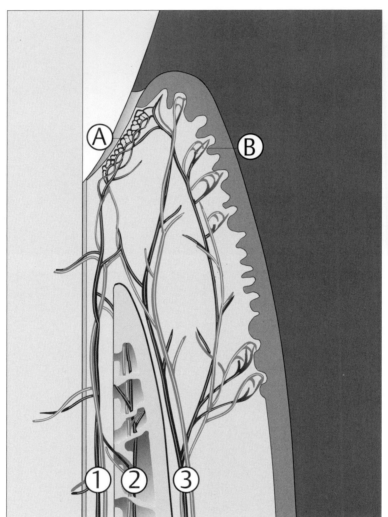

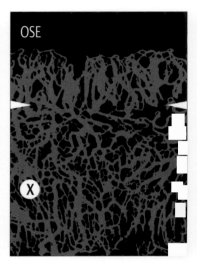

Blood Supply Pathways

1 Periodontal
2 Alveolar
3 Supraperiostal/mucogingival

A Post-capillary Venous Plexus

B Sub-epithelial Capillary Loops

38 Fluorescence Angiography—Vascular Loops Subjacent to the Oral Epithelium
Following intravenous injection of 2 ml of sodium fluorescein solution (20 %), the vessels (capillaries) subjacent to the oral epithelium can be rendered visible by UV light.
Some small vascular loops are visible in the connective tissue rete pegs (**B,** also in Fig. 37).

Courtesy W. Mörmann

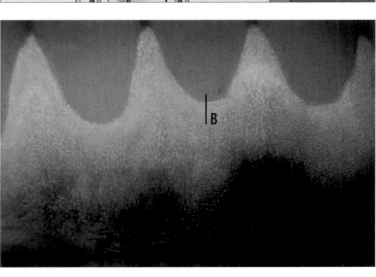

Innervation of the Periodontium

The sensory innervation of the maxilla occurs via the second branch of the trigeminal nerve, and that of the mandible via the third branch. The following description of the neural distribution within the periodontal structures is based upon investigations by Byers (1985), Linden et al. (1994) and Byers & Takeyasu (1997).

The periodontium, especially the gingiva and periodontal ligament, contains "Ruffini-like" *mechanoreceptors and nociceptive nerve fibers,* in addition to the ubiquitous branches of the sympathetic nervous system.

The functions of these innervations are coordinated with those of the dental pulp and the dentin. The stimulus threshold of the mechanoreceptors, which react to tactile (pressure) stimulus, as well as to the stretching of the periodontal ligament fibers, is very low. In contrast, the pain-sensing nociceptive nerve endings have a relatively high threshold. It is via these two separate afferent systems that "information" about jaw position, tooth movements, speech, tooth contact during swallowing and chewing, minor positional alterations (physiologic tooth mobility), pain during unphysiologic loading, as well as injuries are

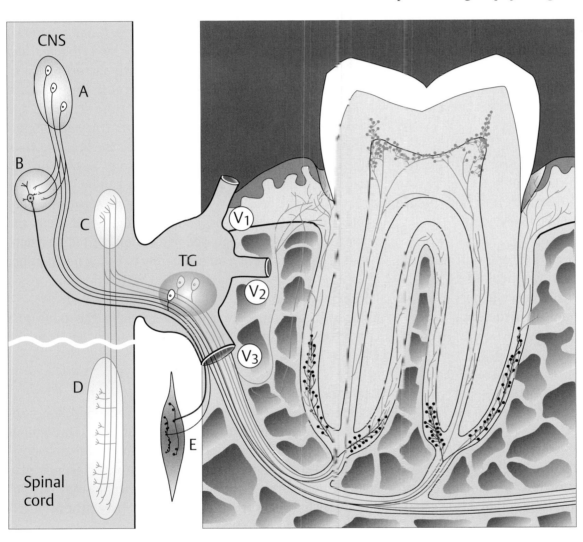

39 Innervation of a Mandibular Molar
Innervation of gingival and periodontal structures is via the mandibular nerve, the third branch of the trigeminal nerve.

Modified from *M. Byers*

A   Mesencephalic sensory neurons of the trigeminal nerve
B   Motor nucleus of the trigeminal
C   Sensory nucleus of the trigeminal
D   Spinal sensory trigeminal nucleus
E   Fibers of the masticatory musculature

TG Trigeminal ganglion (Gasserian ganglion) with its three branches:

V_1 Ophthalmic
V_2 Maxillary
V_3 Mandibular

CNS Central Nervous System

transmitted. In this way, various mechanoreceptors transmit "conscious reactions" via trigeminal ganglia to the sensory nucleus of the trigeminal in the central nervous system, while unconscious reflexes transmit to mesencephalic sensory neurons. These various receptors are localized in varying regions of the periodontal structures: At the level of the middle of the root, one finds more receptors for up-take of "conscious reactions," whereas in the apical region there are more receptors for the unconscious reflexes whose signals transmit to the mesencephalic sensory neurons.

The junctional epithelium as well as the epithelia of the free and attached gingiva, neither of which are vascularized, are served by a dense network of nociceptive and tactile nerve endings. The same is true for the subepithelial, supracrestal gingival connective tissue.

Somatosensory perception in certain gingival diseases (e.g., ulcerative gingivoperiodontitis), as well as pressure and pain sensation during probing of the healthy gingival sulcus or periodontal pockets are the clinical manifestations of the innervation of gingival tissues.

The Coordinated Functions of the Periodontal Structures

Turnover—Adaptation—Defense—Healing

Within the healthy periodontium, there is a constant *turnover* of all tissues, except cementum. The term *tissue homeostasis* was coined to characterize the process by which the composition of the various structures, i.e., the balance of their volumes, their integrity vis-à-vis each other, and their mutually interwoven functions (Williams et al. 1997). The apposition and/or resorption of the various tissues can vary even in the healthy condition, depending upon several factors; for example, the periodontal tissues undergo a process known as *adaptation*, or in cases of reduced occlusal loading (afunction, hypofunction) or increased loading (hyperfunction, parafunction). This concept is not limited only to an adaption to masticatory forces, but is broader in the sense of all "insults" that the periodontal tissues may encounter, including the always present—although in very differing degrees—infection.

Host defense against all "attacks" refers primarily to the immune system (p. 41), but also to the healthy tissue. Disease (periodontitis) will ensue if the demands upon the tissues are larger than their capability to reactively adapt.

The adaptability of the tissues, i.e., their ability to vary the rate of turnover in response to various mediators (e.g., cytokines) also plays an important role in *healing*, for example following injury or after mechanical periodontal therapy (scaling and root planing—S/RP).

Primary Functions of the Periodontal Tissues

Epithelium

The epithelium of the attached gingiva (OE, oral epithelium) is referred to as masticatory mucosa. Like the palatal mucosa, it is keratinized. Keratinization is a mechanism for *protection against all mechanical challenges, but also against thermal, chemical and infectious attack.*

The turnover rate of the gingival epithelium has been variously reported between 6 (Schroeder 1992) and 40 days (Williams et al. 1997). Probably it is influenced by "chalones" (substances which inhibit mitosis) on the one hand and by cytokines (Fig. 95), e.g., epidermal growth factor (EGF) and transforming growth factor (TGF-β) on the other.

The junctional epithelium exhibits a faster turnover rate than gingival epithelium. Cell division occurs in the basal cell layer. All of the daughter cells migrate in the direction of the gingival sulcus, where they are rapidly sloughed.

Through this constant flow of junctional epithelial cells, sulcus fluid, and active migration of granulocytes (PMN), the sulcus is effectively cleared of invading bacteria and their metabolic products. In addition to immunocompetent cells, it is also primarily the dynamics of the resident tissue cells and the coronally streaming flow of tissue fluid that is responsible for the *prevention of infection* and therefore also for the maintenance of health of the marginal periodontal structures.

Gingival Connective Tissue

The circumstance for the periodontal connective tissue is similar to that of the epithelial structures. It has a turnover rate of only a few days, orchestrated by cytokines and growth factors (platelet-derived growth factor/PDGF; fibroblast growth factor/FGF, among others). In this matrix, it is the fibroblasts that are responsible for the synthesis and breakdown of collagen matrix. The matrix metalloproteinases (Fig. 102) that are responsible for the breakdown of collagen depend upon divalent cations (e.g., Zn^{+2}). The balance between synthesis and breakdown can be "shifted" to a certain degree toward synthesis in the presence of pathogenic influences. However, if the pathogenic insult is too great, the process of increased resorption (or reduced synthesis?) can occur and lead ultimately to tissue destruction.

Periodontal Bone

Bone synthesis and resorption, especially the bone loss characteristic of periodontitis, is covered in detail in the chapter "Pathogenesis" (see pp. 60–61).

Cementum

In contrast to epithelium, connective tissue and bone, cementum is not subject to continuous turnover. Throughout life, cementum tends to increase in thickness due to apposition. Local resorption observed as resorption lacunae may result from trauma, orthodontic forces, or they may be idiopathic. Such defects are often "repaired" by synthesis of cellular intrinsic-fiber cementum.

Summary

The healthy periodontal structures have the capacity to mount a certain defense potential even before the actual immune response is mounted; the latter, of course, also introduces certain destructive elements into the milieu.

Etiology and Pathogenesis

The most common diseases of the tooth-supporting apparatus are plaque-induced, usually chronic, inflammatory alterations in the gingiva and the subjacent periodontal structures.

Gingivitis may persist for many years without progressing to periodontitis. With good oral hygiene and effective professional removal of plaque and calculus, gingivitis is completely reversible.

Periodontitis usually develops out of a more or less pronounced gingivitis. Periodontitis is only partially reversible (see periodontal healing, p. 205/regenerative therapies).

The reasons why gingivitis develops into periodontitis (or does *not*) are still incompletely understood. As with all *infections*, it appears that the proliferation of pathogenic microorganisms, their toxic potency, their capacities to invade tissues, and above all the individual host response to such infections are the determining factors (p. 55; Kornman et al. 1997, Page & Kornman 1997, Salvi et al. 1997).

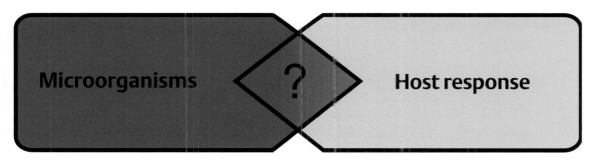

40 Bacterial Attack vs. Defense Reactions by the Host
The virulence of bacteria, their capability to invade into tissues, their number and composition, as well as their metabolic products elicit reactions by the host (immune response). Whether periodontal disease will occur, and its severity, depends only partially upon the bacterial insult. Transition from gingivitis to periodontitis involves factors such as host response, risk factors, and local factors.

An absolutely plaque-free condition in the oral cavity, with prevention of any biofilm formation on tooth surfaces is unachievable, and illusion, and probably even unphysiologic. Nevertheless, gingival and periodontal health can be maintained if the accumulation of plaque is small and if the biofilm contains only weakly virulent organisms (gram-positive, facultative anaerobes), and if an effective host response is mounted.

If the bacterial flora takes on periodontally pathogenic characteristics (e.g., certain gram-negative microorganisms), the result will be inflammation and specific immunologic responses; these responses may represent not only defense mechanisms, but—especially in long-term chronic infec-

tion—also destructive potential (cytotoxic, immunopathologic; p. 34).

Inflammation-inducing products of bacteria include enzymes, antigens, toxins, and "signal" substances that activate macrophages and T-cells (Birkedal-Hansen 1998). It is likely that bacterial enzymes, other metabolic products and toxins can directly elicit injury to the periodontal tissues even *without* immediate host response (inflammation). Bacterial products including hyaluronidase, chondroitin sulfatase, proteolytic enzymes, as well as cytotoxins in the form of organic acids, ammonia, hydrogen sulfide and endotoxins (e.g., lipopolysaccharides, LPS) have been demonstrated in periodontal tissues.

Periodontitis—A Multifactorial Disease

In recent years, the conceptual view concerning the etiology of periodontitis has evolved. Early on, it was the bacteria that were viewed as the determining factor. Certain pathogenic microorganisms were shown to be associated with various forms of periodontal disease, as well as the speed of progression. However, the existence and distribution of pathogenic bacteria did not always correlate with the inception and clinical progression of periodontitis. Furthermore, it was demonstrated that the presence of pathogenic bacteria in a periodontal pocket is not necessarily the *cause* of that pocket; rather, it seemed much more important that

the pocket milieu presents a favorable environment for the existence and proliferation of pathogenic organisms. The stage would then be set—like a vicious cycle—for the progression of the disease processes (Mombelli et al. 1991).

Nevertheless, the old adage *"no bacteria = no periodontitis"* still holds true, but on the other hand it is also a fact that bacteria, including periodontopathic bacteria, do not without exception cause periodontitis.

**41 Etiology of Periodontitis—
Interaction between Dental
Plaque and the Host**

Bacteria
1 The primary etiologic factor for the existence of periodontitis is pathogenic microorganisms within the subgingival biofilm.

Host
2 The genetically determined non-specific and specific immune responses, as well as systemic syndromes and diseases influence the existence and the clinical course of periodontitis.

3 "Habits" and the patient's own approach to general health will influence plaque formation and host immune response, both systemically and particularly with regard to oral health.

4 Social circumstances influence the systemic and psychic well being of the patient. Problems in the socioeconomic arena lead to negative stress.

5 Psychic burdens and stress influence the immune status.

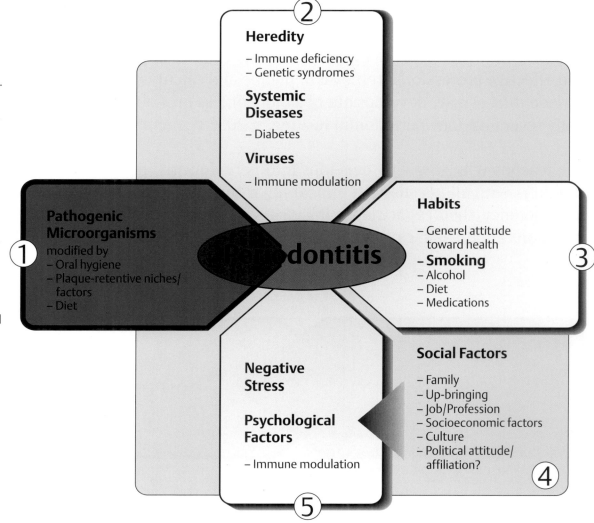

In addition to specific microorganisms, diverse *host factors* are critical for the development of periodontitis from a pre-existing gingivitis (cf. Fig. 41, modified from Clarke & Hirsch 1995). Such factors include the immune responses triggered by pathogens, and these are well understood today. Such defense reactions may be disproportional to the insult, resulting in immunopathologic tissue injury.
Recently, however, in addition to the genetically determined immune reactions, a great number of other individual risk factors have been identified, which may be responsible for the initiation and the degree of severity of the clinical course of periodontitis (p. 51).

Of the risk factors listed in Figures 41 and 104, only a few are capable of damaging the periodontium directly (e.g., smoking); of much greater importance is the influence of such factors on the patient's own immune system. The delicate balance between "attack/destruction" (bacteria) and defense (host response) is disturbed. It is only logical to assume that the most severe, early-onset and aggressive forms of periodontitis will occur when particularly virulent bacteria are present in a weak (immunodeficient) host.

Microbiology

Bacteria are present throughout life in a myriad of sites on and in the human body. The bacteria may be beneficial for the host, or of no consequence (commensal), or injurious. In the oral cavity, over 530 different species of microorganisms have so far been identified; fortunately, for the most part these organisms remain in ecological balance and do not cause disease. Certain facultatively pathogenic ("opportunistic") bacteria are occasionally observed in high numbers, e.g., in cases of disease (periodontitis, mucosal infection). It remains unclear whether these bacteria alone represent the cause of the diseases, or whether they simply find favorable living conditions in the disease milieu. *Non-specific* supragingival plaque (mixed flora) will elicit gingivitis within ca. seven days. If the plaque is removed, gingivitis regresses in a short period of time ("reversibility"). On the other hand, for the various forms of periodontitis, especially the aggressive, rapidly-progressing forms, *specific* bacteria are associated.

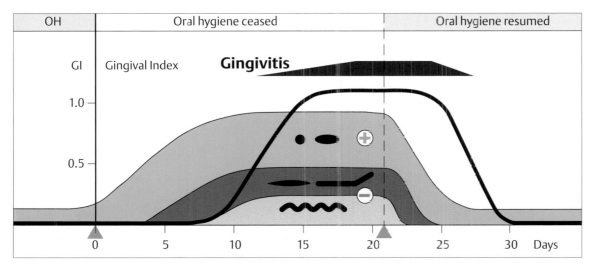

42 Experimental Gingivitis
In 1965, *Löe et al.* published the classic experimental proof of the *bacterial etiology of gingivitis*. In plaque- and inflammation-free subjects, plaque begins to accumulate if all oral hygiene is ceased. For the first few days, this plaque is composed of gram-positive cocci and rods, then later of filamentous organisms and finally spirochetes (gram-negative). Within a few days, a mild gingivitis ensues. If the plaque is removed, the gingiva quickly returns to a state of health.

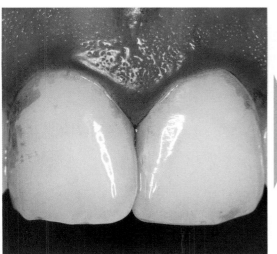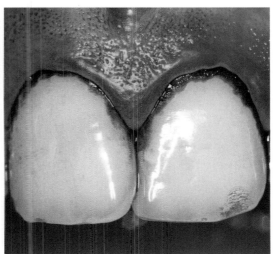

43 Healthy Gingiva and Initial Gingivitis
Left: "Almost" clean central incisors. An extremely thin biofilm is compatible with clinically healthy gingiva. A few bacteria may even serve to maintain the "memory" of the immune system (p. 55).

Right: Plaque accumulation following seven days without oral hygiene. Gingivitis has developed. The proliferation and relative increase in numbers of gram-negative microorganisms are responsible for the gingivitis.

Biofilm—Plaque Formation on Tooth and Root Surfaces

The oropharynx is an open ecosystem wherein bacteria are always present; bacteria attempt to colonize in all favorable locations. Most bacteria, however, can only persist after the formation of a biofilm upon desquamation-free surfaces, i.e., hard substances (tooth and root surfaces, restorative materials, implants, prostheses etc.). In the presence of healthy dental and gingival relationships, there is a balance between the additive and retentive mechanisms of biofilms vis-à -vis the abrasive forces that tend to reduce biofilm formation, e.g., self-cleansing by the cheeks and tongue, diet and mechanical oral hygiene measures.

The existence of a biofilm results within a matter of hours or days, in the phases described below (Darveau et al. 1997, Descouts & Aronsson 1999, Costerton et al. 1999).

The establishment and stabilization of bacteria within a biofilm are important not only for the etiology of periodontitis, but also for adjunctive systemic and topical medicinal treatment for periodontitis (p. 287): Biofilm bacteria imbedded within a matrix of extracellular polysaccharides are more than 1,000 times less sensitive to antimicrobials (e. g., antibiotics) than free-floating ("planktonic") bacteria.

44 Dental Plaque—Development

Within minutes after completely cleansing the tooth surface, a *pellicle* forms from proteins and glycoproteins in saliva.

A *Association*: Through purely physical forces, bacteria associate loosely with the pellicle.

B *Adhesion*: Because they possess special surface molecules (adhesins) that bind to pellicle receptors, some bacteria become the "primary colonizers," particularly streptococci and actinomyces. Subsequently, other microorganisms adhere to the primary colonizers.

C Bacterial *proliferation* ensues.

D *Microcolonies* are formed. Many streptococci secrete protective extracellular polysaccharides (e. g., dextrans, levans).

E *Biofilm ("attached plaque")*: Microcolonies form complex groups with metabolic advantages for the constituents.

F *Plaque growth—maturation*: The biofilm is characterized by a primitive "circulatory system." The plaque begins to "behave" as a *complex organism*! Anaerobic organisms increase. Metabolic products and evulsed cell wall constituents (e. g., lipopolysaccharides, vesicles) serve to activate the host immune response (p. 38). Bacteria within the biofilm are protected from phagocytic cells (PMN) and against exogenous bacteriocidal agents.

X Pellicle
Y Biofilm—"Attached Plaque"
Z Planktonic Phase

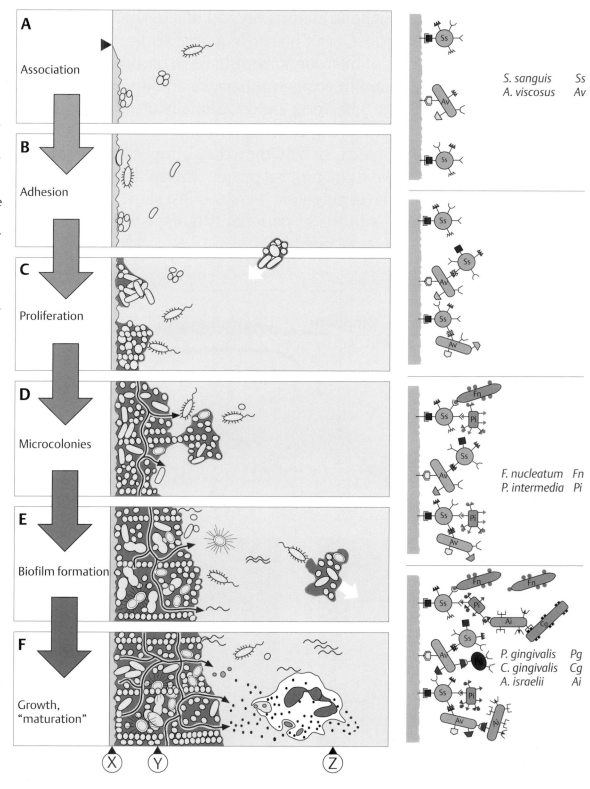

Association

Adhesion

Proliferation

Microcolonies

Biofilm formation

Growth, "maturation"

S. sanguis   Ss
A. viscosus   Av

F. nucleatum Fn
P. intermedia Pi

P. gingivalis Pg
C. gingivalis Cg
A. israelii   Ai

X   Y   Z

Supragingival Plaque

... and its Initial Subgingival Expansion

The first bacteria that accumulate *supragingivally* on the tooth surface are mostly gram-positive (*Streptococcus* sp, *Actinomyces* sp.). In the course of the following days, gram-negative cocci as well as gram-positive and gram-negative rods and the first filamentous forms begin to colonize (Listgarten et al. 1975, Listgarten 1976). By means of a variety of *metabolic products*, the bacterial flora provoke the tissue to increased exudation and migration of PMN leukocytes into the sulcus ("leukocyte walls" against the bacteria).

The increase in PMN diapedesis and the flow of sulcus fluid lead to initial disintegration of the junctional epithelium. This makes it possible for bacteria to more easily invade between the tooth and the junctional epithelium, and invade the subgingival area (gingivitis, gingival pocket formation). In the total absence of oral hygiene, plaque formation and an initial host defensive response within gingival tissue occur. With optimum—including interdental—oral hygiene, the formation of biofilm is repeatedly disrupted and gingival health is maintained.

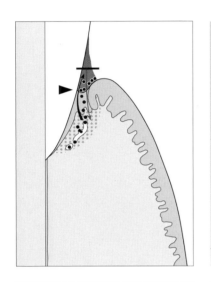

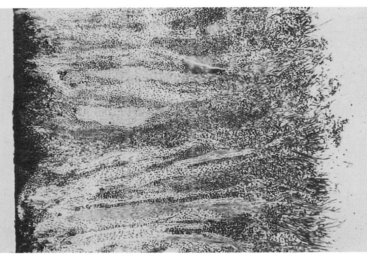

45 One-week-old Plaque—Interactions
Thick zone of early colonizers on the enamel surface and the column-like structures that result from rapid proliferation of streptococci. On the plaque surface, one observes rods and filaments.

Left: Interaction between host and plaque. Chemotactically regulated immigration of polymorphonuclear granulocytes (PMN, arrow). The black horizontal line indicates the level from which this sample of plaque was taken.

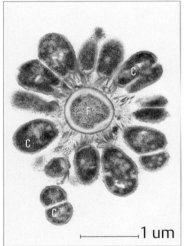

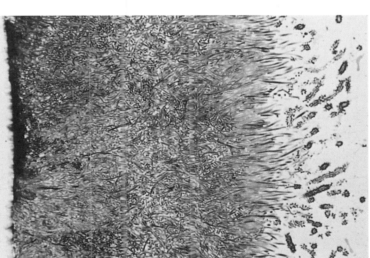

46 Three-week-old Plaque
The composition of the supragingival plaque has changed markedly. Filamentous organisms now predominate. Conspicuous forms resembling "corn cobs" are observed at the plaque surface.
Left: In this transmission electron photomicrograph, the structure of such a "corn cob" is revealed. At the center is a gram-negative filamentous organism (**F**), surrounded by gram-positive cocci (**C**).

Histology and TEM courtesy *M. Listgarten*

1 um

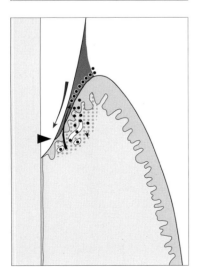

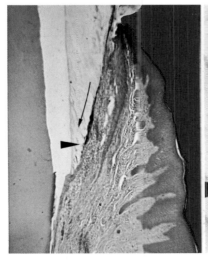

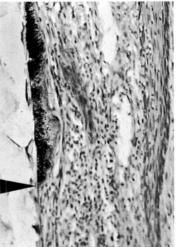

47 Expansion of Supragingival Plaque—Gingival Pocket
Middle and Right: Weakening of the epithelial attachment to the tooth permits apical migration of gram-positive plaque bacteria in a thin layer between the tooth and the junctional epithelium (thin arrow). Gram-negative bacteria colonize subsequently, and a *gingival* pocket forms (Fig. 150).
Histology courtesy *G. Cimasoni*

Left: Schematic representation of the interaction between plaque and host tissue.

Natural Factors Favoring Plaque Retention

The formation of a plaque biofilm can be enhanced by natural retention factors, which can also render biofilm removal by means of oral hygiene more difficult. These retention factors include:

- Supra- and subgingival calculus
- Cementoenamel junctions and enamel projections
- Furcation entrances and irregularities
- Tooth fissures and grooves
- Cervical and root surface caries
- Crowding of teeth in the arch.

By itself, *calculus* is not pathogenic. However, its rough surface presents a retention area for vital, pathogenic bacteria. At the microscopic level, the *cementoenamel junction* is very irregular, and offers retentive roughness. Enamel projections and "pearls" also inhibit soft tissue attachment.
Furcation entrances, fissures, etc. are retentive niches for plaque. *Carious lesions* represent a huge bacterial reservoir. *Crowding of teeth* reduces self-cleansing and renders oral hygiene more difficult.

48 Supragingival Calculus
Lingual surfaces of mandibular incisors and buccal surfaces of maxillary molars near the orifices of salivary ducts often exhibit massive accumulations of supragingival calculus.

Right: TEM of old supragingival calculus. Calcified plaque (**A**) close to the tooth surface. Note the accumulation of cell-free hexagonal monocrystals (**B**) upon the calcified plaque.

Courtesy *H. Schroeder*

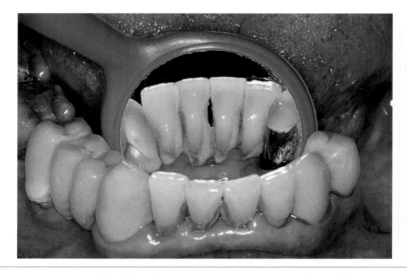
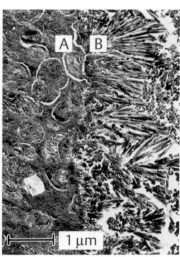

49 Subgingival Calculus
In this patient with long-standing periodontitis, the gingiva has receded. Calculus that was formerly subgingival is now supragingival.

Right: Subgingival calculus is observed clinically after reflecting the gingival margin. Subgingival calculus is usually dark in color (Fe minerals) and harder than the more loosely structured supragingival calculus (calcium phosphates). The cementoenamel junction is indicated by the dashed line.

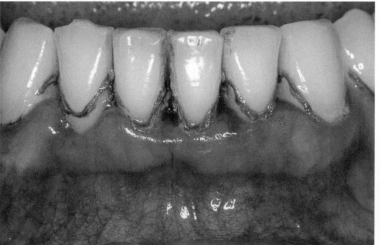
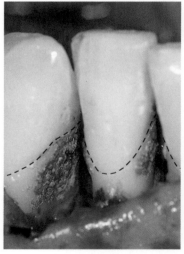

50 Crowding, Enamel Projection (Enamel "Pearl")
The lingually displaced mandibular incisors do not benefit from the natural self-cleansing action of the lower lip. Oral hygiene is also rendered more difficult.

Right: The furcation on this molar is filled by a projection of enamel that ends in a bulbous pearl, extending into the interradicular area. When a pocket forms in such an area, plaque control is particularly difficult.

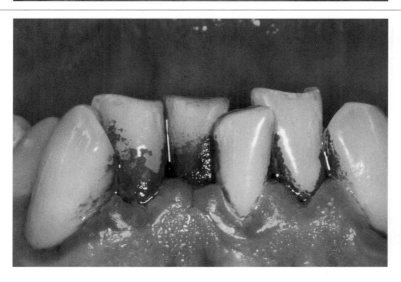
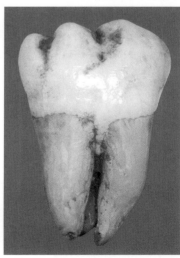

Iatrogenic Factors Favoring Plaque Retention

Restorative dentistry—from a simple restoration to a full-mouth reconstruction—can do more harm than good to the patient's oral health if performed improperly! Placing only optimum restorations is synonymous with preventive periodontics (tertiary prevention, p. 198).

Fillings and crowns that appear to be perfect clinically and macroscopically almost always exhibit deficiencies at the margins when viewed microscopically. When margins are located subgingivally, they always present an irritation for the marginal periodontal tissues.

Overhanging margins of restorations and crowns accumulate additional plaque. Gingivitis ensues. The composition of the plaque changes. The number of gram-negative anaerobes (e.g., *Porphyromonas gingivalis*), the organisms responsible for initiation and progression of periodontitis, increases rapidly (Lang et al. 1983).

Gross iatrogenic irritants such as poorly designed *clasps* and *prosthesis saddles* may exert a direct traumatic influence upon periodontal tissues.

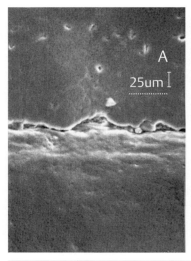 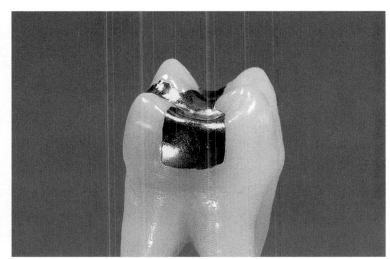

51 Amalgam Restoration—Clinical View and SEM

Left: Viewed in the scanning electron microscope, a clearly visible margin defect is observed. Such a defect is a perfect niche for the accumulation of plaque. The amalgam restoration (**A**) is at the top of this figure, the adjacent enamel below. The white dot under the 25 μm legend are representative of the size of coccoid microorganisms (ca. 1 μm).

Courtesy *F. Lutz*

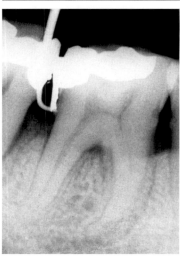 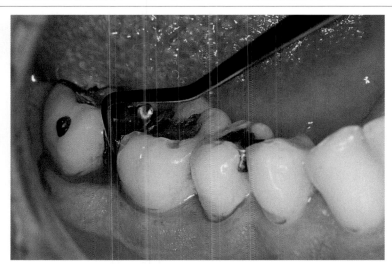

52 Amalgam—Proximal Overhang

Gross overhangs such as this, located subgingivally, invariably lead to plaque accumulation and to gingivitis (note hemorrhage). Pathogenic, gram-negative anaerobes are frequently observed. In contrast to amalgam and especially gold restorations, composite resin restorations are particularly retentive of bacteria.

Left: Radiograph of the same case.

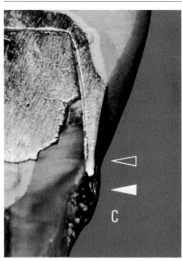 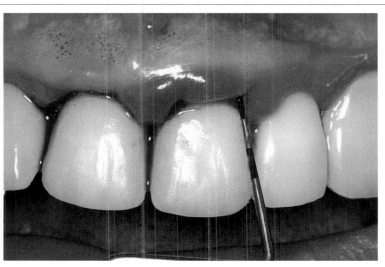

53 Crown Margin Overhang and Open Margins

The cement that was used to cement this crown has begun to extrude from the open margin. The massive retention of plaque between the crown and the prepared tooth leads to severe gingivitis and establishment of a pathogenic bacterial flora.

Left: Section through a porcelain-fused-to-metal crown with a margin that is both overhanging (arrows) and open. Calculus (**C**) and plaque have accumulated apically.

Subgingival Plaque

Extending apically from the supragingival region, a subgingival plaque biofilm will often form within the existing gingival sulcus/pocket; this was previously called the "adherent" plaque. In addition to gram-positive bacteria such as streptococci, actinomyces, etc., as the probing depth increases so does the number of anaerobic *gram-negative* bacteria (p. 36).

This subgingival biofilm can also calcify. A dark, hard and difficult to remove calculus ("serum calculus") accumulates. In addition, the gingival pocket also contains loose agglomerates of non-adherent, often mobile bacteria (with a high concentration of gram-negative anaerobes and spirochetes). In acute phases, *periodontopathic* bacteria often increase dramatically. These include *Actinobacillus actinomycetemcomitans, P. gingivalis, T. forsythia,* spirochetes etc. (pp. 30, 33, 38). Despite these alterations in the subgingival plaque, periodontitis, even in the acute stage, cannot be characterized as a "highly specific" infection because large differences have been reported in the bacterial composition between patients and even within different pocket locations in the same patient (Dzink et al. 1988, Slots & Taubmann 1992, Lindhe 1997).

54 Subgingival Pocket Flora
This is a relatively thin adherent biofilm (blue-violet). One observes loose accumulations of gram-negative, anaerobic, and also motile bacteria. Formations resembling test tube brushes, consisting of filamentous bacteria are also observed (inset).

Histology courtesy *M. Listgarten*

Right: As pocket depth increases (arrow), the resident flora becomes increasingly gram-negative and anaerobic.

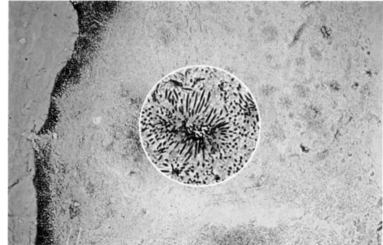
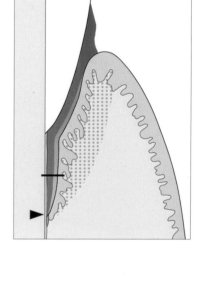

55 Surface of the Biofilm on the Root
Within a pocket, the root surface of a tooth manifesting periodontitis is covered with a densely intertwined bacterial colonization composed of many different bacterial morphotypes (scanning electron photomicrograph).

The *morphology* of the bacteria permits neither a determination of the species nor any clues concerning pathogenicity.

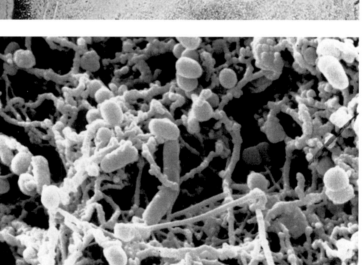

1 um

56 Microorganisms of the Non-adherent Plaque— "Planktonic" Phase
In a dark-field preparation, motile rods and small to larger spirochetes predominate, while cocci and filaments are rare: Typical signs of an active pocket (exacerbation; cf. p. 63).
Right: Intact phagocytes (PMN) in the pocket exudate do not lose their capacity for phagocytosis. The arrow depicts a spirochete being engulfed.

Courtesy *B. Guggenheim*

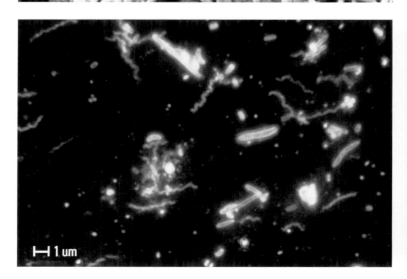
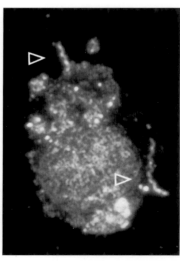

1 um

Bacterial Invasion Into Tissue?

In patients with a compromised immune response, for example in cases of early onset, aggressive periodontitis (p. 96), bacteria with pathogenic potential have the ability to invade the cells of the pocket epithelium and the subepithelial connective tissue, and to remain viable there for varying periods of time. This usually occurs only in the depth of the pockets where the bacteria can avoid the infiltrate (defense), which is usually located close to the gingival margin. The periodontopathic bacteria (p. 33) produce virulence factors (leukotoxins from *Actinobacillus actinomycetemcomitans*, lipopolysaccharides and enzymes), which can initially shut down the chemotactic guidance of defense cells (e.g., PMN) or even kill PMNs. With time, the invading microorganisms are recognized by the activated immune system and killed. If tissue invasion is mild, small areas of necrotic tissue resorption may result, but if the bacterial invasion is massive, acute suppurative abscesses can result (Allenspach-Petrzilka & Guggenheim 1983, Christensson et al. 1987, Frank 1988, Saglie et al. 1988, Slots 1999, Van Winkelhoff & Slots 1999). It is unclear whether oral microorganisms that invade tissue cells actually *colonize*, or whether the individual microorganisms simply invade.

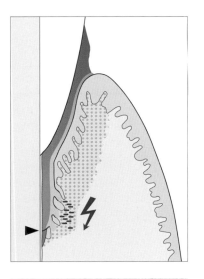

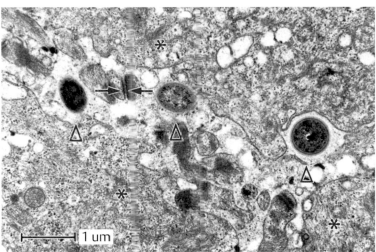

57 Bacteria within the Pocket Epithelium

Bacteria (red triangles) in the widened intercellular spaces of the pocket epithelium. Three epithelial cells (∗) and one desmosome (double arrow) are observed.
The exudate and PMNs have significantly widened the intercellular spaces between the JE cells.

Left: In the depth of the active pocket, one observes ulcerated epithelium, through which bacteria may invade the connective tissue (red bars).

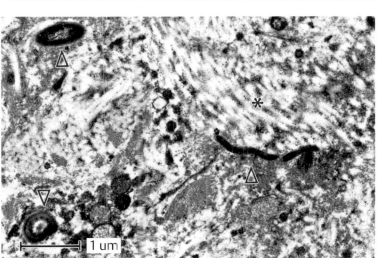

58 Bacterial Invasion—Infection

Bacteria of various species are observed within the connective tissue (arrows) adjacent to a deep periodontal pocket. Tissue damage (∗ = degraded collagen) may result, or tissue may remain completely healthy in appearance.

Left: A gram-negative bacterium (**G**B) is observed in the midst of otherwise essentially intact collagen fibrils

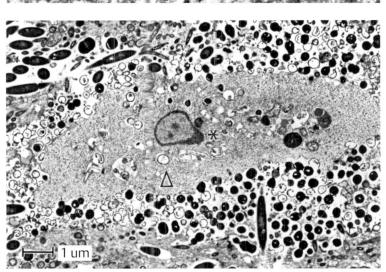

59 Necrosis—Suppuration

Almost the entire photomicrograph is filled by a dead phagocytic cell (PMN, ∗). The cell contains phagolysosomes, some of which exhibit digested material (arrow).
The dead phagocyte is surrounded by dead bacteria and bacterial cell walls. This pus must either be resorbed by the host tissue, or expelled (abscess, fistula).

TEMs courtesy *B. Guggenheim*

Classification of Oral Microorganisms

Thanks to new laboratory techniques (e. g., 16S rRNA analyses), over 500 species and subspecies have been isolated and classified from subgingival and supragingival bacterial samples (Slots & Taubman 1992, Moore & Moore 1994, Socransky et al. 1999). Some of the cultivable species are listed below. Today, only about a dozen microorganisms are classified as *periodontal pathogens*. Foremost among these are gram-negative organisms, including *Actinobacillus actinomycetemcomitans, Porphyromonas gingivalis, Tannerella forsythia* (formerly *Bacteroides forsythus*) and *Prevotella intermedia* (p. 33).

Some of these bacteria possess significant biochemical capacities for the pathogenesis of inflammatory periodontal diseases. For example, they are capable of colonizing root surfaces and cell surfaces, and therefore maintain a secure position in the micro-ecological cosmos of the pocket flora. The microorganisms are usually capable of co-aggregation, i.e., they aggregate with one or more other types of bacteria to form a so-called complex or "cluster" (Socransky et al. 1998, 1999). Such complexes have been characterized as highly pathogenic or only slightly pathogenic.

60 Microorganisms in the Plaque Biofilm and in the Non-adherent Planktonic Phase

	Gram ⊕ positive		Gram ⊖ negative	
Prokaryotes	Facultative anaerobes	Obligate anaerobes	Facultative anaerobes	Obligate anaerobes
Cocci ●	**Streptococcus** – S. anginosus (S. milleri) – S. mutans – S. sanguis • **Ss** – S. oralis – S. mitis – S. intermedius	**Peptostreptococcus** – P. micros • **Pm** **Peptococcus**	**Neisseria** **Branhamella**	**Veillonella** – V. parvula
Rods ▬	**Actinomyces** – A. naeslundii • **An** – A. viscosus • **Av** – A. odontolyticus – A. israelii **Propionibacterium** **Rothia** – R. dentocariosa **Lactobacillus** – L. oris – L. acidophilus – L. salivarius – L. buccalis	**Eubacterium** – E. nodatum • **En** – E. saburreum – E. timidum – E. brachy – E. alactolyticum **Bifidobacterium** – B. dentium	**Actinobacillus** – A. actinomycetem-comitans • **Aa** **Capnocytophaga** – C. ochracea – C. gingivalis – C. sputigena **Campylobacter** – C. rectus • **Cr** – C. curvus – C. showae **Eikenella** – E. corrodens • **Ec** **Haemophilus** – H. aphrophilus – H. segnis	Porphyromonas – P. gingivalis • **Pg** – P. endodontalis **Prevotella** – P. intermedia • **Pi** – P. nigrescens – P. melaninogenica – P. denticola – P. loescheii – P. oris – P. oralis **Bacteroides** – T. forsythia • **Tf** – B. gracilis **Fusobacterium** – F. nucleatum • **Fn** – F. periodonticum **Selenomonas** – S. sputigena – S. noxia

Spirochetes and mycoplasms	**Mycoplasm** – M. orale – M. salivarium – M. hominis		**Spirochetes of ANUG** **Treponema sp.** – T. denticola • **Td** – T. socranskii – T. pectinovorum – T. vincentii

Eukaryotes	**Candida** – C. albicans	**Entamoeba**	**Trichomonas**

Cell Walls of Gram-positive and Gram-negative Bacteria

The technique of *Gram staining* renders differences in the composition of bacterial cell walls visible in the microscope:

- The plasma membrane (phospholipid double membrane; osmotic barrier) which surrounds the cytoplasm of both gram-positive and gram-negative bacteria, as well as the cellular skeleton that provides integrity consists of murein (a peptidoglycan), which represents only a thin layer in gram-negative microorganisms.
- *Gram-positive* bacteria possess only this single, thick cell wall, in the form of a giant netlike molecule ("sacculum"). Antigens such as teichoic acids and proteins emanate

from the murein layer. Penicillin can inhibit or kill gram-positive microorganisms by preventing cell wall synthesis by means of blocking the molecular binding of the polysaccharide chains.

- In *gram-negative* bacteria, especially the external membranes, and particularly the external layer, are highly complex; contained therein is the endotoxin lipopolysaccharide (LPS), which has a two-fold effect upon the host organism: *toxic* via the contained lipid A, and *antigenic* via the O-specific polysaccharide chain (O-antigen; cf. p. 38).

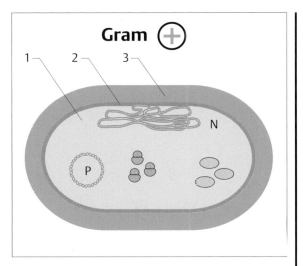

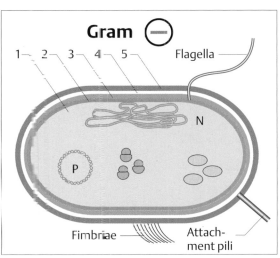

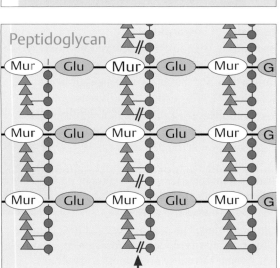

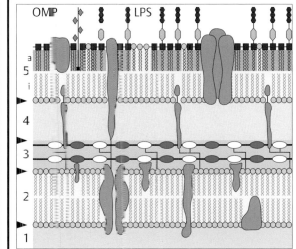

61 Anatomy/Morphology of Gram-positive (*left*) **and Gram-negative** (*right*) **Bacteria**
1 Cytoplasm with organelles: Genome (**N**), plasmid (**P**), ribosomes
2 Cytoplasmic membrane: This phospholipid bilayer functions as an osmotic barrier
3 Peptidoglycan: This large molecule provides protection
4 Periplasmatic space: This is gram-negative specific
5 Outer membrane: Found only in gram-negative organisms, with inner and outer layers

62 Cell Wall Differences
Left: Gram-positive cell walls
P   Cell wall proteins
LTA Lipoteichoic acid
TA Teichoic acids
PS Specific polysaccharides

Right: Gram-negative cell walls
4 Periplasmatic space
5 Inner (**i**) and outer (**a**) layer of the outer membrane with proteins (orange, e. g., **OMP** = outer membrane proteins), lipopolysaccharides (**LPS** in layer **5a**).
1, 2, 3 See legend, Fig. 61.

63 Cell Wall—Details
Left: Gram-positive cell walls. Peptidoglycan consists of alternating units of murein (**Mur**; N-acetyl-muraminic acid) and **Glu** (N-acetyl-glucosamine) and is cross-linked via peptide (blue circles, red triangles). Penicillin blocks this (arrow).
Right: Gram-negative cell wall
LPS = A+B+C, "endotoxin" (p. 38)
A   Lipid A (red, toxic effect)
B   Core polysaccharide
C   O-specific antigen
Modified from *F. Kayser et al.; L. Stryer*

Periodontitis—Classical or Opportunistic Infection?

Classical Infection

In classical infection, upon which the postulates of Henle and Koch are based (see below), the defense capabilities of the host are breached by a *specific, highly virulent* bacterium. The bacterium proliferates within the tissues and elicits typical symptoms of disease. Examples of classical infections include diphtheria, scarlet fever and tuberculosis. Periodontitis is *not* a classical infection. However, those types of periodontitis associated with *Actinobacillus actinomycetemcomitans may* be classified as classical infections.

Opportunistic Infection

Opportunistic microorganisms are only pathogenic in a compromised host. They are regularly found in the natural flora. They normally do not cause damage to the host. However, in patients with reduced resistance, the existence of risk factors or immunosupression, a selective increase in bacteria with *weak virulence factors* may occur, leading to an opportunistic infection. This situation does not fulfill Koch's postulates, but rather those proposed by Socransky for periodontitis (see below, Socransky & Haffajee 1992).

64 Classical Infection

A *Initial situation*: Non-specific, "natural" colonization with gram-positive (blue) and a few gram-negative (red) microorganisms ("resident" flora). The host is healthy (ecological balance).

B *Infection*: An increased number of exogenous specific pathogenic microorganisms (infective dose, violet triangles) penetrates the defense mechanism of the host and begins to proliferate selectively.

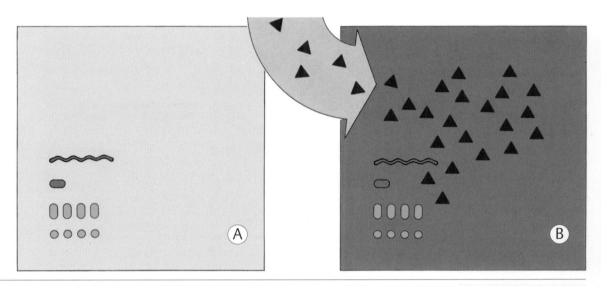

65 Opportunistic Infection

C *Initial situation*: the same non-pathogenic flora is present, as in figure 64A.

D *"Shift"/infection*: Alterations in the micro-ecology and the general resistance of the host leads to a destabilization of the ecological balance. One or more species react to this new situation with selective proliferation as well as altered activity leading to tissue damage (disease).

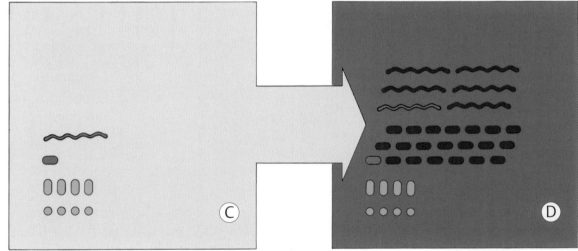

Classical vs. Opportunistic Infection—"Postulates"

In addition to the classical infections with a single pathogen, there is a large group of opportunistic infections in which entire groups of microorganisms can be involved in the initiation and progression of diseases.

Postulates of Henle and Koch

The **causative agent** must always be found in the clinical lesion, and not in healthy subjects.

The putative pathogen must be **cultivable** in pure culture.

The pathogenic characteristics of the causative agent must elicit in **animal models** a disease identical to that in humans, and the agent must be identified in the animal.

In addition: Beyond the postulates of Henle and Koch, there must be clear evidence of the immunological "**pathogen-host relationship**."

Postulates of Socransky

Association: The causative agent must be found in active "sites" in higher numbers than in non-active sites.

Elimination: The elimination of the causative agent must stop the progression of the disease.

Host response: The cellular or humoral immune response must validate the specific role of the causative agent in the disease.

Virulence factors: The causative agent must possess virulence factors that are relevant for the initiation and progression of the disease.

Animal models: The pathogenicity of the causative agent in an animal model must provide conclusive evidence that it can cause periodontitis in humans.

Putative Periodontopathic Bacteria

For almost 100 years, a bacterial etiology for the existence of periodontitis has been sought. Early on, the *non-specific plaque hypothesis* prevailed, but since the 1970s research has indicated specific bacteria as the etiologic agents in periodontal diseases. Nevertheless, it is certain that not all possible periodontopathic microorganisms have yet been identified. With this in mind, Figure 66 (Socransky & Haffajee 1992, Tonetti 1994) presents the most likely periodontopathic microorganisms, but this table makes no claim to completeness; it will certainly be modified and enhanced by future research.

According to Socransky's postulates, the pathogenic potential of a microorganism is determined not only by its association with the disease, but also by:
- Improvement of the disease condition after elimination of the pathogen by therapy
- Activation of the host immune response to the specific infection
- Detection of putative virulence factors (pp. 34–35)
- The elicitation of similar periodontal disease symptoms in animal experiments.

Species		① Association	② Elimination	③ Host Response	④ Virulence Factors	⑤ Animal Studies
Aa	Actinobacillus actinomycetemcomitans	+++	+++	+++	+++	+++
Pg	Porphyromonas gingivalis	+++	+++	+++	+++	+++
Pi	Prevotella intermedia	+++	++	++	+++	+++
Fn	Fusobacterium nucleatum	+++	+	+++	++	+
Tf	Tannerella forsythia*	+++	++	+	+++	+
Cr	Campylobacter rectus	+++	++			
Ec	Eikenella corrodens	+++	+		+	++
Pm	Peptostreptococcus micros	+++	+	+		
Ss	Selenomonas sputigena	+++				
	Eubacterium sp.	++		++		
	Spirochetes	+++	+++	+++	+++	+

66 Frequency of Research Studies That Have Demonstrated the Degree of Pathogenicity of Various Microorganisms According to Socransky's Postulates.
The *number of "plus signs"* indicates the frequency of positive results in the studies.
For all of the microorganisms listed, the direct association with the disease (**1**) was investigated, and in most cases also the other listed criteria (**2–5**).

The intensity of the *background color* (red = gram-negative; blue = gram-positive) depicts the association of the bacteria with the various criteria of periodontitis; and thus, is a measure of their relative pathogenicity.

Association with Periodontitis

+++ Highly pathogenic
++ Moderately pathogenic
+ Slightly pathogenic
no research studies

+++ Highly pathogenic	++ Moderately pathogenic	+ Slightly pathogenic
• Aa Actinobacillus actinomycetemcomitans		S. intermedius
• Pg Porphyromonas gingivalis	P. intermedia	P. nigrescens
• Tf Tannerella forsythia*	C. rectus	P. micros
• Td Treponema denticola (Spirochetes of NUG)	E. nodatum	F. nucleatum
	Treponema sp.	Eubacterium sp.
		E. corrodens

67 Rank Ordering of the Pathogenicity of Individual Bacteria *(Haffajee & Socransky 1994)*

- **A. actinomycetemcomitans**
- **P. gingivalis**
- **Tannerella forsythia*** (2003; formerly **B. forsythus**)
- **Certain spirochetes ...** appear to be the most virulent periodontal pathogenic microorganisms.

Virulence Factors

The destructive potential of bacteria is related to their relative concentration (percentage composition of the total bacterial flora), but also to their so-called *virulence factors*. Bacteria (usually gram-negative) possessing virulence factors are usually found in periodontal pockets when periodontal destruction is actively progressing. Some of these virulence factors have already been mentioned: endotoxin, exotoxin, enzymes, chemotactic substances and antigens. These and other virulence factors that have thus far been demonstrated are listed below.

Virulence Transfer

Virulence factors are transferred to daughter cells following cell division, but such factors can also be transferred from one bacterium to another or to other species of bacteria by means of plasmid transfer.

Plasmids determine various characteristics of bacteria, e.g., the production of toxins (virulence plasmids) and resistance factors (resistance plasmids) against antibiotics.

Bacteriophages are viruses that proliferate within bacterial cells and have the ability to transfer DNA fragments or plasmids between bacteria (Fig. 70; Preus et al. 1987, Haubek et al. 1997, Willi & Meyer 1998).

68 Number (in Percent) of Microorganisms in Active and Inactive Pockets (Dzink et al. 1988)
The course of periodontitis is tooth surface specific and episodic.
The absolute number and the percentage composition of periodontopathic gram-negative bacteria (red) are significantly increased in *active* pockets. In *inactive* lesions, one finds primarily gram-positive "resident" microorganisms (blue), which are less damaging to host tissue and which to a certain degree actually inhibit the pathogens.

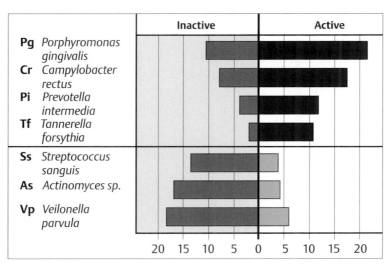

69 Bacterial Virulence Factors
Virulence is multifactorial. It is influenced by the inherent pathogenic potential of a bacterium, its environment, and its interaction with the host. Virulent bacteria require a competitor! In order to elicit periodontitis, microorganisms must
● Establish themselves near the host tissue
● Avoid being eliminated by saliva or exudates
● Find appropriate nutrition
● Avoid the defense mechanisms of the host and other microorganisms
● Be capable of destroying periodontal tissues.
Even though virulent, pathogenic bacteria in the pocket possess a *significant potential for damage*; this potential is small in comparison to that of the host: The clinically detectable destruction of soft and hard tissues is caused mainly by the immune defense mechanisms of the host.

Fact: In order to induce periodontitis, even virulent bacterial strains require partners (complexes: p. 37)
.

Goals	Bacterial Factors	
Adhesion to host tissues **– Surface structures**	– Fimbriae, pili – other adhesins	
Colonization, proliferation	– Nutrition chain development – Proteases for foodstuff metabolism (Host proteins, Fe^{2+}) – Inhibition of inhibitors	
Host response **– Deceiving** **– Inhibiting** **– Eliminating**	– Capsule, mucous – PMN receptor blocker – Leukotoxins (Aa) – Immunoglobulin-destroying proteases (Pg) – Complement-degrading proteases	Microorganisms
Penetration into host tissues, host cells	– Invasins	
Tissue damage – direct *Enzymes* *Bone resorption* *Cellular toxins, poisons*	– Collagenases – Hyaluronidase, Chondroitin sulfatase – Trypsin-like proteases (Pg, Tf, Td) – LPS/lipolysaccharide – LTA/lipoteichoic acids – Capsule-, membrane substances – butyric acid, propionic acid, indoles, amines – ammonia, hydrogen sulfide and other volatile sulfur compounds	
Tissue damage – indirect	– Host inflammatory response to microbial plaque antigens – Sensitive regulation of pro-inflammatory mediators such as TNF, IL-1, IL-6, and thus sensitive regulation of the synthesis of prostaglandin E2 (PGE2), matrix metalloproteinases (MMP) etc.	Host

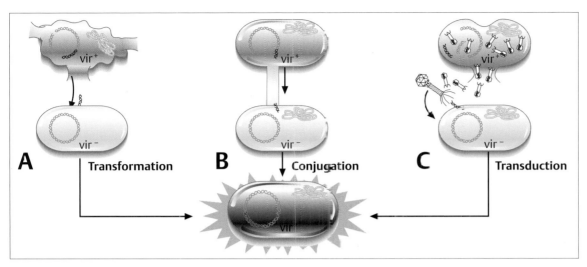

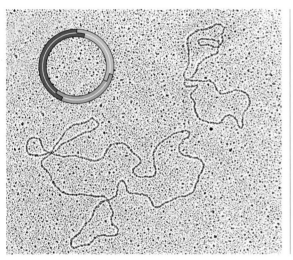

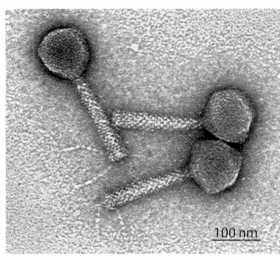

100 nm

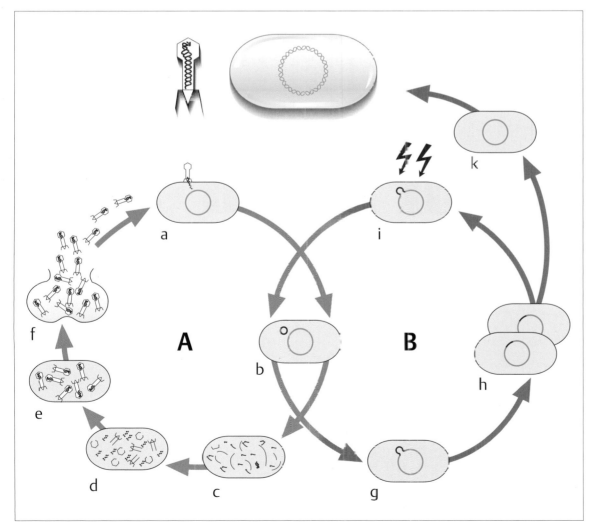

70 Transmission Pathway of Virulence Factors
Circular DNA molecules (plasmids) contain the gene for virulence factors (vir⁺). Three pathways for such DNA transfer are understood:
A *Transformation*: A non-virulent bacterium (vir⁻) takes the free DNA from a dead virulent bacterium.
B *Conjugation:* Two vital bacteria exchange DNA "sexually" by direct cell contact.
C *Transduction:* Phages (viruses) transfer the DNA (Fig. 72).

71 Plasmids and Bacterial Phages
Left: Plasmids are circular DNA molecules consisting of 1,000–450,000 base pairs (2–500 genes). They contain genes for virulence (toxins) as well as resistance factors. In the color schematic (left) three genes are represented.

Right: Bacteriophages are viruses that infect bacteria and propagate within bacteria (transduction).

TEM courtesy J. Meyer.

72 Transduction: DNA Transfer via Bacteriophages
Phages proliferate within bacterial cells by two mechanisms (cycles).
A **Lytic Cycle**:
The bacterium dies.
a The phage injects its genome.
b The injected DNA adopts a ring configuration.
c/d Viral DNA—regulated production of phage components: capsule, genome virulence factor.
e New phages are created (viral morphogenesis).
f Bacteriolysis: Release of innumerable new phages.
B **Lysogenic Cycle**:
The bacterium survives.
b Separate DNA (see above).
g The viral genome is incorporated into the bacterial genome.
h The bacterium is latently infected and divides. The new bacteria are "virulent" and vital (e. g., diphtheria toxin gene).
i Continuous irritation renders the phage genome self-supporting (→ cycle **A**).
k Special cases: the bacterium "loses" the phage genome and remains vital.

Marker Bacteria in Periodontitis

About a dozen bacteria in the oral cavity—so-called "marker" bacteria—have been variously associated with periodontitis. Of these, the best documented "agents of periodontal disease" are:

- *Porphyromonas gingivalis (Pg)*
- *Actinobacillus actinomycetemcomitans (Aa)*
- *Tannerella forsythia (Tf)*

All of the other bacteria within the ecosystem of the oral cavity produce far fewer virulence factors.

Virulence Factors of the Marker Bacteria

- *Toxins*: Best characterized are the leukotoxin from various *Aa* clones, and the special lipopolysaccharide from *Pg* (LPS; p. 38).
- *Ability to invade*: *Pg* and *Aa* can penetrate host *cells* and thus have the ability to avoid the non-specific immune response, the "first line of defense" (p. 42).
- Enzymes and proteases: Upon contact of *Pg* with epithelial cells, numerous enzymes (e.g., extracellular proteases) as well as "gingipains" that reduce host immune response are set free.

73 Virulence Factors of *Porphyromonas gingivalis (Pg)*
Pg requires many of these factors to exist, i. e., to acquire its nutrition, and to maintain itself within the ecology of the periodontal pocket. Its most significant "weapon" against the host organism is its toxic and antigenically effective LPS (p. 38).

Right: Pg smear. Note the numerous vesicles.

TEM Figs. 73 & 75 courtesy *B. Guggenheim*

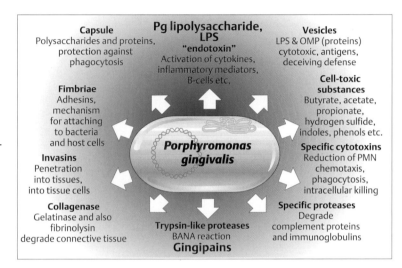
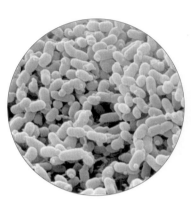

Capsule
Polysaccharides and proteins, protection against phagocytosis

Pg lipolysaccharide, LPS
"endotoxin"
Activation of cytokines, inflammatory mediators, B-cells etc,

Vesicles
LPS & OMP (proteins) cytotoxic, antigens, deceiving defense

Fimbriae
Adhesins, mechanism for attaching to bacteria and host cells

Cell-toxic substances
Butyrate, acetate, propionate, hydrogen sulfide, indoles, phenols etc.

Invasins
Penetration into tissues, into tissue cells

Specific cytotoxins
Reduction of PMN chemotaxis, phagocytosis, intracellular killing

Porphyromonas gingivalis

Collagenase
Gelatinase and also fibrinolysin degrade connective tissue

Trypsin-like proteases
BANA reaction
Gingipains

Specific proteases
Degrade complement proteins and immunoglobulins

74 The Pocket as "Reservoir"
The deeper the *(anaerobic)* pocket, the larger the average number of pathogenic bacteria (*Pg* and *Aa*/serotype b).

In order to initiate disease, a critical number of pathogenic microorganisms is required. For the three microorganisms depicted here, this number varies considerably. The critical number is, for example, for *Aa*/serotype a lower than for *Pg*.

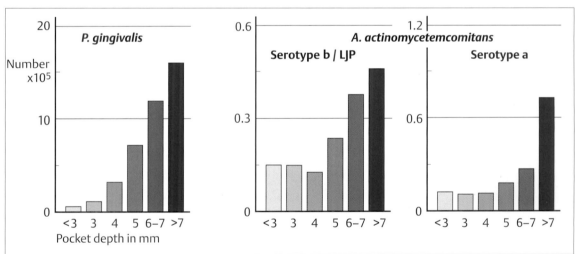

P. gingivalis

Number x10⁵

Pocket depth in mm: <3 3 4 5 6–7 >7

A. actinomycetemcomitans

Serotype b / LJP

Serotype a

75 Virulence Factors of *A. actinomycetemcomitans (Aa)*
The *Aa* leukotoxin is one of the most potent toxins. It has the capability to directly inhibit some of the most important components of the human immune system, e. g., PMNs, immunoglobulins and complement activation. Something over 40 *Aa*-subtypes do not express leukotoxin. One subtype does this in extremely high measure, and it is associated with aggressive periodontitis (LJP). Modified from *J. Lindhe et al. Right:* Smear of *Aa*.

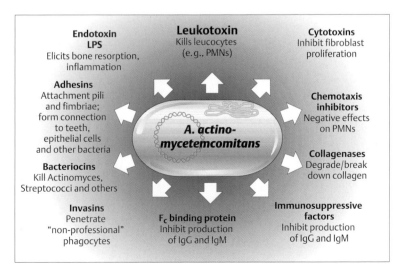
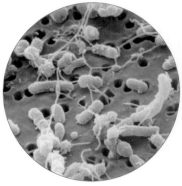

Endotoxin
LPS
Elicits bone resorption, inflammation

Leukotoxin
Kills leucocytes
(e.g., PMNs)

Cytotoxins
Inhibit fibroblast proliferation

Adhesins
Attachment pili and fimbriae; form connection to teeth, epithelial cells and other bacteria

Chemotaxis inhibitors
Negative effects on PMNs

A. actino-mycetemcomitans

Bacteriocins
Kill Actinomyces, Streptococci and others

Collagenases
Degrade/break down collagen

Invasins
Penetrate "non-professional" phagocytes

F$_c$ binding protein
Inhibit production of IgG and IgM

Immunosuppressive factors
Inhibit production of IgG and IgM

Pathogenic "Single Fighters" vs. Pathogenic Complexes?

Just as many microorganisms in the oral cavity profit from the activities of *Aa* and *Pg*, these two organisms are also dependent upon the others: In most cases, plaque formation begins with the "early colonizers" (*Actinomyces naeslundi/viscosus*, streptococcus sp. etc.; p.24); *Aa* and *Pg* enter the biofilm only later. They are capable of colonizing epithelia, but less so hard tooth structure. Pg is a strict anaerobe, and is therefore present in increased numbers in deep pockets (which must be taken into consideration during treatment planning).

As the biofilm "matures," the composition of plaque changes considerably, e.g., from primarily gram-positive to gram-negative bacteria. Socransky and co-workers (1998, 1999) described the so-called "red-complex" of *P. gingivalis, T. forsythia* and *T. denticola* as the "end stage" of the confrontation between pathogenicity and resistance vs. host response.

Conclusion

Actinomyces actinomycetemcomitans, P. gingivalis and the "red-complex" (G; Fig.77) represent the bacterial risk factors for periodontitis in *susceptible individuals* because of their pathogenic virulence factors.

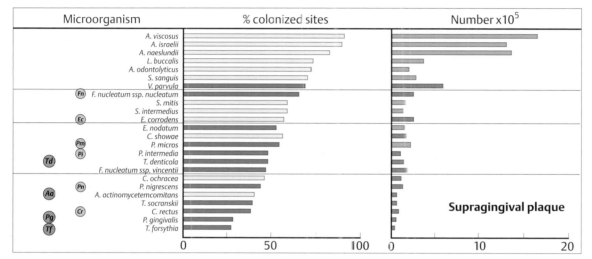

76 Bacteria of the Supragingival Plaque
Percentage of colonized sites (middle) and absolute number (right) of 24 out of 40 tested microorganisms (over 16,000 samples from 213 adults; *Socransky et al.* 1999). The "marker bacteria" are circled on the left.

Bright	aerobe
Dark	anaerobe

Blue	gram-positive
Red	gram-negative

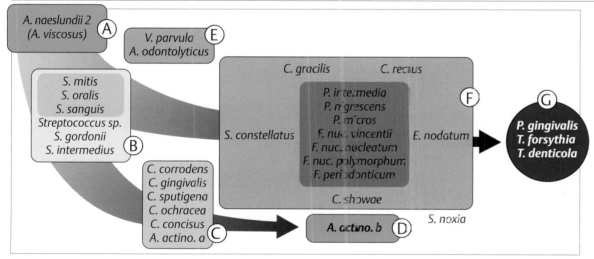

77 Development of Complexes
Dependent upon host response, availability of nutritive substances, and interbacterial competition, the variable "consortium" develops. Bacteria no longer work as single entities: The biofilm acts and reacts as a stable "organism." One pathway (**A → G**) leads by way of several intermediate stages to the "red complex," while another pathway (**A → D**) leads in the direction of *Aa*.
DNA tests permit the identification of such groupings (p. 185)

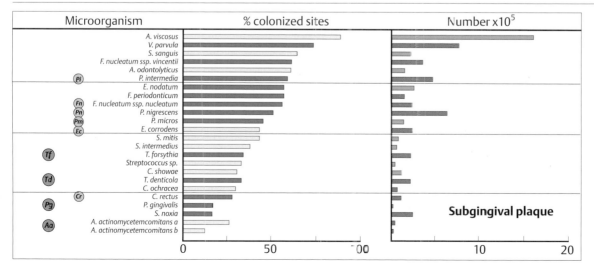

78 Bacteria of the Subgingival Plaque
The data and sources for this information derive from Fig. 76. In the subgingival milieu, the type and number of gram-positive organisms decrease, with an ever-increasing number of various gram-negative organisms. Most of the gram-negative marker bacteria are increased (left).
Relatively seldom, and then in only small numbers, one observes *P. gingivalis* and *A. actinomycetemcomitans*: "quality before quantity"?

Endotoxins—Lipopolysaccharides (LPS)

Bacterial endotoxins are some of the most fascinating biological molecules. They are heat-stable (pyrogens!), extremely toxic and therefore responsible for inflammatory processes, fever and shock. Chemically, all bacterial endotoxins are lypopolysaccarides (LPS; Rietschel & Brade 1992).

Lipopolysaccharides are one component of the outer membrane of the cell wall of *gram-negative* bacteria (lipid bilayer, p. 31), and render the membrane relatively impermeable (e. g., to antibiotics).

Every bacterial species and subspecies can be differentiated by their typical LPS. The O-specific chain (C) is the antigenic portion of the molecule (*surface antigen*). Lipid A is exclusively responsible for the toxicity and the activation of the host-immune reaction via macrophages (MΦ); lipid A is found in the LPS of the outer membrane. Only *free* LPS molecules are toxic for the host, not those embedded within the bacterial cell wall. Free LPS occurs:
- Through vesicle formation
- During cell division (proliferation)
- After destruction of the cell wall of dead bacteria.

79 LPS—Structure and Function
The stimulation of macrophages (MΦ) by LPS initiates the inflammatory and the immune defence reactions.
1 LPS, coupled with the LPS-binding protein LBP, activates macrophages via the specific LPS-receptor **CD14**.
2 This produces the following mediators: cytokines, oxygen radicals, lipids (e. g., prostaglandins), which may work singularly or in combination. Cytokines enhance (+) while lipids inhibit (-) their individual synthesis via "autocrine" mechanisms.
3 Dependent upon the concentration of mediators, a broad spectrum of host reactions is initiated.

Right: Configuration of LPS.
A Lipid A: Up to six variable fatty acids, diglucosamine (red), phosphate (green)
B Nuclear Zones 1 and 2: diverse sugars
C O-specific Chains: repeating units; type-specific antigens.

Modified from *E. Reitschel & H. Brade (1992)*

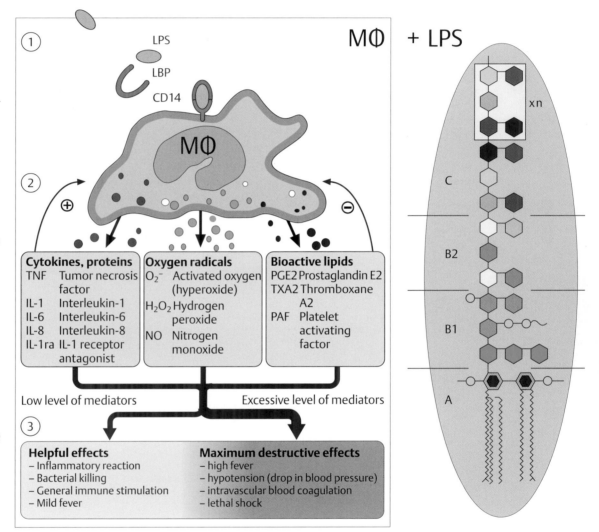

Interaction Between LPS and the Host

Even though metabolism by plaque bacteria results in many biologically active substances (endotoxins, enzymes, chemokines, phlogogens) that may cause *direct* damage, LPS from gram-negative bacteria plays the most important role in the pathogenesis of periodontal diseases: It stimulates macrophages to produce cytokines, activates the *alternative* complement pathway, is antigenically effective and also cytotoxic. With slight plaque accumulation, LPS is present in only low concentrations, but this may "awaken" and activate a dormant host immune system.

The action of LPS is primarily *indirect*: It activates not only macrophages but also endothelial cells and fibroblasts to produce cytokines. LPS molecules from various periodontopathic bacteria induce quite varying amounts of cytokines. LPS from *Pg*, for example, induces much higher levels of cytokines than other microorganisms associated with periodontitis (Takada et al. 1991).
The host may respond to LPS with varying intensity, but the pathogenesis of periodontal disease is primarily determined by the host's immune reaction. This can vary considerably from person to person (Pathogenesis, p. 39).

Pathogenesis—
Reactions and Defense Capabilities of the Host

Periodontal diseases represent a family of related, usually chronic, and very often aggressive infectious bacterial diseases.

The etiologic agents, the *primary pathogens*, are several virulent bacteria found in dental plaque and in the oral cavity. The most important ones are *Aa, Pg* and *Tf,* although other species may play enhancing roles (cf. p. 33). Bacteria *must* be present if periodontitis is to be initiated and propagated, but bacteria are not *solely* responsible for this disease.

Host factors in combination with additional risk factors (smoking, stress etc.) have been shown by recent research to significantly influence the susceptibility, expression (e. g., type and severity) and progression of periodontitis. For this reason it is absolutely necessary to achieve an understanding of the possible reactions of the host organism to the bacterial challenge.

This chapter is therefore structured as follows:

- New concepts concerning pathogenesis—a paradigm shift

- Host defense: mechanisms and participants—cells and molecules

- Non-specific, congenital and specific, acquired immunity—interactive relationships

- Surface molecules, markers (CD), receptors

- Regulating molecules, mediators: cytokines—eikosanoides—matrix metalloproteinases

- Risk factors: genetics—environment—life style

- Pathogenesis I—initial inflammatory reactions, PMN diapedesis

- Pathogenesis II—histologic stages

- Pathogenesis III—molecular niveau

- Attachment loss: breakdown of connective tissue and bone

- The transition from gingivitis to periodontitis—cyclic course of destruction

- Periodontal infections and systemic diseases

- Etiology and pathogenesis—summary and conclusions

New Concepts of Pathogenesis

Research on the etiology and pathogenesis of periodontitis has provided so much new knowledge in recent years that it is reasonable to speak of a *paradigm shift*. This is based primarily on new knowledge concerning biofilms (microorganisms), molecular biology, host susceptibility, risk factors and genetics.

Biofilm

The adherent bacterial flora—dental plaque—is a highly organized biofilm. Bacteria within the biofilm are well protected from the host response as well as from antimicrobial agents. The only effective therapy is purely physical destruction and elimination of the biofilm by means of scaling (tooth and root surface cleaning, supra- and subgingivally).

Molecular Biology

New knowledge about molecular and cellular mechanisms has led to better understanding of the processes by which bacteria in the biofilm elicit immune and inflammatory reactions in the host, leading to connective tissue destruction and resorption of the alveolar bone.

Host Sensitivity and Risk Factors

In order for the aforementioned mechanisms to occur, leading to the initiation and establishment of periodontitis, a susceptible host must be present. The microorganisms, by themselves, *cannot* cause the disease process. Environmental factors and risk factors such as smoking or inherited (unfavorable) host defense mechanisms modify the host reaction and are primarily responsible for the destruction, progression, severity and clinical picture of periodontitis.

Genetics

The various molecular biological mechanisms, the host susceptibility to inflammatory damage, and congenital risk factors are determined for the most part by genetics (p. 51). Therefore heredity assumes a much larger significance today than was previously assumed; humans are born with their predisposition towards periodontitis!

80 Pathogenesis of Human Periodontitis
The disease cannot be phenotypically homogeneous because of the many influences upon the host reactions.

A	Microbiology	pp. 23–40
B	Host reactions	pp. 41–45
C	Metabolism	pp. 60/61
D	Clinical Symptoms	pp. 62/63
E	Genetics	pp. 51–53
F	Risk Factors	pp. 51–54

PMN Polymorphoneuclear Granulocytes (p. 42)
LPS Lipopolysaccharide (p. 38)

Modified from *R. Page & K. Kornman, 1997*

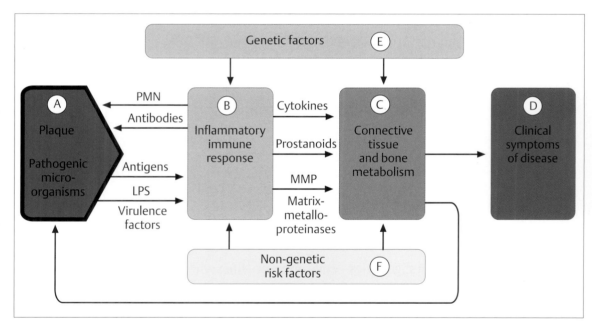

Therapeutic and Diagnostic Consequences

Since the 1960's, prevention and therapy have consisted primarily in the removal or reduction of the infectious bacteria. In the future, attempts will be made to utilize the host response diagnostically and to influence it in therapy; for example, progressive periodontitis is characterized not only by elevated levels of bacterial substances, above all lipopolysaccharides (LPS), but also by *pro-inflammatory* mediators. These include the cytokines TNFα, IL-1 and IL-6, as well a prostaglandins (especially PGE2) and matrix metalloproteinases (MMP).

In contrast, in periodontal health or in a case of a stable lesion, the level of bacterial substances (LPS) is low and the *inflammation-reducing* cytokines such as IL-10, TGFβ as well as MMP- inhibitors (TIMP) are higher.

In the future, therapeutic measures will include attempts to reduce disease-eliciting factors, and to stimulate resistance factors. In addition, it will be necessary to maintain and even increase our efforts to eliminate or reduce other risk factors such as diabetes, smoking, stress and environmental factors.

Host Response—Mechanisms and "Participants"

Various mechanisms within the host organism inhibit bacterial infection. In addition to physical and chemical barriers (skin/keratinization; mucosa/mucous; saliva with mucins, lysozmes, histozines, etc.) the human immune system plays the most important protective role.

One can differentiate between:

- Non-specific, naturally present, "congenital" immunity (p. 42)
- Specific, acquired immunity (p. 43)

First Axis of the Defense System

This consists of cells of non-specific immunity (phagocytes, natural killer cells) and also diverse molecular effectors (complement, C-reactive protein, etc.)

Second Axis of the Immune System

This consists of specific immunity, above all the lymphocytes (T- and B-cells, as well as antigen-presenting cells, e. g., macrophages/MΦ) as well as the various immunoglobulins.

Cellular components of the host response

- **Inflammatory cells**
  - PMN polymorphonuclear granulocyte (p. 42)
    Neutrophils
    Eosinophilic granulocytes
    Basophilic granulocytes, mast cells
  - Thrombocytes

- **Resident cells**
  - Fibroblasts, endothelial cells, epithelial cells

- **Antigen-presenting cells (APC)**   (p. 42)
  - Monocytes/macrophages
  - Langerhans cells, dendritic cells

- **Lymphocytes**   (p. 43)
  - T-cells
    T-helper cells T_H1 and T_H2 = T4-cells
    T-cytotoxic cells   Tc   = T8-cells
  - B-cells, plasma cells (PC)
  - NK = "natural killer cells"

81 Cellular Components of the Immune System
The important cell types for immune response include inflammatory cells, resident cells, antigen-presenting cells and lymphocytes. These are described in detail in the following pages.

Modified from *R. Sanderink 1999*

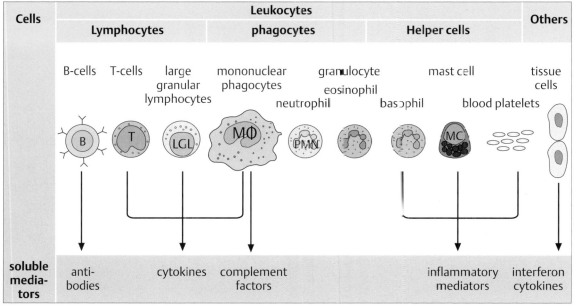

Cells	Leukocytes			Others
	Lymphocytes	phagocytes	Helper cells	

B-cells T-cells large granular lymphocytes	mononuclear phagocytes	granulocyte eosinophil neutrophil basophil	mast cell blood platelets	tissue cells

| soluble mediators | antibodies | cytokines complement factors | inflammatory mediators interferon cytokines | |

82 Components of the Immune System—Cells and Soluble Mediators
A large percentage of the soluble mediators such as complement factors, acute phase proteins (C-reactive protein) etc. are produced in the liver.
Each and every cell that is involved in the maintenance of the structure of the periodontium also synthesizes a large spectrum of cytokines (p. 47) and other mediators. It is important to recognize that even the resident (non-mobile) cells are active in the immunologic process.

Modified from *M. Roitt et al. 1995*

Effectors and regulatory cellular surface molecules

- **Ig   Immunoglobulins**   (p. 43)
  - 5 classes: IgA, IgM, IgG, IgD, IgE
    Subclasses: IgA1 and A2, IgG1 through G4

- **C   Complement**   (p. 42)
  - C 1-9 cascade
  - MAC/major attack complex / C9

- **Cytokines**   (p. 47/48)
  - Interleukins (IL)
  - Cytotoxic factors (TNF)
  - Interferon (IFN)
  - Colony-stimulating factors (CSF)
  - Growth factors (GF)

- **Chemokines**   (p. 48)
  - "class c," α- and β-Chemokines

- **Eicosanoids**   (p. 49)
  - Prostaglandins (e. g., PGE2)
    Leukotrienes (e. g., LTB4)

- **Other mediators**   (p. 50)
  - Matrix metalloproteinases

- **Receptors, surface antigens**   (p. 46)
  - MHC classes I and II (HLA)
  - CD antigens (classification)
  - Receptor molecules
  - Adhesins

83 Humoral Components of the Immune System
Included in this table are also receptors and surface antigens (markers), without which the cell-cell relationships would not be possible (signal formation, antigen presentation etc.).

Modified from *R. Sanderink 1999*

Non-specific, Congenital Immunity—the First Line of Defense

Non-specific immunity represents the quite potent first line of defense. It is phylogenetically ancient, quick to respond, and involves the mechanisms of *phagocytosis* (killing and digesting of microorganisms) and *acute* inflammation.

The *cellular components* of the non-specific immune system consist of the phagocytic cells (neutrophilic granulocytes [PMN] and monocytes/macrophges [MΦ]) as well as the natural killer cells [NK]).

Soluble effector molecules include complement (C) and acute phase proteins (C-reactive proteins), which are synthesized for the most part in the liver.

The inflammatory reaction is highly regulated by *mediator molecules.* Among these is bradykinin, but above all the pro-inflammatory cytokines (pp. 47–48), prostaglandins (p. 49), and many other components of the primary defense axis:

- Polymorphonuclear granulocytes (PMN)
- Monocytes/macrophages (MΦ)
- Natural killer cells (NK)
- Complement (C)
- Additional inflammatory mediators

Non-specific immunity possesses no "memory."

84 Polymorphonuclear Granulocytes (PMN)

PMNs represent the first line of defense. They can be constantly recovered from the gingival sulcus.

A Adhesion to the blood vascular walls and penetration into the tissues

B Chemotactic movement

C Capture of opsonized microorganism (MO)

D Phagocytosis of the MO

E Formation of phagosomes

F Phagolysosomal killing

G Exocytosis (release of killing mediators)

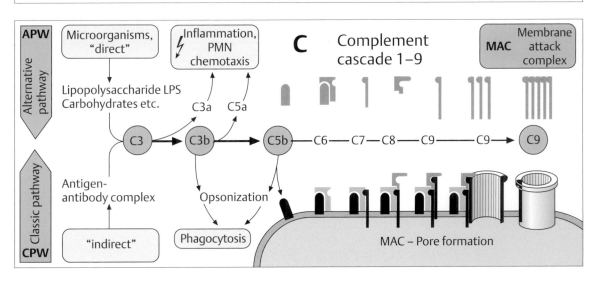

85 Macrophages (MΦ)

The most important component of specific host defense system: They present to the T-lymphocytes the antigens of the phagocytized microorganisms (APC).

LPS Lipopolysaccharide
LBP LPS-binding proteins
CD14 Receptors for the LPS-LBP complex
FcR Immunoglobulin receptor
MHC II Major histocompatibility complex II, p. 46

Modified from *Gemsa et al. 1997*

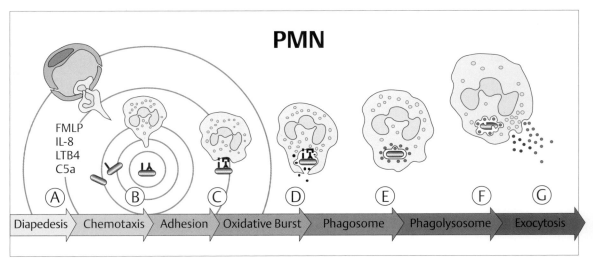

86 Complement (C)

Soluble complement factors C-1 through C-9 circulate in the blood. Most of the C-components are proteins possessing enzyme functions and can be activated through two different pathways.

- Chemotactic activity: **C5a** stronger than **C3a**.
- C3b opsonizes initially, followed by **C5b** etc.
- Pore formation is bacteriocidal through the **MAC**

Modified from *Koolman & Röhm 1998*

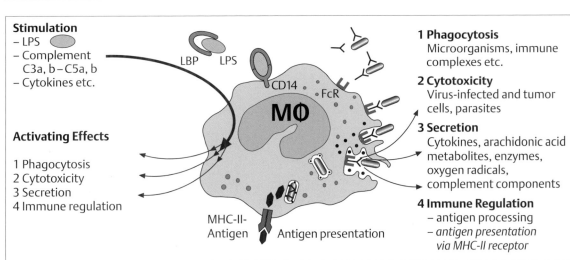

Specific, Acquired Immunity—the Second Line of Defense

- T-Lymphocytes
- B-Lymphocytes/plasma cells
- Immunoglobulins

The phylogenetically younger, specific immunity is responsible for the fine regulation of host defense. Lymphocytes are the key cells of the immune system: They monitor the various immune responses. Two main cell groups can be distinguished: T-cells and B-cells.

It requires more time to set the second line of defense into motion, but specific immunity possesses a "memory" function (immunization!)

- *T-lymphocytes* fulfill numerous functions:
  - Cytotoxic T-cells (T_c-, T8-, CD8 cells) eliminate foreign cells as well as damaged host cells (pore-forming "lymphotoxin" = TNFβ);
  - T-helper cells (T_H-, T4-, CD4 cells)—the subclasses T_H1 and T_H2 secrete various groups of cytokines and thereby program various pathways of the immune reaction (T_H1 → MΦ or T_H2 → Ig).
- *B-cells* as well as immunoglobulin-forming *plasma cells* are responsible for the opsonization of foreign bodies (pp. 44–45), which is regulated mainly by the T_H2 pathway.

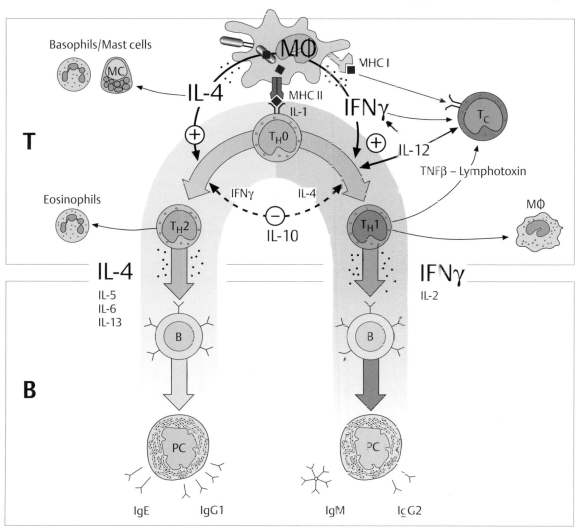

87 T-Cells/T-Lymphocytes
These cells are activated following direct cell contact of antigen-presenting MHC-I and -II molecules (upon MΦ and B-cells), with the T-cell receptor complex (p. 46). T-helper cells (T_H0) differentiate via IL-4 and other cytokines (p. 47) to T_H2 cells, via IFNγ to T_H1 cells; this T-cell subpopulation enhances the differentiation of B-cells in addition to the other defense cells (gray). T-cells (right) synthesize cytotoxins such as lymphotoxin (= tumor necrosis factor, TNFβ).

88 B-Cells, Plasma Cells (PC)
B-cells are activated by cytokines from the T-helper cells (IL-4 and IFNγ) as well as antigens. Mature B-cells express numerous surface-fixed **Ig** (= B-cell receptor) and under the influence of cytokines evolve into plasma cells (**PC**), which release massive amounts of Ig molecules. Cytokines from the T_H1 and T_H2 cells enhance the "switch" from IgE and IgM to the IgG subclasses of immunoglobulins.

Modified from *Zinkernagel 1998*

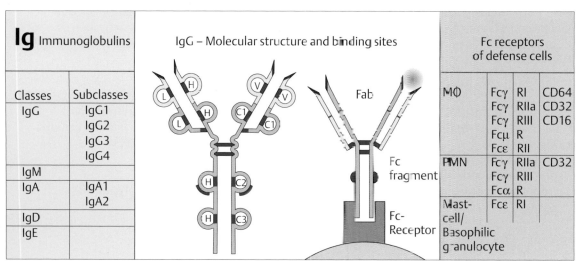

89 Immunoglobulins (Ig)
Left: Ig classes and subclasses.

Middle: Ig molecules are Y-shaped glycoproteins with heavy (**H**) and light (**L**) chains, as well as constant (**C**) and variable (**V**) domains.

Right: The **Fab** fragment contains the antigen-binding site. **Fc** fragment binds on Fc receptors of various defense cells and on complement (CPW, Fig. 90).

Modified from *Roitt et al. 1995*

90 Cellular and Humoral Components

Components of the Immune System—Summary

Cell Type /Molecules

Characteristics

Functions, Effects

Polymorphonuclear granulocyte (PMN, Microphage)

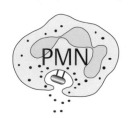

- Differentiation, maturation and clonal expansion in bone marrow
- Lifespan: 2-3 days
- 10-20 µm diameter
- **Fc, C3- C5-receptors**
- Enzyme-containing granules

- Diapedesis, chemotaxis
- Phagocytosis: Adherence, phagolysosome formation, digestion, "oxidative burst"
- Release of lysosomal enzymes
- Release of inflammatory mediators: prostaglandins (e. g., **PGE$_2$**), leukotrienes (e. g., **LTB4**), cytokines

---

Complement system; cascade C1–C9

CPW—classical pathway
- Classical activation pathway, elicited by antibody/ immunoglobulins (Ab/Ig), which aggregate with antigens (Ag): **Ag/Ab** complex

APW—alternative pathway
- Alternative activation — independent of antibodies — via bacterial mucopolysaccharide (e. g., **LPS**); leads to separation of **C3** into **C3b** (and **C3a**) and to activation of **C5**

- Immune adherence: binds to the **Fc** fragment of antibodies
- Elevated capillary permeability
- Anaphylatoxin
- PMN chemotaxis (see also **C5a**)
- Opsinization of bacteria
- Irreversible, structure-dependent and functional membrane damage via formation of the **MAC** ("membrane attack complex"), which leads to pore formation and ultimate cell lysis

---

Monocyte / Macrophage (MΦ)

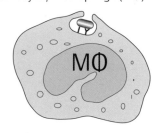

- Differentiation, maturation and clonal expansion within bone marrow
- Lifespan: months
- 12—25 µm diameter
- Diverse receptors:
  - **Fc** for immunoglobulins
  - **CR** for complement (**C3**)
  - **CD** 14 for lipopolysaccharide (p. 40)

- Phagocytosis, antigen processing
- Antigen presentation (for **T**- and **B**-cells)
- Production and secretion of bioactive substances:
  - Cytokines (p. 47-48): **IFNα** (anti-viral), **TNFα, IL-1, IL-6, IL-8**
  - Components of the complement system
  - Lysosomal enzymes
  - Arachidonic acid metabolites (p. 49)
  - Oxygen and nitrogen radicals (p. 42)

T-lymphocytes
T-helper and cytotoxic T-cells

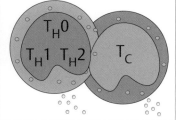

- Stem cells from bone marrow
- Maturation: Thymus-dependent (**T**)
- Lifespan: Months
- 6-7 µm diameter; activated: 10 µm
- Antigen recognition: T-cell receptor (**TCR**)
- Surface antigens / Marker molecules:
  - **CD4** on helper cells (T$_H$0; T$_H$1, T$_H$2)
  - **CD8** on cytotoxic cells (T$_c$)
- **T**-memory cells

"Cell-mediated immunity"

- T-helper cells: Assist with antibody production and the cytotoxic T-cell response (**T$_c$**-cells); activation of macrophages
- Suppression of an immune response
- Release of cytokines of various subclasses (T$_H$0, T$_H$1, T$_H$2): **IL-2, IL-3, IL-4, IL-5, IL-6, IL-7, IL-8, IL-10, IL-12, IL-13; IFNγ, TNFβ**
- Memory function of memory cells

B-lymphocyte/plasma cell

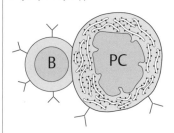

- Stem cells from bone marrow (**B**)
- Maturation: fetal liver, bone marrow, Peyer's patches
- Lifespan: Months
- 6-7 µm diameter
- Activated (plasma cell, **PC**): 10-15 µm diameter
- Surface **Ig** as antigen receptor
- **B**-Memory cell

"Humoral Immunity"

- Immunoglobulin synthesis
- B-lymphocyte: **Ig** antigen-specific, variable class
- Plasma cell: **Ig** antigen- and class-specific
- Clonal expansion following activation
- Memory function of memory cells

Antibody (Ab) =
Immunoglobulin (Ig)

	Molecular weight	percentage
IgG	150 000	80%
IgM	900 000	13%
IgA	300 000	6%
IgD	185 000	1%
IgE	280 000	0.02%

- 5 classes: **IgA, IgD, IgE, IgG, IgM**
- Subclasses: **IgA1, IgA2, IgG1, IgG2, IgG3, IgG4**
- Basic molecule:
  - Heavy (H) and light (L) polypeptide chains
  - Constant (C) and variable (V) domains: Millions of antigen-specific variations are possible

- Opsinization of microorganisms
- Antigen binding: Antigen-antibody complex
- Complement activation (**CPW**)
- Toxin neutralization
- Neutralization of viruses
- Hypersensitivity reaction (**Types 1-3**)

Interactions Between Non-specific and Specific Immunity

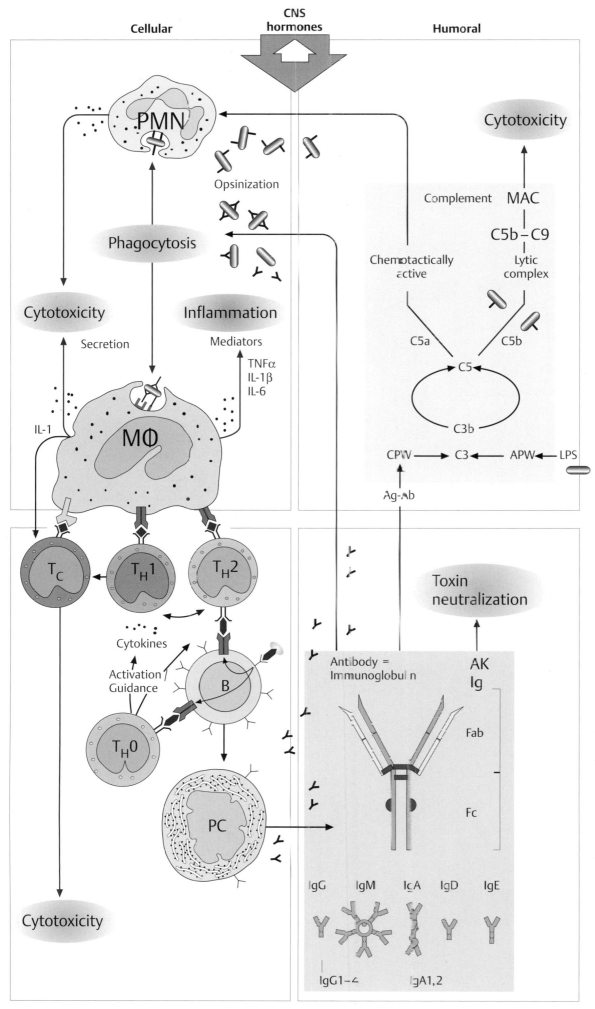

91 Interactions

Non-specific Immunity— First Line of Defense
Modified from *Roitt et al. 1985*

- *PMN granulocytes*: The cells represent the first and most important defense reactions within the junctional epithelium and gingival sulcus (phagocytosis). As PMNs are destroyed, lysozomal enzymes and toxic radicals are set free, which leads to cytotoxicity.
- *Complement*: Activated initially independent of antibodies by way of the initial, alternative pathway (APW); later it is dependent on antibodies via the classical pathway (CPW): Opsonization, chemotaxis, membrane destructive (MAC, Fig. 86) → cytotoxicity.
- *Macrophages (MΦ)*:
  – phagocytosis
  – release of cytokines and inflammatory metabolites and enzymes
  – antigen presentation: MΦ regulates T- and B-cells

Specific Immunity— Second Line of Defense

- *T-lymphocytes*: These are responsible for cell-mediated immunity
  – T-helper cells (T$_H$) work to regulate and/or activate via their cytokines
  – T$_C$-cells are cytotoxic
  – Memory cells of both types provide the immunologic "memory" of the T-cells
- *B-lymphocytes/plasma cells*: These are responsible for humoral immunity. Upon contact with antigens and activation via T$_H$ cells, B-lymphocytes differentiate into antibody-producing plasma cells; "memory" cells of the B-lymphocytes
- *Antibodies (Immunoglobulins)*:
  – Classes: IgG, IgM, IgA, IgD, IgE
  – Subclasses: IgG1–4 and IgA1–2 are immunoglobulins that are serum proteins, which bind specific antigens and are induced by these antigens. They have opsonization functions, neutralize toxins and activate complement (CPW).

Regulatory Cell Surface Molecules: Markers, Receptors

- MHC—major histocompatibility complex
- CD—cluster of differentiation
- Receptor molecules
- Adhesins and ligands

MHC molecule groups (classes I and II) make possible the differentiation between "self" and "non-self" (rejection reaction after organ transplantation).

CD4-marker: Lymphocytes and leukocytes express marker molecules ("antigens") on their surface, which permits a classification of the cell populations.

A systematic and individualized nomenclature, the CD-system, was developed for these markers.

Receptor molecules: Receptors are found on the surfaces of all cells, and most of these can receive bioactive molecules that either enhance or inhibit cell functions, e.g., cytokines, chemokines, complement factors, antigens and antibodies.

Adhesins serve as co-receptors, stabilize the primary receptor binding, and are responsible for the important "second signal" (general activation).

92 Antigen Presentation

By means of its MHC-II receptors, the macrophage presents foreign substrates, e.g., bacterial antigens (red) to a T-helper cell via the T-cell receptor complex (TCR+ CD3+ CD4).

MHC-II complexes (orange in the figure) are found on the antigen-presenting cells (MΦ, dendritic cells, as well as B-cells).

Support for this primary binding is provided by co-receptors, which also are important for the so-called "second signal" (definitive activation of the target cells).

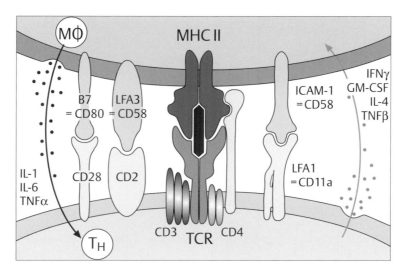

Receptor Binding, MΦ—T$_H$

Supportive and signal-building co-receptors with their CD numbers. The old names indicate their functions, e.g.:

LFA   leukocyte function-associated antigens
ICAM Intercellular adhesion molecule

Release of cytokines following activation by...
- *MΦ:*   TNFα, IL-1, IL-6
- *T-cells:* INFγ, GM-CFS, IL-4, TGFβ etc.

93 Immunoglobuin Gene Super Family

This family of surface molecules (receptors) contains numerous important members:

- MHC-I and –II molecules
- T-cell receptors (TCR) with their co-receptors; these are necessary for T-cell activation (see above)
- Immunoglobulins (pictured: membrane-bound IgG = "B-cell receptor")
- Fc receptors (Fig. 89)
- Diverse ICAM (adhesins)

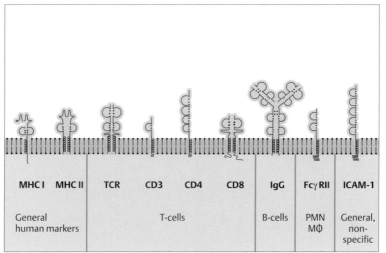

Family of Adhesins

Contained within this family of accessory surface molecules are:

- Integrins
- Lectins
- Selectins
- ICAM of the Ig-gene super-family.

Adhesins increase the avidity of cell-cell binding. This is especially important for the "ordered" diapedesis of inflammatory cells out of the blood vessels (p. 55).

94 Most Important Surface Markers of T-cells and MΦ

Macrophages interact with numerous biologically active molecules such as immunoglobulins (via Fc receptors), complement (via C-receptors, CR) as well as bacterial LPS (via CD14).

T-cells require fewer receptors: Following activation (antigen presentation by MΦ), they are effective through their repertoire of cytokines (p. 47). The subpopulations of cytotoxic T-cells (T$_C$) carry the CD8-receptor; T-helper cells (T$_H$) carry the CD4-receptor.

TCR   T-cell receptor
MHC   Major histocompatibility complex (classes I and II)
FcR   Receptors of the Fc fragments of immunoglobulins (Fig. 89)
CR   Complement receptor
CD14 Receptor for lipopolysaccharide (LPS)

CD Classification

So far, over 130 surface molecules have been classified and their functional significance described.

Cytokines

Cytokines are hormone-like, small molecular weight peptides or glycopeptides. They regulate all of the important biological processes, such as *cell proliferation, cell growth, cell activation, inflammation, immunity* and *repair*. Some cytokines (e.g., IL-8, MCP-1) have a chemotactic effect on immune cells. Members of the cytokine family include:

- Interleukins (formerly "lymphokines")
- Cytotoxic factors (tumor necrosis factor α and β)
- Interferons (anti-viral IFNα and β, "immune-IFNγ")
- Colony stimulating factors (CSF)
- Growth factors (GF)

In combination with other mediators, the cytokines build a large network, which is responsible not only for normal *tissue homeostasis* but also for every type of immune response. Most of the cytokines are local, a small group is also effective systemically (TNF, IL-1, IL-6). Specific receptors for these molecules are present on the target cells (for IL-1 through IL-10, e.g., CD121 through CD130; p. 46).

During the inflammatory reaction, which is a component of natural immunity (p. 42), the pro-inflammatory cytokines (IL-1β, IL-6, IL-8, TNFα, IFNγ) do battle with the inhibitory "immune-regulating" molecules (IL-1ra, IL-10, TGFβ; p. 48).

Cytokines

P = pro-inflammatory
A = anti-inflammatory
C = chemotactic

Interleukins IL

P	**IL-1α**	interleukin 1α
P	**IL-1β**	interleukin 1β
	IL-2	interleukin 2
	IL-3	interleukin 3
	IL-4	interleukin 4
	IL-5	interleukin 5
P	**IL-6**	interleukin 6
	IL-7	interleukin 7
C	**IL-8**	interleukin 8
	IL-9	interleukin 9
A	**IL-10**	interleukin 10
	IL-11	interleukin 11
P	**IL-12**	interleukin 12
A	**IL-13**	interleukin 13
	... and others	

Cytotoxic Factors

P	**TNFα**	tumor necrosis factor α
	TNFβ	tumor necrosis factor β = "lymphotoxin"

Interferon IFN

	IFNα	interferon α
	IFNβ	interferon β
P	**IFNγ**	interferon γ

Colony Stimulating Factors CSF

G-	**CSF**	granulocyte-CSF
M-	**CSF**	macrophage-CSF
GM-	**CSF**	granulocyte/MΦ-CSF
Multi-CSF = IL-3		

Growth Factors GF

A	**TGFα**	tissue growth factor α
A	**TGFβ**	tissue growth factor β
	EGF	epithelial GF
	FGF	fibroblast GF
	PDGF	platelet-derived GF
	IGF	insulin-like GF
	BMPs	bone morphogenetic protein
	PTHrP	parahormone-related protein

Chemotactically Active Cytokines

α-chemokines
IL-8   interleukin 8
β-chemokines
RANTES   regulated on activation, normal T-cell expressed and secreted
MCP-1 monocyte-chemotactic protein
MIP   macrophage-inflammatory protein

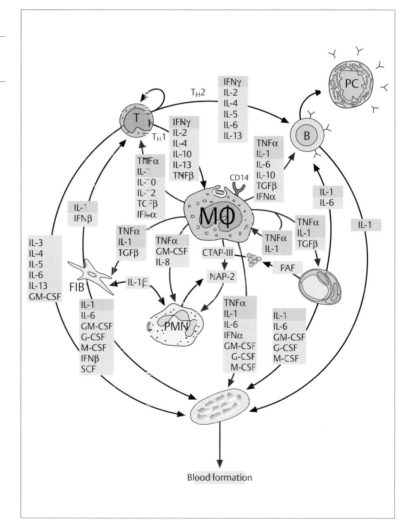

Blood formation

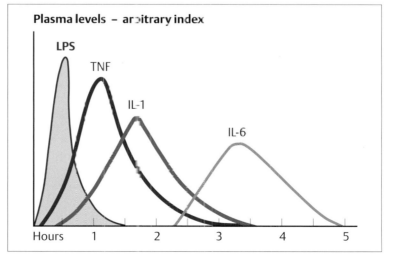

Plasma levels – arbitrary index

LPS
TNF
IL-1
IL-6

Hours   1   2   3   4   5

95 Cytokine Network

The cytokine-producing cells and their target cells exchange signals continuously. This supports primarily tissue homeostasis ("cellular internet").

A high degree of regulation can be achieved over certain physiologic or exceptional functions, for example immune defense, inflammation, healing, growth and cellular proliferation. TNF and IL-1 are important *cytokine inductors* that exert local as well as systemic effects (e. g., effects on the neuroendocrine system, pituitary hormones, liver).

In addition to the *pro-inflammatory* cytokines, one also observes their antagonists: *anti-inflammatory* cytokines (IL-1 receptor antagonist IL-1ra, IL-10, TGFβ).

CTAP-III	connective tissue activating protein III, precursor of NAP-2
NAP-2	neutrophil activating peptide 2
PAF	blood platelet activating factor
SCF	stromal cell factor

Modified from *Gemsa et al. 1997*

96 Cytokine Cascade

Following injection of lipopolysaccharide (filled curved) the blood plasma always reflects the sequence TNF, IL-1 and IL-6: "without TNF, no IL-1; without IL-1, no IL-6" (cascade-like production of these cytokines of the inflammatory process; cf. Fig. 95, pink-highlighted areas)!

Cytokines are not stored, rather they are constantly produced.

Modified from *Abbas et al. 1996*

Cytokines and Their Effects

97 Inflammatory Cytokines

Periodontitis is characterized by an increased secretion of pro-inflammatory and catabolic cyto-kines, mainly the major activators IL-1 and TNFα.

These activate the release of additional cytokines such as IL-6, inflammatory mediators such as the prostaglandins (PGE2, p. 49) and of tissue destructive enzymes such as matrix metalloproteinases (MMP, p. 50).

Especially IL-1 and TNF enhance the net loss of bone because they inhibit synthesis while supporting resorption (disturbed homeostasis; p. 61).

98 Chemokines

The α- and the β- chemokines of the host are differentiated in their sequence of amino acids: between the two cystein residues (-C-C- in the β-chemokines) there is an additional amino acid (X in -C-X-C-) in the α-chemokines.

The receptors of these chemokines upon MΦ and T-cells are "misused" by the HI-virus (p. 148)!

99 Immunoregulatory Cytokines

Control mechanisms including activation, inhibition and selective mechanisms attempt to combat foreign substances and organisms such that the least possible tissue destruction occurs.

Not listed in this table is IL-1ra (anti-inflammatory), the receptor antagonist of IL-1.

100 Cytokines of the Second Line of Defense

Listed here are only three of a long list of cytokines that are responsible for the recruitment, differentiation and activation of target cells (colony stimulating factor CSF and others, including those for mediation of wound healing).

Modified from *Abbas et al.* 1996

Mediators / Cytokines of Non-specific Immunity – The Acute Inflammatory Reaction			
Cytokine	Origin	Target cells	Effects on target cells
TNF(α) *Gene polymorphism*	Monocytes / MΦ T-lymphocytes	MΦ PMN Osteoclasts Hypothalamus Liver	Phagocytosis, IL-1 synthesis, general activation, inflammation enhances bone resorption Fever, cachexia, APP (acute phase proteins)
IL-1 IL-1α IL-1β *Gene Polymorphism*	Monocytes / MΦ others	T-cells, CD4+ B-cells Osteoblasts Osteoclasts Endothelial cells Hypothalamus Liver	Stimulates secretion of IL-2 Enhances proliferation Inhibits bone formation Stimulates bone resorption Activation, inflammation Fever APP (acute phase proteins)
IL-6	Monocytes / MΦ Endothelial cells, T-cells	Thymocytes Mature B-cells Liver	Co-stimulation Proliferation APP, fibrinogen etc.
IL-8 *Chemokines*	Monocytes / MΦ, endothelial cells, fibroblasts, T-cells	PMN Leukocytes	Chemotaxis, activation Chemotaxis, activation

Chemokine = „Chemoattractant Cytokines"			Helix Receptors
Chemokine	Type	Target cells	Effect
α-Chemokine **– IL-8** β-Chemokine **– MCP-1** **– MIP-1α** **– RANTES**	– -C-X-C- MΦ, Tissue cells – -C-C- T-cells • MΦ chemoattr. protein 1 • MΦ inflamm. protein 1α • regulated on activation, normal T-cell expressed and secreted	PMN MΦ MΦ MΦ, CD4- Memory cells	Low concentration: Chemotaxis High concentration: Activation Recruiting and activation Recruiting and activation Recruiting and activation

Mediators /Cytokines of Immunologically-elicited Inflammation (Chronic)			
Cytokine	Origin	Target cells	Effects on target cells
IFNγ *Immune-interferon*	T-cells, NK-cells	Mono / MΦ, NK all cells	Activation Enhanced expression of MHC molecules of classes I & II
Lymphotoxin TNFβ	T-cells	PMN, NK endothelial cells	Activation Activation
IL-10	T-cells	Mono / MΦ B-cells	Inhibition Activation
IL-5	T-cells	Eosinophils, B-cells	Activation Proliferation and activation
IL-12	Macrophages	NK-cells, T-cells	Activation Proliferation, activation Differentiation of CD4-/T_H0-cells into T_H1-cells

Mediators / Cytokines of Lymphocyte Activation, Proliferation and Differentiation			
Cytokine	Origin	Target cells	Effects on target cells
IL-2	T-cells	T-cells NK-cells B-cells	Proliferation, cytokine production Proliferation, activation Proliferation, Ig formation
IL-4	CD4+-T-cells Mast cells	B-cells Mono / MΦ T-cells	Isotype change to IgE Inhibition of activation Proliferation
TGFβ	T-cells Monocytes / MΦ	T-cells Mono / MΦ other cells	Inhibition of proliferation Inhibition of activation Inhibition of proliferation

Eicosanoids – Prostaglandins and Leukotrienes

Eicosanoids (C20 molecules) comprise a large group of mediators with a broad spectrum of efficacy. They consist of the 4x unsaturated fatty acid *arachidonic acid* (ARA). ARA is a constituent of the phospholipid plasma membrane of all human cells. ARA is not freely available; rather, it is released from the inner membrane layer by the action of *phospholipase A2* and is subsequently processed further enzymatically (*ARA cascade*), specifically by *lipoxygenases* to leukotrienes (LT), and through *prostaglandin synthases* (= cyclooxygenases 1 and 2; COX-1 and COX-2) to prostaglandins (PG), prostacyclins and thromboxanes.

Especially important in periodontology are:

- The chemotactically effective leukotriene (LTB4)
- Prostaglandin PGE2 (synthesized locally by macrophages), which, in elevated concentration, is one of the most potent inflammatory mediators.
PGE2 is produced via COX-1 (gene on chromosome 9; *MΦ-positive and MΦ-negative = normal phenotype;* see below) as well as through COX-2 (gene on chromosome 1; p. 53).

Arachidonic Acid Cascade

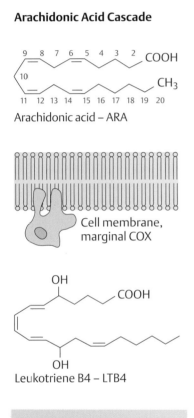

Arachidonic acid – ARA

Cell membrane, marginal COX

Leukotriene B4 – LTB4

Prostaglandin E2 – PGE2

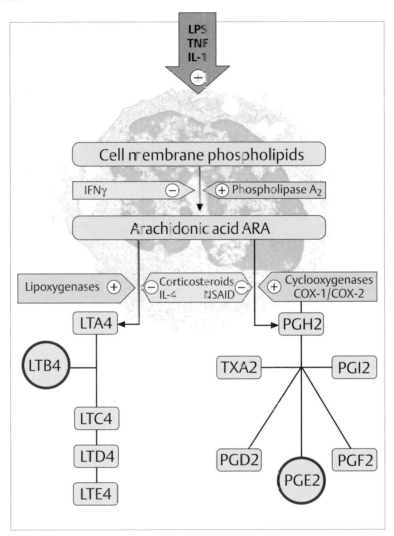

101 Arachidonic Acid Cascade
Macrophages secrete diverse eicosanoids in response to bacterial metabolites such as LPS and/or via cytokines (TNF, IL-1):

- Prostaglandins e. g., **PGD2, PGE2, PGF2**
- Thromboxane, e. g., **TXA2**
- Prostacyclins, e. g., **PGI2**
- Leukotrienes, e. g., **LTA4-LTE4**

These bioactive molecules are not stored in the cells, but are constantly produced.

Prostaglandins exert *physiologic effects* upon stomach mucosa, blood clotting, smooth musculature (vessels, intestines), uterus (contractions, at high dosage even abortion!).

An "overproduction" (inflammation, fever, etc.) is theoretically preventable at various sites by means of inhibitory substances (blue field) of the individual enzymes (red field).
Available today for use in practice are corticosteroids and non-steroidal inflammatory inhibitors (NSAID, p. 294).

COX-1 versus COX-2

COX-1 is responsible for maintaining PGE2 production at a *constant, physiologic level*, essential for the protection of the gastrointestinal mucosa (mucin) and the function of blood platelets (clotting). Through the actions of pro-inflammatory cytokines (IL-1, TNF) COX-1 is *not* up-regulated, in contrast to COX-2, which is largely responsible for the high levels of PGE2 during inflammation.
A different PGE2 secretion by macrophages in response to bacterial stimuli (*MΦ-positive phenotype* to COX-1; Offenbacher et al. 1993) is responsible for a generally elevated ability to mount the inflammatory response (cf. p. 52).

Medicinal Therapeutic Possibilities

The most important inhibitors of PGE2 synthesis are the non-steroidal anti-inflammatory drugs (NSAIDs) such as acetyl salicylic acid (aspirin). These agents block COX-2 as well as COX-1. The threatening side effects of COX-1 inhibition (stomach ulcer; hemorrhage) most often prohibit a high dosage or long-term regimen.
With the development of so-called super aspirins, which are pure COX-2 inhibitors (p. 294), it appears that in the near future it will be possible to suppress the high level of regulation of PGE2 by means of COX-2 molecules.

Enzymatic Mechanisms—Matrix Metalloproteinases

Periodontopathic bacteria in the subgingival plaque, which initiate and propagate the inflammatory process, cause periodontal destruction *directly* (via *bacterial proteolytic enzymes*, e.g., "gingipains"), but especially also *indirectly* by means of the complex stimulation of a large group of proteolytic *host enzymes*, which have the capability to destroy the extracellular matrix of connective tissue and bone.

Most important in this regard is the family of zinc-dependent enzymes, the more than 14 matrix metalloproteinases (MMP; Birkedal-Hansen 1993, Deschner 1998).

The major MMP elements include gelatinases, collagenases, stromelysins, matrilysins and others.

Stimulation and Expression of MMPs

Bacterial products (e.g., LPS) can directly stimulate macrophages to produce the precurser molecules (pro-MMP). The macrophages then synthesize and secrete both cytokines and prostaglandins, which then can stimulate fibroblasts and other tissue cells to increase MMP synthesis and secretion. At the same time, other factors become active

102 Matrix Metalloproteinases—Classes
Activated inflammatory and structural cells synthesize a broad array of zinc-containing proteolytic enzymes (and simultaneously their inhibitors, even TIMP). Matrix metalloproteinases destroy the extracellular matrix of connective tissue; they exhibit overlapping substrate specificity.

Figs. 102 and 103: Modified from *J. Reynolds and M. Meikle 1997*

Enzyme		MMP Number	Substrate
Gelatinases			Collage degradation
	– Gelatinase A	**MMP-2**	Native collagen IV, V, VII, X
	– Gelatinase B	**MMP-9**	Elastin and fibronectin
Collagenases			
	– Fibroblast type	**MMP-1**	Collagen types I, II, III, VII, VIII, X
	– PMN Type	**MMP-8**	
Stromelysins			
	– Stromelysin-1	**MMP-3**	Proteoglycan – nuclear protein
	– Stromelysin-2	**MMP-10**	Fibronectin, laminin
	– Stromelysin-3	**MMP-11**	Collagen IV, V, IX, X and elastin
Matrilysin		**MMP-7**	Fibronectin, laminin, collagen IV
Metalloelastase		**MMP-12**	Elastin
Membrane type		**MMP-14**	Pro-gelatinase A

103 Structure of MMP
MMP molecules A-C are free enzymes; the fourth (D) is a membrane MMP of the cell surface. Non-activated MMP exhibit six primary domains:
1 Propeptide (latent enzymes)
2 N-terminal end, *catalytic portion*, with Zn^{2+}!
3 "Hinge" between 2 and 4
4 C-terminal end
5 Transmembrane domain
6 Gelatin-binding site

MMP is activated by plasmin and other substances.

(growth factors, hormones), which play an indirect role in the synthesis of MMPs and their *inhibitors* (e.g., TIMP, tissue inhibitors of MMP).

Inhibition and Inactivation of MMP

The healthy extracellular matrix of connective tissue and bone undergoes constant turnover. Regulatory mechanisms are targeted toward an equal balance between synthesis and breakdown, i.e., for tissue homeostasis. In the case of inflammation, particularly in periodontitis, this balance is altered in favor of the catabolic enzymes.

Natural inhibitors of MMP expression, and therefore also of destruction, are regulated both *locally* (TIMP, IL-10, TGFβ) and *systemically* (steroidal inhibitors).

Non-steroidal, synthetic inhibitors are of great interest for periodontal therapy. Most important here are the *chemically modified tetracyclines* (CMT 1–10; Ryan et al. 1996).

One of these agents, an MMP-blocking modified doxycycline (DOX), has recently reached the commercial market as a long-acting LDD (low-dose DOX: *Periostat*™; p. 294).

Risk for Periodontitis—the Susceptible Host

Microorganisms as the Agents of Disease

The role of bacterial plaque as the primary etiologic factor for gingivitis and periodontal diseases is unquestioned. For the progression of gingivitis to periodontitis, the "marker bacteria" such as *A. actinomycetemcomitans* (*Aa*) and the "red complex" of the BANA-hydrolyzing bacteria *P. gingivalis*, *T. forsythia*, and *T. denticola* (Fig. 77) are always present.

The Host and Its Environment

In addition, a long list of other factors, so-called secondary etiologic factors or "risk factors" co-determine the initiation, the progression and the clinical picture. These risk factors negatively influence the tissue as well as the defense reactions (immunity) of the host; they render the host more susceptible to the disease process. These risk factors may be just as important as the bacteria in the pathogenesis of periodontitis.

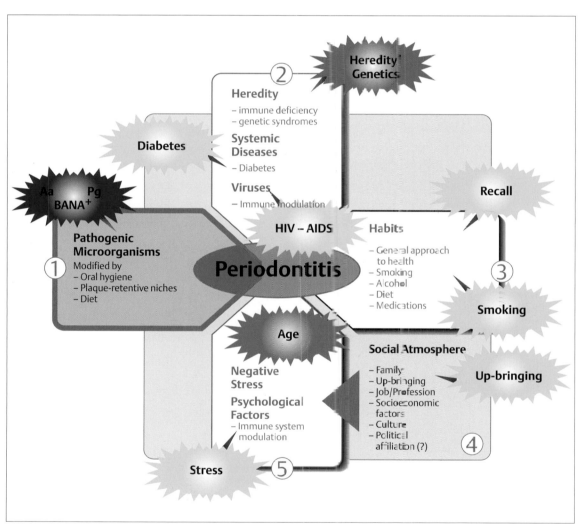

104 Risk Factors and Their Odds Ratios

Primary "risk factors"
– *Specific pathogens from plaque*
- *A. actinomycetemcomitans:*   ×**2**
- *BANA⁺-Complex*:*   ×**3.6** (Pg-Tf-Td)
- *P. gingivalis:*   ×**2.7**

Secondary "risk factors"
– *Non-alterable risk factors*
- Genetic defects   **?**
- IL-1 gene polymorphism: ×**2.7**
- Ethnic origin: **?**
- Gender: **?**
- Age: **?**

– *Alterable risk factors*
- Smoking: ×**2.8–6.7**
- Stress: ×**3–5**
- Up-bringing: ×**3**
- Lack of recall: ×**3.2**
- Diabetes mellitus: ×**2–3**
- HIV / AIDS: **?**

* BANA-positive bacteria hydrolyze N-α-benzoyl-DL-arginine-2-naphthalamide (a synthetic trypsin substrate)

Adapted from *N. Clarke & R. Hirsch* 1995 (p. 22)

Classification of Risk Factors ("Odds Ratios")

In terms of their importance for prognosis and choice of therapy, the recognition and weighing of risk markers or risk factors for the patient, each tooth and each aspect of each tooth are of critical importance during examination and collection of clinical data.

The term *"odds ratio"* refers to a statistically determined multiplier. It expresses the increased risk vis-à-vis normal susceptibility, but it is more of a relative figure than a definitive value.

Risk factors can be classified in many ways (see also p. 54):

- Microorganisms—host
- Host systemic—local
- Genetic or non-genetic (inherited or acquired)
- Avoidable or non-avoidable, etc.

One impressive and practical classification simply discriminates between:

- Risk factors that can be altered (see also p. 54)
- Risk factors that cannot be altered

Genetic Risk Factors—Diseases, Defects, Variations

In the case of periodontitis—a "multifactorial" disease—*genetic* and *non-genetic* factors influence each other, and their effects cannot always be sharply distinguished from each other. Both usually increase the pathogenesis as well as the clinical symptoms of the disease. One example is a low IgG2-blood level (caused by genetics and smoking).

Genetic Diseases—Genetic Defects

A genetic defect (e. g., in Papillon-Lefèvre Syndrome with its mutated cathepsin-C receptors) can be powerful enough to elicit disease by itself. This pertains primarily to single-gene diseases or chromosomal anomalies (Hart & Kornmann 1997). In such genetic diseases, periodontitis often occurs in adolescence, and sometimes even during eruption of the primary teeth. Many patients with pre-pubertal, juvenile or aggressive periodontitis exhibit granulocyte defects (PMN; see below).

Genetic Risk Factors

The majority of diseases are *multifactorial*, with a genetic component as the basis (gene variations: polymorphisms, e. g., the IL-1 gene). Such genetic risk factors may be associated with various loci (multi-gene diseases). The genetic insufficiency, in itself, does not in such cases lead to clinical manifestations of disease; only over the course of time, in adulthood, the clinician may note that a patient has become more susceptible, for example, to chronic periodontitis. Defects, polymorphisms with risk for periodontitis include:

- Fc receptors (FcγRII on PMN granulocytes)
- IgG2 level
- IL-1 gene (+) polymorphisms (p. 189)
- COX-1 (+) gene: elevated PGE2 production
- MΦ (+) phenotype: inflammation/wound healing
- Others: polymorphisms of IL-4, IL-10, TNFα, FMLP, Vit.-D3, cathepsin-C receptors, among many others.

105 Genetic Risk Factors—Influence on Pathogenesis
Demonstrated (red) and probable (yellow) genetically elicited defective immune functions. Their gene loci are portrayed in Fig. 106.

- *Antibodies*: reduced IgG2-level
- *PMN defective function*: LAD type 1 (leukocyte adhesion deficiency); adherence deficiency, FcγRII deficiency.
- *Cytokines*: positive IL-1 genotype
- *Prostaglandins COX-1*: with positive COX-1 genotype, MΦ produce excessive PGE2
- *Inflammation, wound healing*: negative effects with a positive (MΦ+) phenotype

Modified from *T. Hart & K. Kornman 1997*

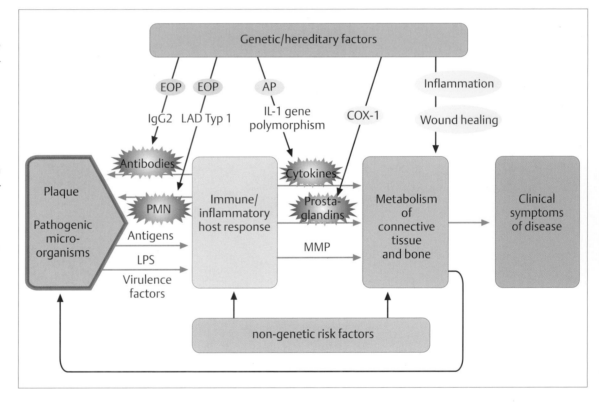

PMN Defects

From family studies, research with twins, as well as DNA analysis, the role of inherited PMN defects in aggressive periodontitis has long been acknowledged (Michalowicz et al. 1991, Michalowicz 1994, Hart et al. 1994). All of these research studies clearly show the important role of the PMN during host defense against infection. Numerous and diverse PMN functions may be combined or altered: Chemotaxis, peroxide production, phagocytosis, bacteriocidal activity/"killing," LTB-4 production (see also van Dyke 1995).

The following systemic diseases resulting from granulocyte defects are also associated with periodontal diseases (for additional examples: see Hart et al. 1994):

- Leukocyte adhesion deficiency (LAD) type 1
- Chediak-Higashi Syndrome
- Down Syndrome
- Papillon-Lefèvre Syndrome
- Diabetes mellitus
- Chronic granulomatosis
- "Lazy Leukocyte Syndrome"
- Crohn's Disease, others

Genetic Susceptibility to Periodontitis

Leukocyte Adhesion Deficiency, Type 1 (LAD Type 1)

Chemotactically-regulated PMN diapedesis cannot occur because of lacking adhesins on the PMN surface and lacking corresponding ligands on the endothelial cells; despite numerous PMNs in the vessels, one observes only few of these cells in the surrounding tissues. Early-onset, aggressive periodontitis is the result.

Low IgG2 Level

A low IgG2 level, resulting from genetic predisposition or tobacco use is associated with aggressive periodontitis. IgG2 binds to polysaccharide-like antigens, and is therefore important for defense against gram-negative bacteria.

PMN Receptors for IgG—FcγRII

Affinity and avidity for bacteria (the initiation of phagocytosis) are high when these bacteria are *opsonized*, for example, via immunoglobulins. The Fc-domain of IgG (Fig. 89) binds to the FcγRII receptors of the PMN. Defective or lacking receptors leads to aggressive periodontitis.

Gene Polymorphisms—IL-1-positive Genotype

The positive genotype (p. 189) sets the stage for stimulation of macrophages, with four-times the IL-1 content; this is associated with chronic adult periodontitis.

Gene for Cyclooxygenase 1 (COX-1)

The macrophage gene COX-1, which is responsible for the physiologically *constant* prostaglandin production, produces excessive amounts of PGE2, one of the most powerful inflammatory mediators (p. 49), when appropriately stimulated (TNFα, IL-1).

MΦ (+) Phenotype

Not all MΦ react equally to the same level of stimulation (e. g., LPS). The positive phenotype synthesizes and secretes the cytokine-inductors TNF and IL-1 in elevated levels, which have major effects on *inflammation* and *wound healing*.

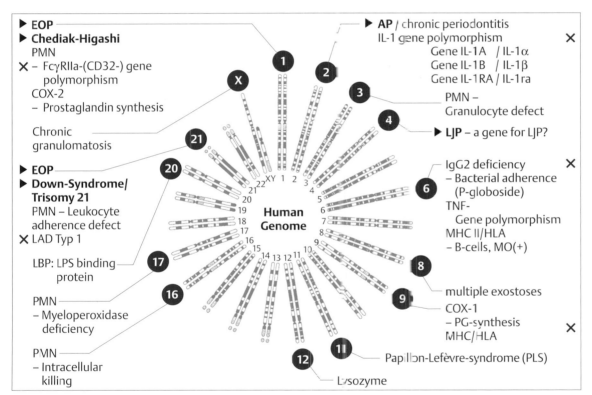

106 Human Chromosomes with Genes That May be Associated With the Periodontium or With Periodontitis (as of 1998)
To date it is primarily single-gene defects and gene polymorphisms by which the gene loci and the corresponding functional disturbances are understood (gene defects, gene variants; gene alleles).

Note: nomenclature change, 1999

AP → chronic periodontitis, type II/CP

EOP ⎱ → Aggressive periodontitis,
LJP ⎰   type III/AP

The Human Genome

The ambitious goal of the Human Genome Project was to decipher the entire DNA sequence (ca. 30 billion base pairs) of the human genome by the year 2003. Because of the intensive competition from private researchers, the goal was accomplished in the year 2000, although several gaps remain. It will require much more time until the function of the individual genes (ca. 25,000—30,000?), and their coded proteins and their functions and structures of the domain (estimated at 1,000—5,000 3D structures) will be clarified.

For this project (Structural Genomics Project), several scientific consortia in the USA and Germany have combined to found, for example, the "Protein Structure Factory" in Berlin. With precise knowledge of the structure and function of important human proteins, it will eventually be simpler to understand the complicated interplay of normal or defective genes, and to utilize such knowledge for diagnosis and therapy (e. g., for targeted medications).

The likelihood is high that such new and practical knowledge can also be applied to the periodontal diseases.

Alterable Risk Factors, Modifying Co-Factors

Periodontopathic microorganisms are non-alterable risk factors that initiate periodontal diseases (pp. 51–53); however, there is also a large number of alterable risk factors—earlier called co-factors—which influence the course of periodontitis to greater or lesser degree depending on their importance or intensity. It is possible to a certain degree within this group to differentiate between general (systemic) and local risk factors:

Systemic:
- Systemic diseases
  (diabetes, HIV infection, etc.; p. 119)
- Smoking
- Stress
- Medicines
- Education, social circumstances
- Lifestyle
- Environment
- Nutrition

Local:
- Saliva quality and quantity
- Mouth breathing
- Exogenous, mechanical, chemical, thermal, corrosive and actinic irritations
- Allergic reactions
- Function: occlusal trauma
- Orofacial clenching/bruxing phenomena
- Work-related parafunctions.

Serious systemic diseases such as untreated diabetes, blood disorders, hormonal imbalance etc., can be partially responsible for initiation of and accelerating progression of gingivitis or periodontitis. This will be covered in the chapters "Types of Disease" (p. 77) and "Oral Pathologic Alterations" (p. 119).

Smoking is acknowledged today as one of the most important risk factors. Tar products cause local irritation of the gingiva, nicotine is a sympathomimetic which leads to reduced metabolism in the periodontal tissues, and combustion products influence the chemotactic reactions of PMNs. An important risk is the lowering of the IgG2 level (p. 53).

Stress may be elicited by various causes such as work overload, social circumstances, environmental effects etc., and can lead to a negative influence upon the immune system or to increases in the pro-inflammatory mediators; the latter are associated with elevated susceptibility to periodontitis.

Side effects of medicaments can play a role in the initiation or progression of gingivitis or periodontitis, and are described in the chapter "Oral Pathologic Alterations" (p. 119).

Poor up-bringing and a *compromised socioeconomic status* may lead to insufficient appreciation for systemic health as well as oral hygiene, and this can have a negative effect on the periodontal structures.

Negative environmental factors can reduce the efficacy of the immune system and therefore also host defense against infections.

Nutrition can influence the speed of plaque formation as well as its composition. Extreme diets and inadequate nutrition can weaken the immune system and therefore the host's ability to respond to marginal infections.

The *saliva* has protective functions. Salivary mucins (glycoproteins) cover all mucosal surfaces as a protective film. Depending upon its flow rate and viscosity, saliva has a more or less powerful cleansing effect. Salivary content of bicarbonate, phosphate, calcium and fluoride determines its buffering capacity and its remineralizing potential. The antimicrobial activity of saliva is determined by its content of secretory immunoglobulins (sIgA) as well as lysozyme, catalase, lactoperoxidase and other enzymes.

Mouth *breathing* leads to drying out of the mucosa, and the protective effect of saliva is lost.

Exogenous irritants can injure the mucosa, gingiva and periodontium to varying degrees:
- *Mechanical* injuries, e. g. improper use of the toothbrush and other hygiene aids, can lead to injury and acute inflammation.
- *Chemical* irritants such as highly concentrated topical medicaments and acids can lead to lesions of the gingiva and mucosa. The same is true of *thermal* irritants (burns). These lesions are usually reversible, but in serious cases necrosis may result.
- Non-noble materials (e. g., root canal pins) may *corrode* following root fracture and cause damage to the periodontal ligament through corrosion products (Wirz et al. 1997 b)
- *Actinic* irritation: Mucositis and xerostomia may occur following radiation therapy for tumors in the head and neck region.

Allergic reactions may appear as mild erythema all the way to painful blister formation.

Pathogenesis I—Initial Inflammatory Reactions

Reactions in Healthy Tissues

Bacterial plaque metabolites "attract" PMNs. Proteins from bacterial vesicles and LPS, which react with LBP, as well as chemotactically active substances such as formyl peptide (FMPL, p. 58) stimulate tissues and vessels *directly* (A), supported by the mast cells (MC) near the vessels, or *indirectly* (B) by way of the macrophages (MΦ). These cells also produce pro-inflammatory cytokines (IL-1, TNF), MMP, PGE2, and IL-8, a chemokine that is also produced by the junctional epithelial cells near the sulcus. A chemotactically effective concentration gradient is created upon which the de-

fense cells (PMNs) become oriented as they exit the vessels and proceed toward the biofilm ("blue arch").

Vascular Reactions

Post-capillary venules expand in reaction to signal substances (e.g., histamine from mast cells, prostacyclins, NO etc.), and the flow of blood slows. Endothelial cells and host defense cells in the blood stream (primarily PMNs) express adhesins which enhance the adherence of the PMNs to the vessel wall, and subsequently make possible their diapedesis into the irritated tissue.

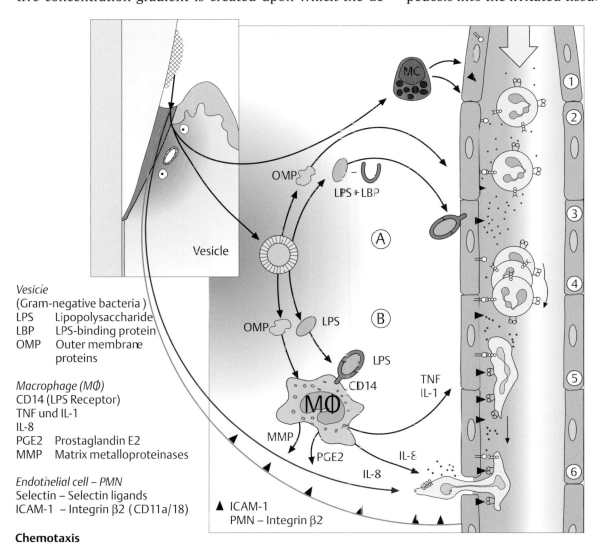

Vesicle
(Gram-negative bacteria)
LPS   Lipopolysaccharide
LBP   LPS-binding protein
OMP   Outer membrane
       proteins

Macrophage (MΦ)
CD14 (LPS Receptor)
TNF und IL-1
IL-8
PGE2   Prostaglandin E2
MMP   Matrix metalloproteinases

Endothelial cell – PMN
Selectin – Selectin ligands
ICAM-1 – Integrin β2 (CD11a/18)

107 Leukocyte Recruiting, Vessel—PMN Interactions

1 *Recruiting*: In the slowed blood stream of the widened venules, PMNs approach the vessel walls.

2 *Contact—selectins*: Molecules of the selectin family upon endothelial cells and PMNs "brake" this movement.

3 *"Rolling"*: The PMNs roll toward the vessel wall guided by the selectins (ELAM-1).

4 *Activation of integrins*: Chemokines from endothelium and tissue activate integrin β2 on PMNs.

5 *Fixation/Adherence*: ICAM-1 on the endothelial cells and integrins (PMN) retain the PMN. The PMN then wanders, by means of chemotactic guidance, toward the expanded intercellular spaces.

6 *Transmigration/Diapedesis*: The PMN leaves the venule. It wanders apically toward the sulcus bottom, i.e., toward the plaque, guided by its chemoreceptors (7-helix receptor, cf. HIV, p. 148)

Chemotaxis

● Classical chemotactic substances   ● α-Chemokine   ● β-Chemokine

Bacteria	FMLP (Formyl peptide, p. 58)		
Host	C5a (Complement)	Interleukin 8 (IL-8)	MCP-1
	LTB4 (Leukotriene, p. 49)		MIF-1α und 1β
	PAF (Platelet activating factor)		RANTES

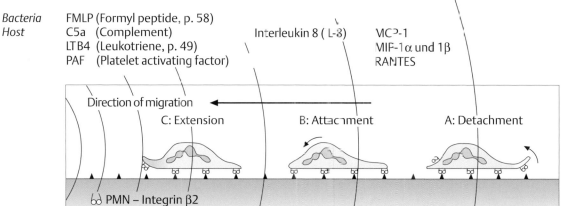

108 Migration of a PMN (from right to left): Detachment—Attachment—Extention

The PMN migrates upon cells and matrix substances along the gradient of the diverse chemokines in contact with their integrin molecules with ICAMs.
ICAMs are adhesins that belong to the superfamily of immunoglobulin genes (p. 46); they can be expressed on all tissue components.

Direction of migration ←

C: Extension   B: Attachment   A: Detachment

◌ PMN – Integrin β2
▲ ICAM-1

Pathogenesis II—Histology

As early as 1976, Page and Schroeder, on the basis of a literature review and their own experiments, described the histologic development of gingivitis and periodontitis. Their now-classic publication differentiated an initial, an early and an established gingivitis, and demarcated these from periodontitis. With today's knowledge "initial gingivitis" is no longer considered to be an early stage of disease, rather as the physiologic response of tissues and the immune system to dental plaque, even when plaque is present only in minute quantities (Schroeder 2000)

Early Gingivitis

Even in clinically healthy gingiva, some polymorphonuclear granulocytes (PMNs) transmigrate the junctional epithelium (p. 55). If this PMN migration becomes accompanied by a gingival sulcus infiltrate containing subepithelial T-cells, the condition is referred to as *early gingivitis*. Only in children can this stage of the disease process be maintained over longer periods of time.

In most adults, this "early lesion" develops quickly into an *established gingivitis*, which can vary considerably.

109 Healthy Gingiva
Very little plaque accumulation (hatched area), normal junctional epithelium (red), minimal sulcus depth (red arrow).
A few polymorphonuclear leukocytes (PMNs, blue dots) transmigrate the junctional epithelium in the direction of the sulcus bottom. Dense collagenous fiber apparatus, intact fibroblasts. This "condition" was earlier described as "initial gingivitis."

110 Early Gingivitis
Heavier plaque accumulation. In this early lesion, PMNs (blue dots) transmigrate the junctional epithelium and create a wall against plaque bacteria in the slightly deepened sulcus (red arrow apical to the plaque border).
In the subepithelial area, an early infiltration of lymphocytes is observed (black dots).

Modified from *R. Page &*
H. Schroeder 1982

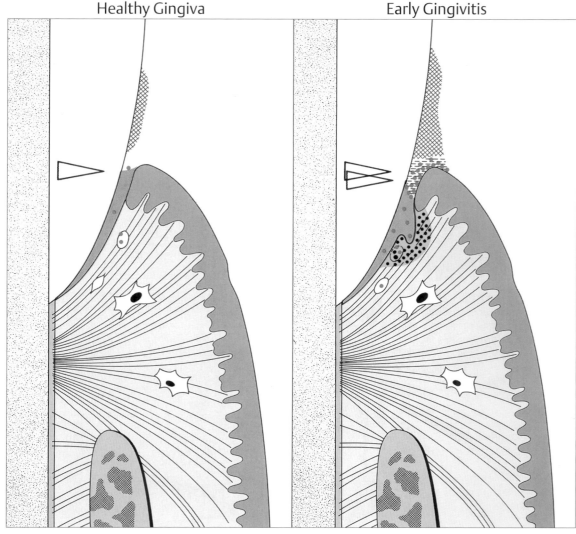

Healthy Gingiva   Early Gingivitis

	Healthy Gingiva	Early Gingivitis
Plaque	Few, mainly Gram-positive aerobes	Mainly Gram-positive aerobes
Junctional Epithelium / Pocket Epithelium	Normal junction epithelium, exhibiting no rete	Initial alteration and lateral proliferation of the junctional epithelium coronally
Vasculature Inflammatory Cells, Infiltrate Exudate	Few PMNs from the subepithelial vascular plexus transmigrate the junctional epithelium. Very little exudate ("sulcus fluid"). No subepithelial round-cell infiltrate	Vasculitis, out-flow of serum proteins, PMN migration, accumulation of lymphoid cells, T-cell dominance, few plasma cells; appearance of immunoglobulins and complement
Connective Tissue Fibroblasts, Collagen	Normal	Cytopathic alterations of fibroblasts; collagen loss in the infiltrated connective tissues
Alveolar Bone	Normal	Normal
Disease Course	–	Early lesion: 8–14 days after uninhibited plaque accumulation

Established Gingivitis

This can persist over many years without developing into periodontitis. It appears not to be caused by any specific microorganisms, but is influenced by their quantity and by the metabolic products from the biofilm.

Periodontitis

The transition from gingivitis into *periodontitis* (*progressive lesion*) is caused on the one hand by changes in the pathogenic potential of the plaque, and on the other hand by an inappropriate or inadequate host response to the infection, as well as the existence of risk factors (p. 55).

It is possible to identify periods of stagnation and exacerbation, which progress slowly (chronic) or rapidly (aggressive) depending on the type of disease (p. 112).

The histopathologic characteristics of the gingival and periodontal lesions cannot explain the myriad of individually varying and therefore difficult to classify forms of the disease (breakdown, progression etc.).

Only the most recent knowledge from molecular biology makes it possible to understand the immunologic processes within the periodontal tissues. These processes will be described in the following two pages.

Established Gingivitis   Periodontitis

111 Established Gingivitis
Increased plaque accumulation leads to massive influences on the constituents of the gingiva. All of the characteristics of gingivitis remain, but these can now also be identified histologically, and may vary in severity. The junctional epithelium—"epithelial attachment"—becomes apically displaced by the advancing plaque front (gingival pocket; arrow), but there is no loss of connective tissue attachment. The differentiated inflammatory infiltrate protects the deeper structures.

112 Periodontitis
The most important histologic differences between gingivitis and periodontitis include progressive connective tissue attachment loss and bone resorption, as well as apical proliferation and partial ulceration of the junctional epithelium (pocket epithelium; the base of the pocket is indicated by the red arrow).
In acute phases there is bacterial invasion of the tissue with resultant micro- or macro-abscesses.

Gram-positive and Gram-negative	Sub-epithelial, mainly anaerobic and Gram-negative	**Plaque**
Lateral proliferation of JE; apical migration; pseudopocket formation	Apical proliferation of the pocket epithelium, ulceration of the pocket epithelium, true pocket formation	**Junctional Epithelium / Pocket Epithelium**
Acute inflammatory alterations; plasma cells; immunoglobulins in connective tissue and sulcus; elevated GCF flow; leukocyte "wall" at plaque front.	Acute inflammatory manifestations as with gingivitis; massive infiltration; plasma cell dominance; copious and partially suppurative exudation; expansion of the inflammation and immunopathology.	**Vasculature Inflammatory Cells, Infiltrate Exudate**
Severe fibroblast damage, further collagen loss, stabilization of the exudates.	Further collagen loss in the infiltrated tissues, simultaneous fibrosis in peripheral gingival areas	**Connective Tissue Fibroblasts, Collagen**
Normal	Resorption of alveolar bone (attachment loss)	**Alveolar Bone**
Manifest 3-4 weeks after plaque accumulation, but can persist for many years without further progress	Periods of stagnation and exacerbation, slowly or rapidly depending upon the type of disease	**Disease Course**

Pathogenesis III—Molecular Biology

More than 20 years after the histologic description of the structural biology of periodontal diseases (Page & Schroeder 1976, pp. 56–57); Kornman, Page and Tonetti (1997) attempted to describe the pathogenesis of gingivitis and periodontitis with consideration for the actual molecular biology and newest genetic knowledge.

They divided their "expanded" pathogenesis into four stages or "momentary pictures," which were related in every case to a significant change in the activity of the immune system:

1 Reactions of the healthy periodontium to plaque
2 Initial acute, local inflammatory reactions
3 High regulation of the inflammation and infiltrate
4 Chronic immune reactions; attachment loss

The primary activities of cells and molecules that participate in the local changes in the marginal periodontium are described briefly in the figures below.

Stage 1

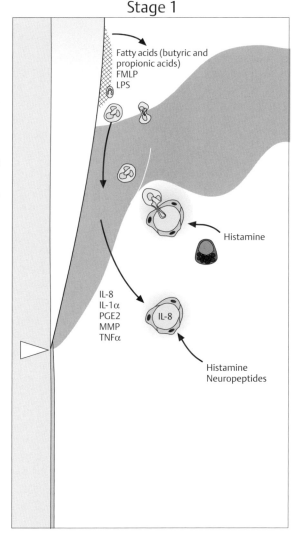

113 Stage 1:
Initial Reactions to the Plaque
Plaque bacteria produce metabolites, e. g., fatty acids (butyric acid, propionic acid), and the peptides FMLP and LPS, which stimulate the cells of the junctional epithelium to synthesize inflammatory mediators (IL-8, TNFα, IL-1α, PGE2, MMP). Free nerve endings produce neuropeptides and histamine, which highly regulate the *local vascular reaction*. Perivascular mast cells release histamine, which causes the endothelium to release IL-8 in the vessels. IL-8 attracts PMNs.

114 Stage 2:
Activation of Macrophages and the Serum Protein System
This vascular reaction (p. 55) causes serum proteins (e. g., complement) to spill into the connective tissues and activate the *local inflammatory reaction*.
Later, leukocytes and monocytes are recruited. Activated macrophages produce inflammatory mediators, e. g., IL-1β, IL-1ra, IL-6, -10 and –12, TNFα, PGE2, MMP, IFNγ as well as chemotaxins such as MCP, MIP and RANTES.

Stage 2

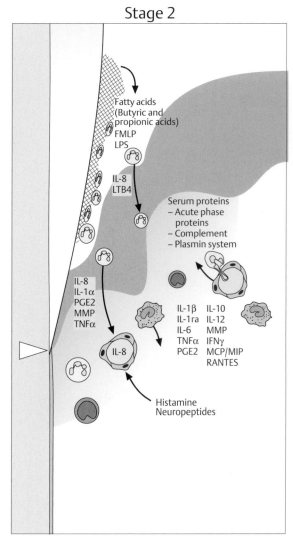

Host Defense Cells

   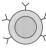

| PMN | Macrophage | T-cell | B-cell | Plasma Cell | Mast Cell | Fibroblast |

Signal and Effector Molecules

Host:
- Cytokines
  * proinflammatory
- Eicosanoids
- Proteases etc.
  ** chemotactically effective

Bacterial:
- Antigens, toxins and chemotaxins**

Abbreviations for molecules A-L
for all stages

FMLP**	N-Formyl-Methionyl-Leucyl-Phenylalanine	**IL-1ra**	Interleukin-1-receptor-antagonist	**IL-10**	Interleukin 10
		IL-2	Interleukin 2	**IL-12***	Interleukin 12
IgG	Immunglobulin G	**IL-3**	Interleukin 3	**IL-13**	Interleukin 13
		IL-4	Interleukin 4		
IL-1α*	Interleukin 1α	**IL-5**	Interleukin 5	**IFNγ***	Interferon γ
IL-1β*	Interleukin 1β	**IL-6***	Interleukin 6		
		IL-8*	Interleukin 8	**LPS**	Lipopolysaccharide

In a healthy individual, the term *local* defense means that plaque-irritated tissues recruit and activate only those cells and substances that are necessary for an effective defense. A network of mediators (cytokines, prostanoids, enzymes) deriving from immigrated immune cells and resident host cells serve to coordinate the actual situation and attempt also to maintain tissue homeostasis as long as possible, without tissue loss.

If the pathogenic microorganisms continue to exert "pressure" over a longer period of time (chronic inflammation), and if the immune response is not sufficiently competent ("susceptible host"), the tissue balance is tipped into a stage of increased breakdown that is enhanced by pro-inflammatory mediators and destructive enzymes.

These molecular and cellular reactions to bacterial metabolites and virulence factors vary considerably from person to person, but nevertheless permit an understanding of the numerous possible clinically relevant forms of gingivitis and periodontitis.

Stage 3

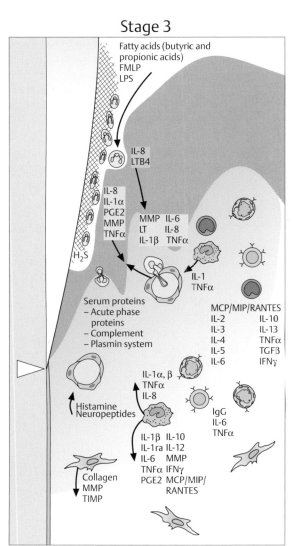

Stage 4

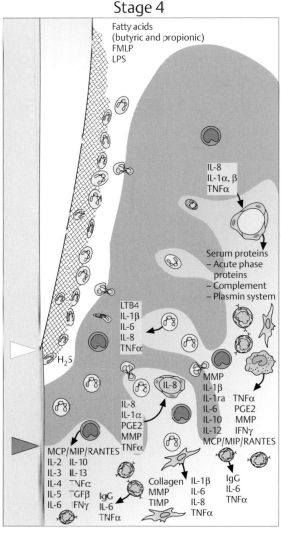

115 Stage 3: Up-regulation of the Activity of Inflammatory Cells—Detachment of the Junctional Epithelium Leads to a Gingival Pocket

The *inflammatory infiltrate* is dominated by lymphocytes. Activated T-cells coordinate the response via cytokines (IL-2 through –6, IL-10 and –13, TNFα, TGFβ, IFNγ). Plasma cells produce Igs and cytokines. Activated PMNs synthesize diverse cytokines, leukotrienes and MMP. Activated fibroblasts produce MMP and TIMP instead of collagen. The infiltrate (blue) expands.

116 Stage 4:
Initial Attachment Loss

In the infiltrated connective tissue, there is elevated activity of macrophages, with highly regulated mediators and host reactions. Immunocompetent cells produce numerous cytokines (IL-1β, IL-6, IL-8, TNFα) as well as PGE2, MMP and TIMP. Plasma cells dominate the infiltrate. The disturbed tissue homeostasis leads to the destruction of collagen, connective tissue matrix and bone. *Periodontitis* is the consequence.

Modified from *K. Kornman et al. 1997* [pinxit *T. Cockerham*]

Host Defense Cells

   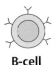

| PMN | Macrophage | T-cell | B-cell | Plasma Cell | Mast Cell | Fibroblast |

Signal and Effector Molecules
Host:
- Cytokines
  * proinflammatory
- Eicosanoids
- Proteases etc.
  ** chemotactically effective

Bacterial:
- Antigens, toxins and chemotaxins **

Abbreviations for molecules L – Z
for all stages

LTB4**	Leukotriene B4	**MMP**	Matrix metallo-proteinases	
MCP**	Monocyte chemo-attractive protein	**PGE2**	Prostaglandin E2	
MIP	Macrophage inflammatory protein	**RANTES****	Regulated on activation, normal T-cell expressed and secreted	

TIMP	Tissue inhibitors of MMP
TGFβ	Transforming growth factor β
TNFα*	Tumor necrosis factor α

Attachment Loss I—Destruction of Connective Tissue

Attachment loss (AL) is one of the primary symptoms in active phases of periodontitis: Extracellular matrix and collagen, e.g., periodontal ligament fibers, are destroyed. The critical milestone in this process is the major change in the activity of resident fibroblasts: Tissue homeostasis is lost, the balance between synthesis and resorption is forced toward more active destruction. This stimulation of tissue resorption may have several different causes:

• In *chronic periodontitis*, it is above all the macrophages (MΦ), activated by bacterial metabolites (e.g., LPS) that stimulate the resident fibroblasts toward secretion of destructive (secondary) mediators such as PGE2 and enzymes (e.g., MMP). On-going efforts in research today are targeted toward reducing such macrophage hyperactivity through use of various medicaments.

• In *acute inflammation and abscesses*, PMNs within the connective tissues are activated by the extremely high chemokine concentrations. During the "respiratory burst" and afterwards, a massive amount of lytic enzymes is set free (acid hydrolases, elastase, neutral proteases etc.), and these have the capacity to destroy host tissue.

117 Connective Tissue—Homeostasis of Apposition and Resorption

Influence of messenger substances (cytokines, primarily growth factors) and secondary mediators such as PGE2, MMP and TIMP on fibroblasts (FIB). Synthesis and resorption of extracellular matrix (collagen fibers and ground substance) remain in balance.
Also the number of cells is regulated by proliferative and apoptotic signals. Apoptosis (genetically determined cell death) is initiated by many mechanisms, for the most part yet to be understood.

⬆ Enhanced
⬇ Reduced

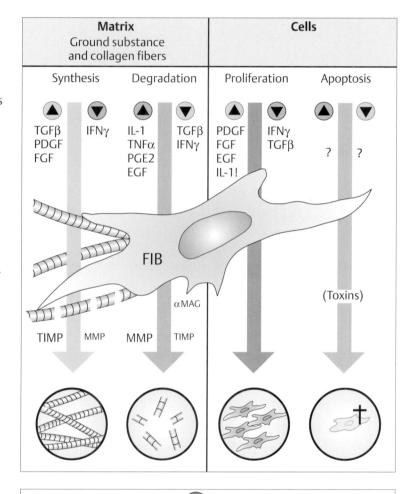

Alphabetical Listing of the Mediators

EGF   Epidermal Growth Factor
FGF   Fibroblast Growth Factor
IFNγ Interferon γ
IL-1 Interleukin 1
αMAG α-Macroglobulin
MMP   Matrix Metalloproteinases
PDGF Platelet-Derived Growth Factor
PGE2 Prostaglandin E2
TGFβ Transforming Growth Factor β
TIMP Tissue Inhibitor of MMP
TNFα Tumor Necrosis Factor α

118 Inflammation-provoked Destruction of Connective Tissue Matrix and Bone

1 Lipopolysaccharide (LPS) activated macrophages (MΦ)
2 Up-regulated inflammatory mediators (IL-1β, TNF, PGE2) and enzymes (MMP) activate fibroblasts, and degrade connective tissue and bone matrix *directly*.
3 Fibroblasts also destroy collagen by means of MMP.
4 Bone resorption results directly (via MΦ) or indirectly through stimulation of osteoclasts.

Modified from *R. Page et al. 1997*

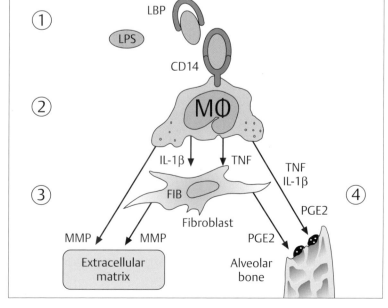

CD14   LPS receptor
IL-1β Interleukin 1β
LBP   LPS binding protein
LPS   Lipopolysaccharide
MΦ   Macrophage
MMP   Matrix Metalloproteinases
PGE2   Prostaglandin E2
TNFα   Tumor Necrosis Factor α

Attachment Loss II—Bone Resorption

The numerous mechanisms that serve homeostasis but also effect increased local synthesis and resorption of the alveolar bone are well-understood: The instigating agents of tissue loss in periodontitis are bacterial substances such as lipopolysaccharides, lipoteichoic acids (LTA) etc. These lead to an increased release of cytokines and mediators such as IL-1, TNFα, IFNγ, growth factors (e.g., bone morphogenetic protein, BMP) and local factors such as PGE2, MMP and others (abbreviations in the figure legend, left).

These factors stimulate the activity of osteoclasts directly, or may work indirectly, first on pre-osteoclasts, and thus increase the "pool" of bone resorbing cells. The mentioned bacterial substances and the host-mediators also demonstrate a direct repression or modulation of the bone-forming osteoblasts (Schwartz et al. 1997).

During acute phases of periodontitis, it appears that a direct initiation of bone resorption by bacterial products such as LPS, LTA and peptidoglycans is possible.

**Stimulatory (+) and
Inhibitory (-) Components
of Bone Resorption**

Gram-negative bacteria:
Ag   Antigens
LPS   Lipopolysaccharides

Gram-positive bacteria:
Ag   Antigens
LTA   Lipoteichoic Acid
E   Enzymes

Host cells:
B   B-cells
PC   Plasma Cells
T_H   T-Helper Cells
MΦ   Macrophages
FIB   Fibroblasts

Host molecules:
C   Complement
IL-1   Interleukin 1
IFNγ   Interferon γ
MMP Matrix Metalloproteinases
PGE2 Prostaglandin E2
TIMP MMP-Inhibitors
TNFα Tumor Necrosis Factor α

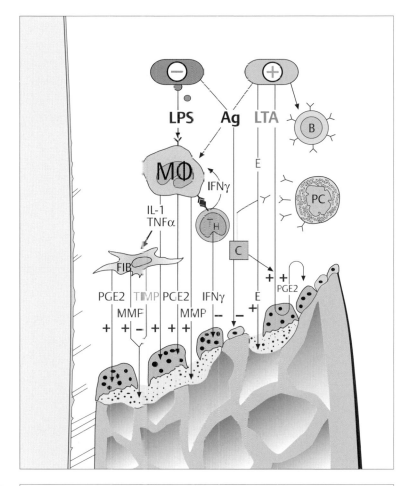

**119 Mechanisms of Local
Periodontal Bone Destruction**
The arrows emanating from the macrophages (MΦ) and from stimulated fibroblasts (FIB) indicate the enzymatic destruction of the *organic* bone matrix (MMP/TIMP).
Activated, multinuclear osteoclasts (red) resorb *inorganic/mineral portions* of the alveolar bone (acid-released calcium phosphate).
Osteoclasts exhibit on their outer surface a "sucker," and within a brush-like border (secretion of acids, resorption of released minerals).

Additional Local (Growth) Factors:
BMP   Bone Morphogenetic
            Protein
TGFβ Transforming Growth
            Factor β

Inhibition of osteoblasts:
A1   Pre-osteoblasts are inhibited in differentiation to osteoblasts
A2   Production of TGFβ, BMP is inhibited
A3   Matrix production is inhibited

Stimulation of osteoclasts:
B1   Osteoclast differentiation is enhanced
B2   Osteoclast activity is enhanced

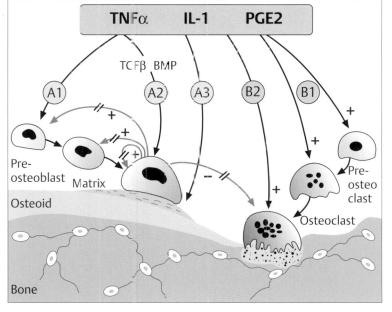

**120 Bone Remodeling During
Progressive Periodontitis—
Local Factors for Inhibition and
Stimulation!**
The local factors released from the inflammatory cells, osteoblasts and osteoclasts alter normal tissue homeostasis: Osteoblasts are inhibited, osteoclasts are stimulated. The differentiation, proliferation and the capability of osteoblasts to synthesize matrix substances and cytokines (e.g., for the auto- and paracrine stimulation) are thereby influenced.

Modified from *Z. Schwartz et al. 1997*

Pathogenesis—Clinical Features: From Gingivitis to Periodontitis

The stages in the pathogenesis of gingivitis and periodontitis have already been described histopathologically (p. 56) and at the molecular level (p. 58).

In 1993, Offenbacher and his coworkers presented a promising concept to explain why the presence of so-called pathogenic bacteria (p. 33) is associated in some patients with gingivitis and in others with periodontitis. A most important role is played by the neutrophilic granulocytes (PMN): If PMNs exhibit a defect in diapedesis, a failure to respond to chemotaxis, inadequate mobility, inability to phagocytose

and "digest" the bacteria, the PMNs are incapable of preventing bacterial invasion or the establishment of the subgingival biofilm. Also, when too few PMNs are present or if the bacteria are capable of avoiding them selectively, a clinically obvious and established gingivitis will develop (Schroeder 1994). The progress of chronic or aggressive periodontitis then depends upon the additional immunologic defense mechanisms and the genetically determined inflammatory response and healing capabilities of the tissue (varying host suceptibility).

121 Clinical Flow Diagram: from Gingivitis to Periodontitis
Biofilm metabolites activate host defense. Host response varies individually and will be more or less severe depending on the inflammatory reaction → gingivitis.

A *Early colonizers* (*Ss* and *Av*) make possible colonization by further bacterial species (*Fn, Pi, Pg*) into the developing biofilm (cf. Fig. 44).
Polymorphonuclear granulocytes (PMNs) are the first defense cells in the sulcus (Miyasaki 1991). If the PMN response is defective or if the bacteria are able to avoid the PMN response, pathogenic bacteria become established in the subgingival area, and elicit a *"limited" periodontitis.*

B A so-called leukocyte wall, formed primarily by PMNs, covers the plaque.
The initial defense axis (*congenital immunity*) consists of phagocytic cells (PMNs), complement and antibodies.
If the first axis fails, the secondary defense axis (MΦ and T-cells) must be activated: *acquired immunity*. The inflammatory process becomes chronic, and periodontitis progresses.
The MΦ/ T-cell reaction varies in intensity: Tendencies toward inflammation and the genetics of healing are different, and the progression of the periodontitis will also vary.

C Host defense mechanisms of the inflammatory infiltrate create this second defense axis.

Modified from *K. Miyasaki 1991, S. Offenbacher et al. 1993*

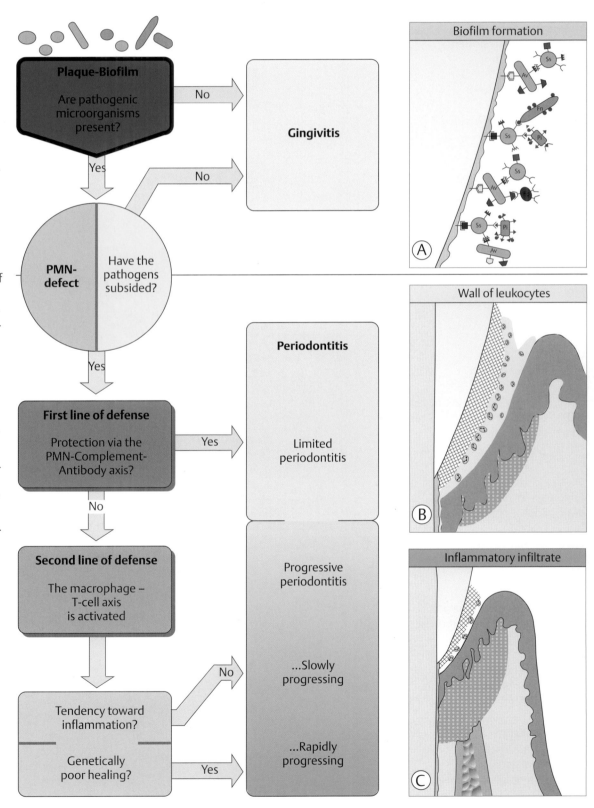

Cyclic Course of Periodontitis

Stable Lesion—Active Progressing Lesion

Periodontitis seldom progresses continuously. Most often, as demonstrated by Goodson et al. (1982) and Socransky et al. (1984), the attachment loss occurs cyclically, in "bursts" on individual teeth or on individual surfaces of teeth. During acute phases, the gram-negative, anaerobic and motile bacteria increase in numbers. Within a very short period of time, direct *microbial invasion* of the tissues can occur. This invasion reacts to acute host defense mechanisms, with the formation of *micronecrosis* or suppurating *abscesses*. Attachment loss occurs via collagen destruction.

Additional mechanisms remain under discussion (Page et al. 1997):

- Changes in the biofilm with high levels of LPS; consequence: Very high levels of IL-1, TNF, PGE2 and MMP, with the already discussed consequences.
- Significant disturbance of the normal chemotactic gradients (IL-8, FMPL): The PMNs "explode" within the connective tissue, which is thereby damaged.
- PMN diapedesis is inhibited by LPS from *P. gingivalis* and various polyamines: PMNs are effectively removed from the acute defense reaction.

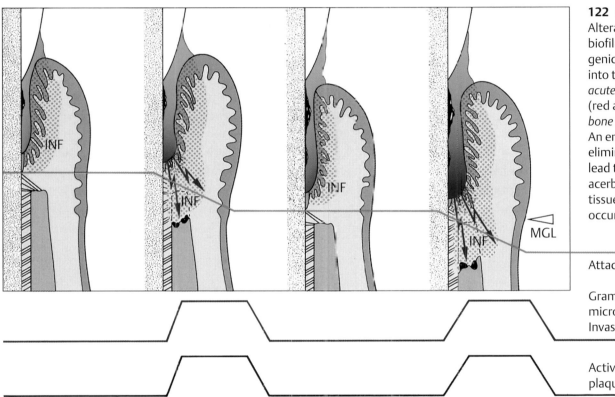

122 Cyclic Nature
Alterations in the subgingival biofilm, the increase in pathogenic bacteria and their invasion into tissues (see text) elicit the *acute inflammatory tissue reaction* (red arrows), *attachment loss* and *bone resorption*.
An enhanced host response can eliminate the bacterial insult and lead to *stagnation* of the acute exacerbation. A certain degree of tissue regeneration may even occur during such stages.

Attachment loss

Gram-negative, anaerobic, motile microorganisms
Invasion/infection

Activity: Exudate, hemorrhage, plaque, PMN, infiltrate, ulceration

Modified from *M. Newman 1979*

123 Regular and Irregular, "Site-specific" Attachment Loss
The chart (below) reveals probing depths to 6 mm. Such pockets can remain inactive for years (**A**). It is only seldom that pocket depth grows deeper *continuously* (**B**). On individual surfaces of teeth, it is much more common to see symptoms of activity (phases **1–4**):

A Probing depth remains constant for years
B Continuous process: 1 mm attachment loss
C Four acute phases: With attachment loss
D Two acute phases: With loss and remission

Modified from *S. Socransky et al. 1984*

Periodontal Infections and Systemic Diseases

Does Periodontitis Make Us Sick?

The strong influence of host factors in the pathogenesis and progression of periodontitis has been previously described. New knowledge from research has shown that the chronic infectious disease "periodontis" may also lead to serious systemic diseases in particularly susceptible individuals. Periodontitis, at the very least, must be viewed as a weighty risk factor for these systemic, and also multifactorial, diseases (Mealey 1999). Interactions have been demonstrated, or are suspected, with the following systemic diseases:

- Cardiovascular diseases:
  angina pectoris, myocardial infarction, endocarditis
- Difficulties during pregnancy: premature birth, low birth weight, increased infant mortality
- Stroke, brain abscess
- Pulmonary infections
- Diabetes Mellitus (DM)

Cardiovascular Diseases:
Angina Pectoris, Myocardial Infarction, Endocarditis

We have known for a long time the "classic" risk factors for this group of diseases: high triglycerides and low density cholesterol, stress, smoking and simply being a male. Beck and coworkers (1996) demonstrated in a large, longitudinal study of over 1100 men that periodontitis with deep probing depths increased the risk of coronary heart diseases, independent of the other risk factors.

In very general terms, *any infection* is a risk factor for atherosclerosis, embolism, and endocarditis. Infections with gram-negative microorganisms are associated with the flowing of inflammatory mediators into the vascular system, including also the systemically active cytokines (TNF, IL-1, IL-6), growth factors and prostaglandins.

Some gram-positive organisms may also be causative for severe cardiovascular diseases: Streptococci from the oral cavity, especially *S. sanguis*, can elicit the feared endocarditis or support it (De Bowes 1998, Herzberg & Meyer 1998, Meyer & Fives-Taylor 1998, Chiu 1999).

Problems in Pregnancy: Premature Birth, Low Birth Weight, Elevated Infant Mortality

Premature births with a birth weight of under 2500 g are the direct consequence of premature contractions and rupture of the membrane. Risk factors include smoking, drug abuse, alcohol, diabetes, high and low age of the mother, and bacterial infection of the urogenital tract.

However, in one out of four cases, other reasons for premature birth and low birthweight were identified (Offenbacher et al. 1996, 1998; De Bowes 1998). The initiation of contractions and subsequent birth are influenced significantly by prostaglandins (PGE2, PGF2α—components of the "morning after pill" RU 486!); these are mediators, of course, that have long been known to be increased in patients with periodontitis.

Stroke, Brain Abscess

Microorganisms from many different infected organs can reach the brain. Organisms from the oral cavity are rare there, and therefore appropriate research is lacking. Ziegler and coworkers (1998) described possible relationships between oral infections (including severe periodontitis) and stroke. Brain abscesses are usually a result of anaerobic infections. Except for individual case reports, no comprehensive research studies are available to definitively conclude that infections of the brain could be caused by oral microorganisms (Saal et al. 1988, Andersen & Horton 1990).

Pulmonary Infections

Oral, nasal and pharyngeal microorganisms frequently contaminate the upper airways (De Bowes 1998, Scannapieco et al. 1998, Scannapieco 1999). Clinic patients and the homebound, especially those in need of constant care, often exhibit poor oral hygiene and a high level of plaque accumulation. Such plaque represents a significant reservoir for potential pathogenic invasion of the respiratory tract (Terpenning et al. 1993).

Diabetes Mellitus (DM)—Type 1, Type 2

Intensive research has demonstrated that diabetes significantly increases the risk for periodontitis and its progression (p. 215). Other studies have asked the question whether periodontitis influences metabolic control in diabetes patients (Yki-Järvinen 1989, Grossi & Genco 1998, Lalla et al. 2000). Rayfield and coworkers (1982) found a direct correlation between the number of acute infections and complications in the control of the blood sugar level. There is a good correlation between acute infections and reduced response to insulin, a condition that can inhibit clinical recovery after prolonged periods of time (Sammalkorpi 1989).

Etiology and Pathogenesis—Summary

Healthy Gingiva

The tissues of healthy gingiva (pp. 8–13) contain within their epithelial and connective tissue structures a certain defense potential against the microorganisms of dental plaque. Even in healthy tissues, one observes the ever-present immunologic defense reactions (interactions between host and bacteria: the human being as "biotope").

Plaque

Dental plaque is a biofilm. Within only hours after thorough cleaning, it is re-formed upon the pellicle of the tooth structure. Plaque also occurs as a bacterial accumulation upon soft tissues (e.g., mucosal surfaces) and is therefore not always removed periodically by common oral hygiene procedures! Initially gram-positive bacteria proliferate and form an organized biofilm. These bacteria do not invade the host tissues and therefore effect such tissues only via their metabolites.

Connective Tissue

The bacterial metabolites recruit mainly polymorphonuclear granulocytes (PMN) from the activated subepithelial venule plexus. The PMNs exit in small numbers from the vessels. In this *clinically healthy stage*, very few if any other inflammatory cells are observed. Immunoregulatory mediators far exceed the pro-inflammatory mediators. There is no damage to fibroblasts or collagen.

Junctional Epithelium/Gingival Sulcus

In addition to blood plasma constituents (sulcus fluid), PMNs wander in small numbers, following the chemotactic gradient, through the intercellular spaces of the junctional epithelium, and enter the gingival sulcus. Here they build a defensive wall against the plaque bacteria, but are not capable of eliminating an organized biofilm via phagocytosis.

With good oral hygiene, the balance between the bacterial presence and the initial, non-specific defense (PMN mediators of inflammation) can be maintained over years. This "condition" was earlier referred to as "initial gingivitis," however with regard to today's knowledge, it cannot be defined as a true "disease."

The "old" periodontologists of the first half of the twentieth century would perhaps define this histologic situation as "physiologic inflammation" of the gingiva.

Established Gingivitis

If, in a patient with healthy gingiva, the biofilm is permitted to grow and mature by cessation of oral hygiene measures, gram-negative bacteria quickly establish a foothold, and their metabolites (e.g., LPS) traverse the junctional epithelium and enter the connective tissue. This leads to the establishment of "*early gingivitis*" (Page & Schroeder 1976). This condition is characterized by elevation in the sulcus fluid flow and PMNs. In the subepithelial area, one observes primarily T-cells. Also observed is initial collagen loss, cytopathic alterations of the resident fibroblasts and early lateral proliferation of the juctional epithelium. This "early gingival lesion" is only a shortly-lived (4–14 days) pre-stage of *established gingivitis*. Only in children can the early gingivitis lesions persist over long periods of time. In adults, one observes almost exclusively the *established gingivitis* lesions, with very different degrees of manifestation.

Plaque

The biofilm persists. The host defense can attack it only superficially, and if oral hygiene is inadequate, it will expand broadly. With time, the gram-negative bacteria increase in percentage.

Connective Tissue

As a result of the continuous diffusion of antigens and toxins (e.g., lipopolysaccharides), more and more macrophages are activated which, via the pro-inflammatory cytokines (TNF, IL-1, IL-6, IL-8) and other secondary mediators of inflammation (above all, PGE2; p. 49) the endothelial cells of the vessels are signaled to now permit other cellular blood-borne substances to exit the vasculature in addition to PMNs and plasma proteins (Expression of specific adhesins). In the rapidly expanding inflammatory infiltrate, both humoral (immunoglobulins from B-cells/plasma cells) and cellular (T-cells) immune reactions occur. The host defense now becomes more targeted via antigen processing and targeted immunoglobulin production: The mounting of the specific, adaptive immunity, the second line of defense (pp. 43 and 62).

Junctional Epithelium/Sulcus/Gingiva

The junctional epithelium proliferates laterally, but not apically.
Inflammatory swelling (edema, hyperplasia) of the gingiva can place segments of the plaque subgingivally, resulting in a situation in which primarily gram-negative, anaerobic bacteria come to reside within the deepened suclus (gingival pocket, pseudopocket). *Established gingivitis* is the result. At this point, there is no attachment loss. With targeted and adequate treatment, this gingivitis is completely reversible.

Chronic and Aggressive Periodontitis

The etiology and the pathogenesis of all forms of periodontitis are essentially similar. However, the various clinical courses of disease (chronic, aggressive, etc.) can be explained by the varying intensity and quality of the bacterial insult on the one hand, and the host response to the infection, as well as the number and type of collateral risk factors on the other hand.

Plaque

Gingivitis develops into periodontitis with attachment loss and formation of true periodontal pockets only if the plaque contains virulent periodontopathic bacteria at a critical level (p. 33), and in response to an inadequate local immune response in a susceptible host individual.

As pocket depth increases, the plaque becomes progressively more gram-negative and anaerobic. Protected within the biofilm, especially in the subgingival region, the bacteria can no longer be eliminated by the host defense mechanisms. Because the biofilm has become established between the tooth root and vital pocket soft tissue, natural restitution of the health of the tissues has been rendered virtually impossible.

The virulent pathogenic bacteria have the capacity to destroy at ever-increasing rates the defense response and the tissue homeostasis, as was described for gingivitis.
High LPS concentrations and the presence of numerous mediators maintain strict control over the both targeted and peripheral host reactions.

Gingiva/Periodontal Ligament/Alveolar Bone

In patients with periodontitis, it is quite common that gingivitis also persists, but its degree of severity can vary widely. In the case of juvenile, aggressive periodontitis (formerly LJP), gingival inflammation may remain quite mild even in the face of pronounced attachment loss (p. 116).

In the presence of non-alterable (e. g., genetic) and/or alterable (e. g., smoking) risk factors, there may occur an increase in pro-inflammatory mediators (inadequate host response), a condition which could force periodontopathic microorganisms apically, and therefore involve deeper regions of the periodontium (*periodontal ligament and alveolar bone*) in the destructive process. The result is destruction of the tooth-supporting apparatus and attachment loss (progressive lesion; periodontitis).

124 The "Bottom Line": Mediators and the Origins of Periodontitis
Periodontal *health* is characterized by few pathogenic bacteria, a low level of pro-inflammatory cytokines, prostaglandin E2 and matrix metalloproteinases MMP and a high level of tissue inhibitors of MMP (TIMP) and cytokines that suppress the immune-inflammatory reaction (IL-1ra, IL-10, TGFβ). In *periodontitis* one observes exactly the opposite!

Modified from *R. Page et al. 1997*

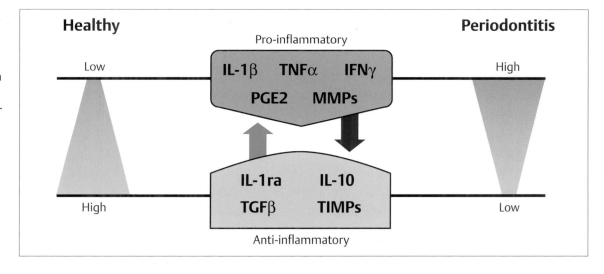

Fact

At the end of the day, all of the previously described clinical, histologic and molecular biologic reactions are steered by signal molecules of the cytokine network ("internet of the tissues"), and by anabolic/anti-inflammatory or catabolic/pro-inflammatory mediators.

Knowledge of the interactions of these guiding factors permits recognition of the individual forms of periodontitis (primarily the aggressive form) and permits diagnosis and ultimately also appropriate treatment. In addition to the classical diagnostic techniques (probing depth, attachment loss, attachment level, radiographic appearance, plaque indices, bleeding indices etc.), specific diagnostic tests are already on the market which modify and enhance the new

knowledge: Bacteriological tests (e. g. DNA tests, p. 183) and tests of the host's reaction (e. g., gene tests: IL-1 gene polymorphism, p. 189). Today, one has hope that in the near future the very bases of the described mechanisms in the complex disease of periodontitis can be stabilized to prevent destruction of periodontal tissues pharmacologically, biochemically or by genetic technology.

There is hope that, in the near future, periodontitis will not simply be treated by means of mechanical therapy, but rather that the clinical diagnosis of still *healthy* individuals at a young age can provide the practitioner with means for primary prophylactic measures to keep the disease process under control or prevent it entirely.

Indices

The inflammatory diseases of gingiva and periodontium, as well as their symptoms and the etiologic agents of these conditions (microbial plaque/biofilm) can be assessed clinically using qualitative and/or quantitative indices. In most instances, indices are used in epidemiologic studies, but they can also be useful during clinical examination of individual patients.

Indices are expressed numerically to describe defined diagnostic criteria: A disease process or its severity is described or classified using numbers (1, 2, 3 etc.). Simple indices record only the presence or absence of a symptom or an etiologic agent with "yes or no" entries, e.g., after sulcus probing: (+) = "bleeding," (–) = "no bleeding."

An appropriate index permits quantitative and qualitative statements about the criteria under investigation (disease, disease etiology), and is simple, objective, reproducible, rapid and practical. It should also be amenable for use by auxiliary personnel. Indices must provide data that are amenable to *statistical evaluation*.

Although indices for the most part were developed for *epidemiologic studies*, international standardization among various research groups has proven to be impossible: Many investigators use various indices or employ no indices whatever in periodontitis studies, rather they collect data on pocket probing depth and/or attachment loss in millimeters, which are then attributed to certain degrees of severity. Severity grades I–III: for probing depths up to 3 mm (I), between 4 and 6 mm (II) and those of 7 mm and greater (III). Other epidemiologists may assess these three severity grades using different millimeter measurements. Therefore it is scarcely possible to precisely compare the results of various studies to each other. Nevertheless, approximate conclusions can be drawn, e.g., concerning the worldwide incidence of periodontitis (p. 75).

Indices are also used in the *private practice with individual patients*: Especially plaque and gingivitis can be readily assessed in numerical fashion.

Repeated determination of an index during the course of preventive or active therapy can help ascertain the degree of patient motivation/compliance and treatment success or failure.

In this chapter, only a few of the many indices will be briefly described, primarily those which have been used for international epidemiologic studies, as well as some that are indicated for use on individual patients in private practice.

Plaque Indices
- Plaque index (PI)—O'Leary et al. 1972
- Approximal plaque index (API)—Lange 1986
- Plaque index (PI)—Silness & Löe 1964

Gingivitis Indices
- Bleeding on probing (BOP)—Ainamo & Bay 1975
- Papilla bleeding index (PBI)—Saxer & Mühlemann 1975
- Gingival index (GI)—Löe & Silness 1963

Periodontal Indices
- Periodontal disease index (PDI)—Ramfjord 1959
- Community periodontal index of treatment needs (CPITN)—WHO 1978
- Periodontal screening and recording (PSR)—ADA/AAP 1992

"Gingival Recession Index"
- Recession is measured in mm from the cementoenamel junction to the gingival margin (Jahnke et al. 1993, p. 162) or classified according to Miller (1985, pp. 162–163).

Plaque Indices

125 Plaque Index simplified, PI—Plaque Control Record, PCR (PI; PCR—O'Leary et al. 1972)

This precise index records the presence of supragingival plaque on all four tooth surfaces. For this test, the plaque is disclosed. The presence (+) or absence (–) of plaque is recorded in a simple chart, and the plaque incidence in the oral cavity is expressed as an exact percentage.

● PI is an index for the practice.

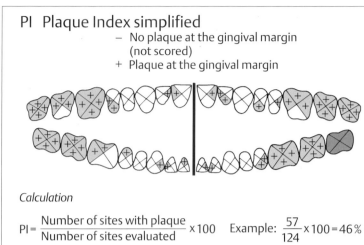

PI Plaque Index simplified
  – No plaque at the gingival margin (not scored)
  + Plaque at the gingival margin

Calculation

$$PI = \frac{\text{Number of sites with plaque}}{\text{Number of sites evaluated}} \times 100 \quad \text{Example:} \quad \frac{57}{124} \times 100 = 46\%$$

Abbreviation	Grade
PI=PCR	$\oplus$ & $\ominus$

126 Approximal Plaque Index— API (Lange 1986)

Following application of disclosing solution, a simple yes/no decision is made concerning whether the examined *interproximal surfaces* are covered by plaque (+) or not (–). The proportion of plaque-covered interproximal spaces is expressed as a percentage. Usually, analogous to the papilla bleeding index (PBI, Fig. 129), in a given quadrant the interproximal spaces are scored from only one aspect, i. e., from the facial (Q2 and Q4) or from the oral aspect (Q1 and Q3). The API is indicated for individual patient data collection and for motivation. It correlates with the PBI and is calculated as shown in the following formula:

$$API = \frac{\text{No. of plaque (+) sites}}{\text{No. of sites examined}} \times 100$$

Right: The problem of missing teeth (dark): If only one tooth is missing (above), the measurement site remains intact; if two adjacent teeth are missing (below) one measurement site is lost. In the depicted quadrants (2 and 3) the API is 69 %.

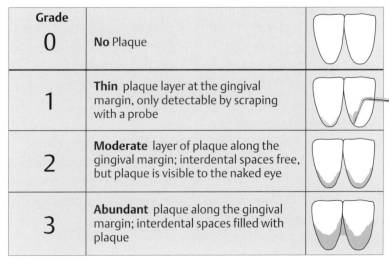

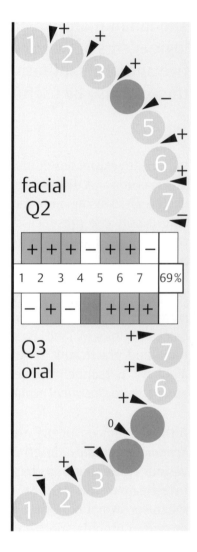

127 Plaque Index (PI; Silness & Löe 1964)

This index ascertains the *thickness* of plaque along the gingival margin; only this plaque plays any role in the etiology of gingivitis. To visualize plaque, teeth are dried with air. Plaque is not stained.

The PI is indicated for epidemiologic studies in which the gingival index (GI) is recorded simultaneously. It is less useful for routine dental office charting.

Grade		
0	**No** Plaque	
1	**Thin** plaque layer at the gingival margin, only detectable by scraping with a probe	
2	**Moderate** layer of plaque along the gingival margin; interdental spaces free, but plaque is visible to the naked eye	
3	**Abundant** plaque along the gingival margin; interdental spaces filled with plaque	

Abbreviation	Grade
PI	0–3

Gingival Indices

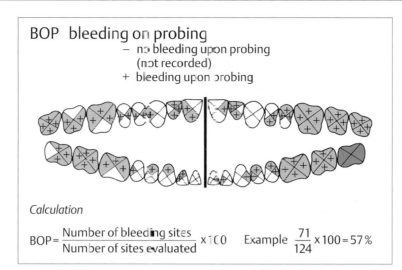

BOP bleeding on probing
- no bleeding upon probing (not recorded)
+ bleeding upon probing

Grade	Abbreviation
$\oplus$ & $\ominus$	BOP

Calculation

$$BOP = \frac{\text{Number of bleeding sites}}{\text{Number of sites evaluated}} \times 100 \qquad \text{Example} \quad \frac{71}{124} \times 100 = 57\%$$

128 Bleeding on Probing – BOP (Ainamo & Bay 1975)

As in the PI (Fig. 125), all four surfaces of all teeth are assessed with regard to whether probing elicits bleeding (+) or not (−). The severity of gingivitis is expressed as a percentage.

Because more than 100 sites must be measured, the BOP is indicated only for individual patient examinations (e. g., data collection, recall).

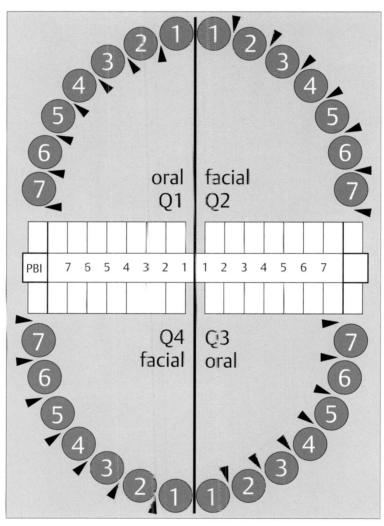

Grade	Abbreviation
0–3	GI

Grade	
0	Normal gingiva; no inflammation; no discoloration (erythema); no bleeding
1	Mild inflammation; slight erythema; minimal superficial alterations. **No bleeding**
2	Moderate inflammation; erythema; **bleeding on probing**
3	Severe inflammation; severe erythema and swelling; **tendency to spontaneous bleeding;** possible ulceration.

129 Papilla Bleeding Index—PBI (Saxer & Mühlemann 1975)

The PBI discriminates four *different degrees (intensities) of bleeding* subsequent to careful probing of the gingival sulcus in the papillary region (see p. 70). Probing is performed in all four quadrants. To simplify the recording of the PBI, quadrant 1 is probed only from the oral aspect, quadrant 2 from the facial, 3 again from oral, and from the facial in quadrant 4 (see black arrows in diagram). Bleeding scores are entered into the chart (middle).

The PBI can be reported as the *bleeding number* (= sum of all values) or as an index (average severity, as in this formula:

$$PBI = \frac{\text{Bleeding Number}}{\text{Number of sites measured}}$$

- The PBI is valuable for the practitioner, who can compare values over time (patient motivation, risk factors).

Left: In this example (quadrants 2 and 3), the PBI is 2.1; the bleeding number is 27. Missing teeth? Compare Fig. 126, right.

130 Gingival Index—GI (Löe & Silness 1963)

The GI records gingival inflammation in three grades. It is measured on six selected teeth (16, 12; 24 and 36, 32; 44; cf. Fig. 127) on facial, oral, mesial and distal sites. The symptom of *bleeding* comprises a score of 2.

- The GI was developed for epidemiologic studies. It is less applicable for individual patients because the differences between the scoring levels are too gross.

Papilla Bleeding Index—PBI

The PBI was developed for use in the private practice and not for epidemiologic studies. It is a *sensitive indicator* of the severity of gingival inflammation in individual patients. The PBI does not require a great amount of time, since only 28 measurement sites in the complete dentition are evaluated (Saxer & Mühlemann 1975).

The PBI has proven to be particularly useful for assessing inflammation in the interdental papillae by recording bleeding on probing in the interdental areas during the course of treatment. The index therefore offers an excellent means for patient *motivation* (p. 222). While the patient watches in a mirror, the practitioner can score the intensity of papillary inflammation. The patient can see when the gingival tissue bleeds, which helps him to realize where the diseased sites in the mouth are located.

The patient will realize and experience the reduction in inflammation during the course of therapy as the index is repeated at each visit, and this is a good motivator for thorough and continuing patient compliance.

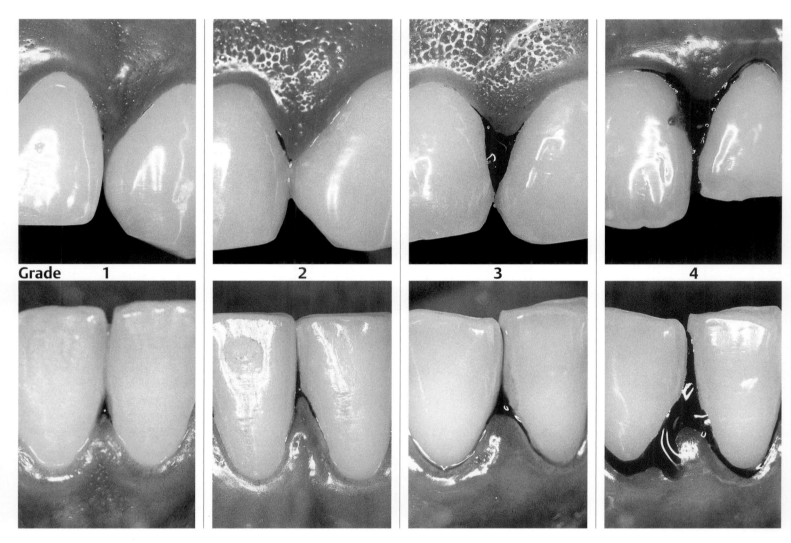

Grade   1   2   3   4

131 Grade 1—Point
20–30 seconds after probing the mesial and distal sulci with a periodontal probe, a single bleeding point is observed.

132 Grade 2—Line/Points
A fine line of blood or several bleeding points become visible at the gingival margin.

133 Grade 3—Triangle
The interdental triangle becomes more or less filled with blood.

134 Grade 4—Drops
Profuse bleeding. Immediately after probing, blood flows into the interdental area to cover portions of the tooth and/or gingiva.

Recording the PBI

Bleeding is provoked by sweeping the sulcus using a blunt periodontal probe under light finger pressure from the base of the papilla to its tip along the tooth's distal and mesial aspects. After *20–30 seconds*, when a quadrant has been completely probed, the intensity of bleeding is scored in four grades and recorded on the chart.

The sum of the recorded scores gives the "*bleeding number.*" The PBI is calculated by dividing the bleeding number by the total number of papilla examined.

Periodontal Indices

The determination of the *severity* of periodontitis through use of an index is really impossible. In contrast to a gingivitis index, which must only record the intensity of inflammation, any periodontitis index must, above all, measure the pocket probing depths and the degree of loss of tooth-supporting tissues (attachment loss). Periodontal indices find their most important use in epidemiologic studies. In private practice, a periodontal index may provide a quick overview of a patient's condition.

Many years ago numerous epidemiologic studies were performed using the *Periodontal Disease Index* (PDI) of Ramfjord (1959). More recently the CPITN has been recommended by the World Health Organization (WHO; p. 72). The CPITN was modified by the American Dental Association (ADA 1992) and the American Academy of Periodontology (AAP 1992) for a triage-type rapid diagnosis in general dental practice (PSR, p. 73).

Periodontal Disease Index (PDI)

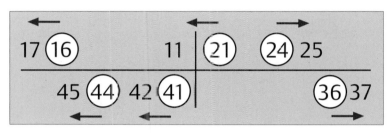

Grade	
0	Inflammation-free. No gingival alterations
Gingiva	
1	Mild to moderate gingivitis at isolated sites on the gingiva surrounding the tooth
2	Mild to moderate gingivitis surrounding the tooth
3	Severe gingivitis, visible erythema, hemorrhage, gingival ulcerations
Periodontium	
4	Attachment loss to 3 mm, measured from the CEJ
5	3–6 mm attachment loss
6	Attachment loss greater than 6 mm

135 Measurement of the PDI Using Ramfjord Teeth— Replacement Teeth
Ramfjord demonstrated that for epidemiologic purposes six teeth (circled) could be taken as representative of the entire dentition. If any of the "Ramfjord teeth" are missing, the replacement teeth (not circled) are substituted.

136 Periodontal Disease Index (PDI)—Degree of Severity
Within the PDI, grades 1, 2 and 3 represent a *gingivitis index*, while grades 4, 5 and 6 represent an index for the extent of periodontal destruction (*attachment loss*) independent of gingivitis and probing depths.

The PDI is not indicated for private practice but for epidemiologic studies.

Periodontal Disease Index (PDI)

The PDI does not include examination of all 28 teeth (third molars are excluded in almost *all* indices), but rather a sample of six teeth that are representative of the entire dentition. These teeth were chosen so that each tooth type, both jaws and each quadrant are taken into account: teeth 16; 21, 24; 36; 41 and 44. These are the so-called "Ramfjord teeth." If one of these teeth is missing, its distal neighbor (17, 11; 25; 37; 42 or 45, respectively) may be substituted (Marthaler et al. 1971).
The PDI evaluates these selected teeth for both gingivitis and attachment loss, with three gradations for each. For

periodontitis grades 4, 5 and 6, probing depth ("pocket depth") is *not* measured, rather the distance from the cementoenamel junction to the bottom of the pocket is recorded (attachment loss).

An average PDI score (e. g., 2.8) *cannot* be taken to indicate that only gingivitis (to grade 3) is present, or whether attachment loss has already occurred on individual teeth. For example, mild gingivitis and slight attachment loss on individual teeth could lead to an average value of < 3. Grades 1–3 and grades 4–6 must there be evaluated separately.

Community Periodontal Index of Treatment Needs—CPITN

The CPITN was developed in 1978 by the World Health Organization (WHO, 1978; Ainamo et al. 1982). It is used primarily for epidemiologic studies (p. 76). The major difference between the CPITN and other indices is that it determines not only the severity of gingivitis (bleeding) and periodontitis (pocket probing depth), but also provides information concerning the type of disease process and therefore also the extent of therapy that is necessary. Thus the CPITN provides not only conclusions about the incidence of gingivitis and periodontitis in a population, but also about the necessary expense, in both time and money, that will be necessary for treatment of a population group.

The CPITN does not consider the attachment loss on individual teeth, rather only the clinical situations requiring treatment:

- Gingival inflammation
- Bleeding
- Calculus
- Pocket probing depth

The CPITN is measured and ascertained using a *special probe* on all teeth, and the most severe areas in each *sextant* is noted in the chart.

137 Special Probes and the Codes 0–4 for Recording the CPITN and PSR
These probes are characterized by a small sphere of 0.5 mm diameter and a black band between 3.5 and 5.5 mm.
For use in the practice, additional grooves at 8.5 and 11.5 mm may be included. Probing is performed with a ca. 0.25 N force. The highest code in each sextant is entered into a simple form (see below).

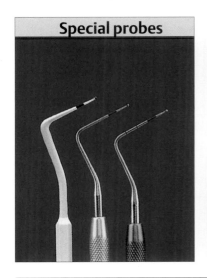

Special probes

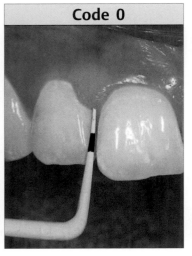

Code 0

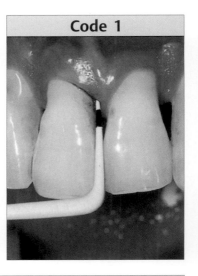

Code 1

138 CPITN and PSR Codes— Definitions
Codes 0–4 define health (0) or disease in gingiva and periodontium (1–4). In principle they are identical for both indices. Because it was developed for private practice, the PSR is somewhat more detailed than the CPITN, because in addition to the actual codes, an asterisk (*) can be added as an indication that the case is more complicated, e. g., by …

- Furcation involvement
- Elevated tooth mobility
- Mucogingival problems (e. g., lack of attached gingiva)
- Recession > 3 mm

Table for recording the PSR:

4*	1	3
3	2*	3

Comments:
- Pocket-free sextant in the anterior region, but severe recession in the mandibular anterior sextant (*)!
- Pockets up to 5 mm in sextants 3, 4, 6
- Sextant 1: Furcation involvement and pockets of 7 mm.

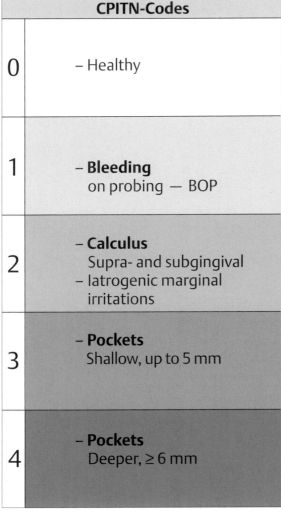

	CPITN-Codes		PSR-Codes	
0	– Healthy		– No bleeding – No calculus – Band 100% visible	0
1	– **Bleeding** on probing — BOP		– **Bleeding** – No calculus or defective restorations – Band 100 % visible	1
2	– **Calculus** Supra- and subgingival – Iatrogenic marginal irritations		– Bleeding – **Calculus** – Band 100 % visible	2
3	– **Pockets** Shallow, up to 5 mm		– **Band only partially visible** Probing depths 3.5–5.5 mm	3
4	– **Pockets** Deeper, ≥ 6 mm		– **Band no longer visible** Probing depths greater than 6 mm	4

Periodontal Screening and Recording—PSR

The PSR is a modified CPITN, developed by the American Academy of Periodontology (AAP 1992) and the American Dental Association (ADA 1992). As with the CPITN, taking the PSR is a relatively quick procedure, not requiring extensive forms to be filled out (no "paper war"!). This index serves for early detection of periodontitis.

The index reveals for the practitioner the current state of the gingiva (bleeding) as well as previously occurring pathologic processes in the form of pocket depth and the as-

sociated attachment loss. Further, the PSR provides indication as to whether additional, more-detailed examinations are necessary: If a code 3 or 4 is diagnosed on any tooth surface, a complete periodontal examination must be performed and a panoramic radiograph or a full-mouth radiographic series taken.

The PSR assists the general practitioner in the decision concerning whether a patient should be referred to a specialist for more complex periodontal therapy.

Code 2	Code 3	Code 4
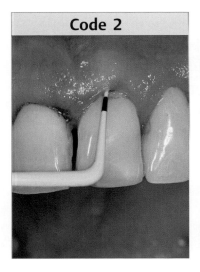	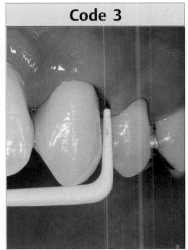	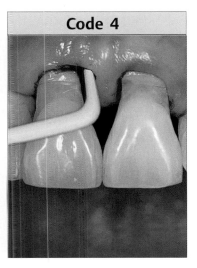

139 Clinical Definition of Codes 0–4

0 Probing elicits no bleeding; healthy

1 BOP (plaque, but no calculus)

2 The probe encounters supra- and subgingival calculus; bleeding

3 Probing depths between 3.5 and 5.5 mm, i. e., the black band remains at least partially visible

4 Probing depths 6 mm or more, the black band disappears subgingivally (bleeding, plaque, calculus)

	CPITN – Treatment need		PSR – Treatment need	
0	– Home care		– Preventive treatment only	0
I	– OHI (oral hygiene instruction)		– OHI – Plaque and debris removal	1
II	I + calculus removal and scaling		– OHI – Subgingival plaque and calculus removal	2
			– As in 2 + Complete periodontal exam and radiographs ⇨ Possible referral to specialist	3
III	I + II + complex therapy		– As in 2 and 3 + More extensive treatment, possibly surgery ⇨ Refer to specialist	4

140 CPITN and PSR— Treatment Needs

In contrast to the "codes," the treatment needs deriving from them diverge somewhat:

● In contrast to the CPITN, in the PSR even with healthy gingiva (**Code 0**) preventive measures are advised (oral hygiene instruction, prophylaxis)

● With **Code 1**, professional plaque removal (PSR) should be performed in addition to the patient's own oral hygiene (CPITN).

● At **Code 2**, both indices recommend supra- and subgingival plaque and calculus removal.

● At **Code 3**, both the diagnosis and the therapy are somewhat extended: complete periodontal charting, panoramic radiography or full-mouth series.

● The same holds for **Code 4**. The suggestion "refer to a specialist," is used in the PSR mostly as an aid in the general practice.

Epidemiology

Descriptive epidemiology deals with the occurrence, the severity and the distribution of diseases, as well as physical and/or mental incapacity, or mortality, in any selected population.

Analytical epidemiology seeks furthermore to discern the cause(s) of a disease. During the comprehensive examination of patients with periodontitis, in addition to the primary etiologic agent—plaque biofilm—other important factors such as heredity, socioeconomic status, behavior patterns, systemic diseases, risk factors as well as ethnic origin should also be ascertained as closely as possible. From this data, one can derive the likely consequences of prophylaxis and treatment, also from a public health standpoint (Albandar & Rams 2002).

In the field of periodontology, epidemiologists deal primarily with the dissemination of and the etiologic factors for gingivitis and periodontitis.

Not all results of the classic epidemiologic studies of the previous decades enjoy unquestioned acceptance today, however. The early studies did not consider all etiologic factors (see above), nor the varying forms of the disease, symptoms of activity and localization of the disease process. Furthermore, many studies did not draw conclusions concerning the treatment needs of the populations under study (AAP 1996).

Epidemiology of Gingivitis

Numerous epidemiologic studies have been performed worldwide, especially in children and adolescents. Their results reveal enormous differences. The morbidity rates (percent affected in the studied population) range from about 50 to almost 100% (Stamm 1986, Schürch et al. 1991, Oliver et al. 1998).

Further, the reported degrees of severity of gingivitis vary greatly among the studies. These differences can be explained primarily by the use of non-standardized examination methods (various indices) and the constantly changing classifications of the diseases themselves. Other etiologic considerations that could explain the large differences include the quite varied status of prevention (plaque control) in the population groups studied, as well as geographic, social and ethnologic factors.

The incidence and severity of gingivitis may even vary in the same patient group with short-term repeated examinations (Suomi et al. 1971, Page 1986). In addition, the degree of severity of gingivitis over the course of one's life can vary enormously: It achieves its maximum in adolescents reaching puberty, then recedes somewhat, exhibiting a slight tendency to increase in adults as age increases (Stamm 1986, Fig. 178 right).

The existence of gingivitis cannot be taken as evidence that periodontitis will eventually develop (Listgarten et al. 1985, Schürch et al. 1991). The *public health significance* of gingivitis epidemiology may therefore be called into question.

In studies in which both gingivitis and plaque were considered, a clear positive correlation between oral hygiene and severity of gingivitis emerged (Silness & Löe 1964, Koivuniemi et al. 1980, Hefti et al. 1981).

Epidemiology of Periodontitis

Many new epidemiologic studies of periodontitis have been published from many countries (Ahrens & Bublitz 1987, Fig. 142; Miller at al. 1987; Miyazaki et al. 1991a, b, Fig. 143; Brown & Löe 1993, Fig. 141; Papapanou 1994, 1996; AAP 1996; Oliver et al. 1998). As was the case with gingivitis studies, the results must be carefully interpreted. It is very difficult to compare the results of various studies when different parameters and different measurement techniques were employed without calibration. Up until now, epidemiologic studies, especially of elderly patients, have not even considered the causes of tooth loss all the way to edentulousness (caused by periodontitis?).

Furthermore very little attention has been given to fact that the measured parameters are applicable only to individual sites around individual teeth, and cannot be taken as a generalization, for example as an indication of the loss of tooth-supporting tissues in the entire dentition.

Most epidemiologic studies are really only "momentary" studies of the extent of disease (mean values).

Only Löe et al. (1986) studied the course of attachment loss over many years *longitudinally*, in a group of Norwegian students and academics on the one hand and tea plantation workers in Sri Lanka on the other hand. They also compared the ethnic and socioeconomic differences between these two very different population groups. The results demonstrated that in the Norwegian group the mean attachment loss in the entire dentition was 0.1 mm per year, while this figure was 0.2–0.3 mm in those subjects examined in Sri Lanka! The molars were most often affected in both groups.

Forms of Periodontitis

Epidemiologic studies rarely differentiate between the rare, early forms of the disease which can progress very rapidly even in young adults (aggressive periodontitis), and the more widespread, usually slowly-progressing chronic periodontitis. True aggressive forms are probably quite rare (2–5 % of all cases) in Europe and the USA.

More precise figures are available concerning aggressive, localized periodontitis (formerly: LJP, p. 118): In Europe, about 0.1 % of young people are affected, while in Asia and Africa high morbidity rates up to 5 % have been reported (Saxen 1980; Saxby 1984, 1987; Kronauer et al. 1986).

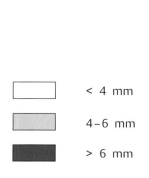

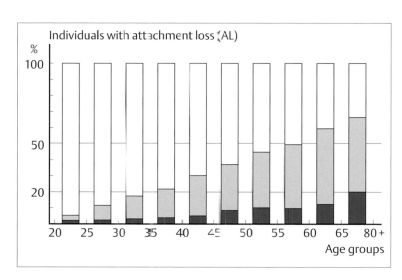

141 Attachment Loss in 15,000 Employed Individuals in Various Age Groups in the USA
After recording attachment loss (distance from the cementoenamel junction to the bottom of the pocket) approximately 30 % of all subjects exhibited 4–6 mm of attachment loss, while only 7.5 % had more than 6 mm of attachment loss.
In the same study, pocket probing depths were measured, and were distinctly less than the attachment loss figures, because probing does not evaluate recession.

Attachment Loss—Studies in the USA

Miller et al. (1987) and Brown & Löe (1993) examined over 15,000 employed persons in the USA, ranging in age from 18 to 80 years. In addition to other parameters, most important in the studies was the measurement of attachment loss. Approximately 76 % of all subjects exhibited attachment loss 2 mm or more, but only 7.6 % had attachment loss of more than 6 mm. Both studies showed that loss of tooth-supporting tissues increased with age, but contended that periodontitis (and recession) cannot be termed a "disease of the elderly."

CPITN Studies

In recent years, the CPITN was used most frequently the world over for epidemiologic studies. During the examination of 11,305 subjects in Hamburg (Fig. 142), the use of this index revealed that only 2.8 % were totally periodontally healthy (Code 0) and required no treatment. Nine percent exhibited bleeding on probing (Code 1) and 44 % had pocket probing depths up to 5.5 mm (Code 3). These patients required supra- and more importantly subgingival scaling, which could be performed by qualified auxiliary personnel (dental hygienist). Only in 16 % of the subjects were probing depths of 6 mm and greater detected (Code 4). These patients

required additional complex therapy beyond simple scaling (root planing, surgical procedures) by the dentist. Severe periodontitis (Code 4) increased with age; mild periodontitis was correspondingly less often recorded in elderly patients.

WHO Studies

In a literature review of numerous investigations from Europe, the USA and Latin America, Miyazaki et al. (1991 a, b) encountered inconsistent results. Despite significant differences among the various countries, severe forms of periodontitis (CPITN Code 4) were observed at a level of only 10–15 %.

One overall conclusion can be drawn: In Europe, the USA and Latin America, gingivitis and mild periodontitis are quite common. Profound manifestations of attachment loss are only observed in ca. 10–15 % of these populations.

It is important to note, however, that scored codes or millimeter measurements do not mean that periodontitis is generalized throughout the mouth: A patient is classified as "affected" even if only a single tooth surface of the entire dentition has a single pocket depth measurement of 6 mm, corresponding to Code 4! This fact relegates the published "10–15 %" affected rate to a somewhat lower level.

Periodontitis is likely more widely distributed in Asia and Africa compared to the populations described here.

142 CPITN Study of 11,305 Subjects in Hamburg, Germany
Percentage distribution of the degrees of severity (Codes 0–4) for periodontal diseases (above) and the treatment needs and types of therapy that derive from the data (TN I-III, below).

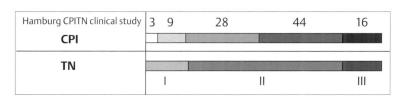

143 Forty-two (!) CPITN Studies from America and Europe
The large differences between the clinical studies in various countries are clearly obvious. But even sequential epidemiologic studies in a single country, e. g., in France or in Germany, exhibit enormous differences that can hardly be explained by true differences in the severity of the disease. One must therefore assume that the individual degrees of severity as recorded by the CPITN were interpreted quite differently by the various examiners.

Despite these limitations, this summary of numerous studies can be viewed positively, because severe periodontitis (Code 4) and "treatment need" III (= complex therapy) were diagnosed in "only" ca. 10–15 % of all subjects.

One must consider, however, that a single patient, e. g., with a "Code 4," that may be present only in a single quadrant or on a single tooth or a single site on a tooth, does not indicate that complex therapy (TN III) should be performed on a single tooth nor in the entire dentition. Such information does indicate that such a patient is likely more susceptible to periodontitis.

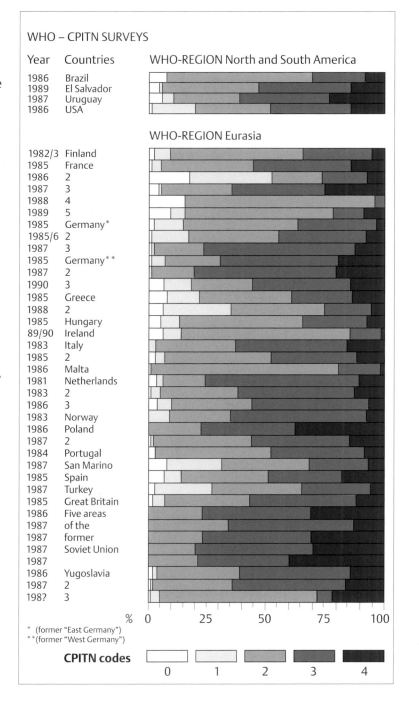

Types of Plaque-associated Periodontal Diseases

Gingivitis — Periodontitis

The general term "periodontal diseases" encompasses inflammatory as well as recessive alterations within the gingiva and the periodontium (Page & Schroeder 1982; AAP 1989, 1996; Ranney 1992, 1993; Lindhe et al. 1997; Armitage 1999).

While gingival recession may have various etiologies, including morphologic, mechanical (improper oral hygiene) and even functional (p. 155), gingivitis and periodontitis are plaque-associated diseases. Today it is becoming more and more clear that bacteria alone, including even the so-called periodontopathic bacteria, can always elicit gingivitis, but *not* periodontitis in every case. The initiation of periodontitis, its speed of progress and the expression of its clinical picture also involve the responsibility of negative host factors and additional so-called risk factors (Clark & Hirsch 1995). One of the most important are defects of the acute host response resulting from functional disturbances of polymorphonuclear granulocytes (PMN), other insufficient immunologic reactions, and the predominance of pro-inflammatory mediators, many of which are genetically determined. The now well established alterable risk factors include, particularly, "unhealthy" habits such as smoking, alcohol consumption and a less than well-rounded diet (p. 22).

Furthermore, systemic disorders and syndromes are usually *un*alterable, obligate or facultative risk factors for periodontitis. In this regard, especially Diabetes mellitus is viewed as prejudicial (p. 132). Finally, the entire social environment of an individual can play an important role for the initiation and propagation of periodontitis (pp. 22 51).

All of the factors discussed in the chapter "Etiology and Pathogenesis" (p. 21) enhance the occurrence of all diseases, including periodontitis. Thus, periodontitis is considered to be of multifactorial etiology. It remains difficult in the face of a manifest disease process to differentiate the "etiologic weight" of bacteria on the one hand and the host response and risk factors on the other hand, or to differentiate between and among such etiologic factors. The contemporary, on-going search for responsible "risk markers" is therefore very important.

Today, clinicians can use additional clinical parameters such as bleeding on probing, the severity of the disease in relation to patient age, as well as microbiologic and genetic tests in order to establish some semblance of a proper diagnosis and prognosis (p. 165).

In the future, more precise research into the reduced host defense occasioned by immunologic defects, as well as the type and quantity of participating cytokines and inflammatory mediators (e. g., in sulcus fluid, blood or saliva) will simplify diagnosis and permit more definitive predictions about the probable course of the disease, as well as indicating more targeted therapy.

Classification of Periodontal Diseases—Nomenclature

Most recent research results and clinical knowledge have led the nomenclature of the periodontal diseases into a state of constant change. Indeed, because of varying interpretations of scientific results, it has often led to conflict between authors and scientific societies.

Relatively recently, the new nomenclature from the *American Academy of Periodontology* (AAP, 1989) was generally accepted. This classification distinguished between gingivitis (G) and adult periodontitis (AP) of the following types: Early-onset periodontitis (EOP) with further subclassifications (PP, JP, RPP), periodontitis associated with systemic diseases (PSD), the acute necrotizing, ulcerative gingivoperiodontitis (ANUG/P), and the therapy-resistant, refractory periodontitis (RP).

After only a few years, however, this "new" classification was no longer satisfactory! The *European Federation of Periodontology* (EFP) proposed in 1993 a new classification, and even *this* was modified in 1999/2000 during an international workshop in collaboration with the AAP (Armitage 1999).

The "old" classification from 1989 was criticized because it placed too much weight upon the age of the patient vis-à-vis the initiation of the disease process. For example "adult periodontitis" (AP) as a chronic disease could also be observed in adolescents; rapidly-progressing periodontitis (RPP) was observed not only in young individuals (EOP) but also could appear "suddenly" in older patients; the localized, juvenile form (LJP) was not observed *only* in young patients. Furthermore, "refractory periodontitis" (RP) cannot be viewed as a specific disease entity, because following treatment for periodontitis the disease might recur or the disease might simply not respond to the therapy.

Classification 1999/2000

This *Color Atlas* of *Dental Hygiene* consistently utilizes the most recent nomenclature (1999/2000), but several "old" and well-known terms are used for occasional clarification, e. g., LJP, which is now classified as "Type III, aggressive periodontitis A, localized."

The table below is a brief summary of the new nomenclature to assist the hygienist. The complete and extremely comprehensive "Classification of Periodontal Diseases and Conditions" can be found in the appendix (p. 327). Some view the new classification as too expansive and comprehensive, while others criticize it as incomplete!

Classification of Periodontal Diseases (International Workshop of the AAP/EFP, 1999)

Type I	**Gingival Diseases**	
	A	Plaque-Induced Gingival Diseases
	B	Non-Plaque-Induced Gingival Lesions
Type II	**Chronic Periodontitis**	
	A	Localized
	B	Generalized
Type III	**Aggressive Periodontitis**	
	A	Localized
	B	Generalized
Type IV	**Periodontitis as a Manifestation of Systemic Disease**	
	A	Associated with Hematological Disorders
	B	Associated with Genetic Disorders
	C	Not Otherwise Specified (NOS)
Type V	**Necrotizing Periodontal Disease**	
	A	Necrotizing Ulcerative Gingivitis (NUG)
	B	Necrotizing Ulcerative Periodontitis (NUP)

Types VI–VIII   Further forms as well as transitions and "status pictures" of the diseases described, as well as the strengths and weaknesses of the new classifications are described in detail (pp. 327–330) and in the original publications.

Gingivitis

Plaque-induced Gingivitis, Gingivitis Simplex, Type I A 1

Gingivitis is ubiquitous. It is a bacterially-elicited inflammation (non-specific mixed infection) of the marginal gingiva (Löe et al. 1965).

In the chapter "Etiology and Pathogenesis," the development and progression of gingivitis from healthy tissue to an early lesion and on to established gingivitis was described (pp. 56–59; Page & Schroeder 1976, Kornman et al. 1997). In children, the early lesion (gingivitis) with T-cell dominance can persist for many years; on the other hand, in adults, the persistent lesion is almost exclusively *established* gingivitis (with plasma cell dominance), which can assume quite variable clinical severity. It is possible, clinically and pathomorphologically, to differentiate gingivitis into mild, moderate and severe, although this classification is relatively subjective.

For a more precise diagnosis of gingival inflammation, it is prudent to employ accepted indices that quantitate bleeding upon probing of the gingival sulcus.

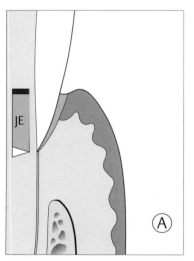
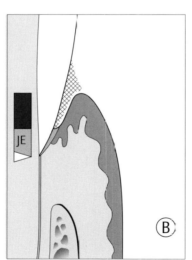
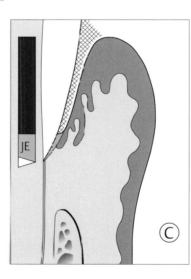

144 Sulcus and Gingival Pocket

A **Sulcus:** Histologically, in healthy gingiva the sulcus is maximally 0.5 mm deep. However, upon probing, the probe may penetrate the junctional epithelium up to 2 mm.

B **Gingival Pocket:** In gingivitis, the coronal portion of the junctional epithelium detaches from the tooth. There is no true attachment loss.

C **Pseudopocket:** With swelling of the gingiva, a pseudopocket may develop.

The borderline between healthy gingiva and gingivitis is difficult to ascertain. Gingiva that appears to be clinically healthy will nevertheless almost always exhibit *histologically* a mild inflammatory infiltrate. If there is an increase in clinical and histologic inflammation, one observes lateral proliferation of the junctional epithelium. The JE becomes detached from the tooth at its marginal aspect, as the bacterial front progresses between the tooth surface and the epithelium. The result is a *gingival pocket*.

In cases of severe gingivitis with edematous swelling and hyperplasia of the tissues, a clinical pseudopocket often forms.

Gingival pockets and pseudopockets are not *true* periodontal pockets because no connective tissue attachment loss has occurred, nor has there been *apical* proliferation of the junctional epithelium. However, because the milieu of pseudopockets is an oxygen-poor environment, periodontopathic anaerobic microorganisms can thrive.

It is true that gingivitis may develop into periodontitis. However, even without treatment, gingivitis can persist over many years in a stationary manner, exhibiting only minor variations in intensity (Listgarten et al. 1985). With treatment, gingivitis is fully reversible.

Histopathology

The clinical and histopathologic pictures of established gingivitis are well correlated (Engelberger et al. 1983).

The mild infiltration that occurs even in clinically healthy gingiva may be explained as a host response to the small amount of plaque that is present even in a clean dentition. Such plaque is composed of non-pathogenic or mildly pathogenic microorganisms, primarily gram-positive cocci and rods.

As plaque accumulation increases, so does the severity of *clinically* detectable inflammation, as evidenced by the quantity and expanse of inflammatory infiltrate. The sub-epithelial infiltrate consists primarily of differentiated B-lymphocytes (plasma cells), with a smaller number of other types of leukocytes.

With increasing inflammation, more and more PMN granulocytes transmigrate the junctional epithelium. As a consequence, the junctional epithelium takes on the characteristics of a pocket epithelium (p. 104, Fig. 209; Müller-Glauser & Schroeder 1982), but without any significant apical proliferation.

145 Healthy Gingiva (left)
Even in clinically healthy gingiva (GI = 0, PBI = 0), one can observe a very discrete sub-epithelial inflammatory infiltrate. Scattered PMNs transmigrate the junctional epithelium, which remains for the most part intact (HE, x10).

146 Mild Gingivitis (right)
As clinical inflammation increases (GI = 1, PBI = 1) the amount of inflammatory infiltrate increases and collagen is lost (Masson stain, x 10).

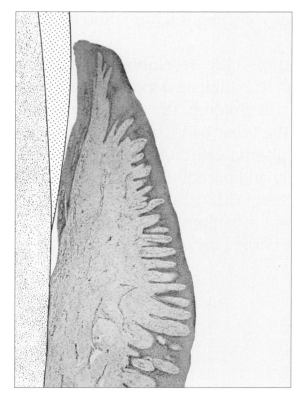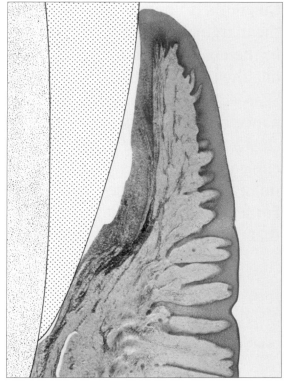

147 Moderate Gingivitis (left)
When gingivitis is clinically apparent (GI = 2, PBI = 2), the infiltrate becomes more dense and expansive. Collagen loss continues. The junctional epithelium proliferates laterally; a gingival pocket develops. **P** = subgingival plaque. (Masson stain, x 10)

148 Severe Gingivitis (right)
Pronounced edematous swelling (GI = 3, PBI = 3–4). The inflammatory infiltrate is expansive; collagen loss is pronounced. The junctional epithelium is transformed into a pocket epithelium (gingival pocket). Only in the apicalmost area are any remnants of intact junctional epithelium observed. Apical to the JE, the connective tissue attachment is intact (no loss of attachment; HE, x10).

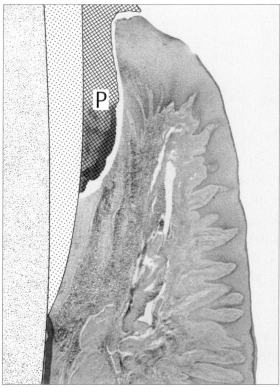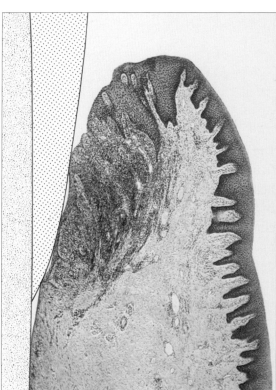

Clinical Symptoms

- Bleeding
- Erythema
- Edematous and hyperplastic swelling
- Ulceration

The earliest clinical symptom of an established lesion is *bleeding* subsequent to careful sulcus probing. This hemorrhage is elicited by the penetration of the probe tip through the disintegrating junctional epithelium and into the highly vascular sub-epithelial connective tissue. At this stage of the inflammatory process (PBI = 1), *no gingival erythema* may be visible clinically. Clinical symptoms of advanced (established) gingivitis include profuse bleeding after sulcus probing, obvious *erythema* and simultaneous *edematous swelling*. In the most severe cases, spontaneous bleeding and eventually *ulceration* may occur. The *chronic* types (and severities) do not elicit pain; pain occurs only in *acute* gingivitis (e.g., NUG, p. 85).

Even severe gingivitis may *never* progress to periodontitis. With proper treatment, gingivitis is reversible.

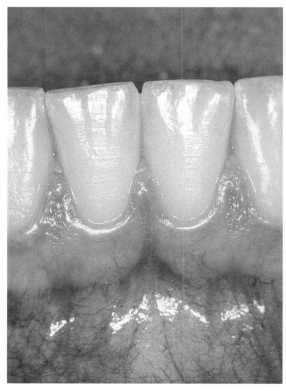

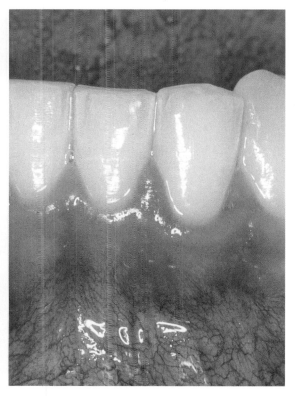

149 Healthy Gingiva (left)
The gingiva is pale salmon-pink in color, and stippled. The narrow free gingival margin is distinguishable from the attached gingiva. After gentle probing with a blunt periodontal probe, no bleeding occurs.

150 Mild Gingivitis (right)
The localized erythema is scarcely visible, and one observes slight edematous swelling. Some of the former stippling is lost, and there is minimal bleeding upon probing.

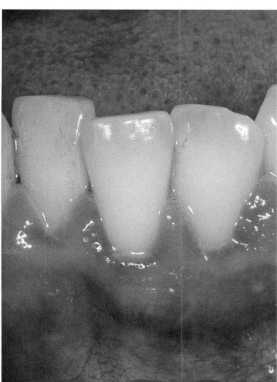

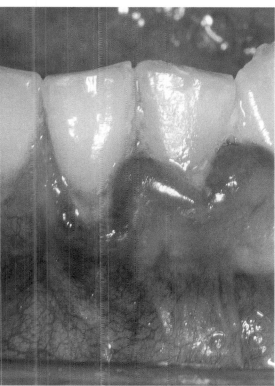

151 Moderate Gingivitis (left)
Obvious erythema and edematous swelling. No stippling is apparent, and there is hemorrhage following probing of the sulcus.

152 Severe Gingivitis (right)
Fiery redness, edematous and hyperplastic swelling; complete absence of any stippling; interdental ulceration, copious bleeding on probing, and spontaneous hemorrhage.

Mild Gingivitis

A 23-year-old female came to the dentist for a routine check-up. She had no complaints and was not aware of any gingival problems, although in her medical history she indicated that her gingiva bled occasionally during tooth brushing. Her oral hygiene was relatively good. She had received tooth brushing instructions from a dentist once, but no subsequent OHI. The patient was not on a regular recall schedule. Calculus removal had been performed sporadically in the past during routine dental check-ups, and several restorations placed.

Findings:

API	(Approximal Plaque Index): 30%
PBI	(Papilla Bleeding Index): 1.5
PD	(Probing depths): ca. 1.5 mm maxilla, ca. 3 mm mandible
TM	(tooth mobility): 0

Diagnosis: Gingivitis in initial stage
Therapy: Motivation, OHI, plaque and calculus removal
Recall: Prophylaxis at 6-month intervals
Prognosis: Very good

153 Mild Gingivitis in the Anterior Area
In the maxilla, one observes no overt signs of gingivitis, except for a mild erythema.
In the mandible, especially in the papillary areas, slight edematous swelling and erythema can be detected (arrows).

Right: Radiographically there is no evidence of loss of interdental bone height. The maxillary central incisors exhibit short roots.

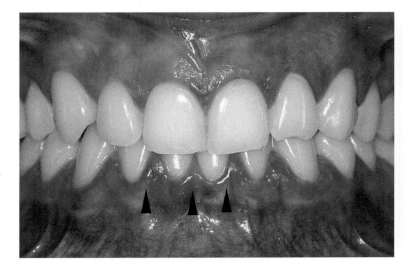
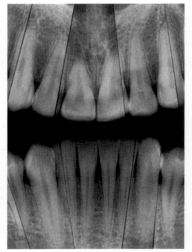

154 Papilla Bleeding Index (PBI)
After gentle probing of the sulci with a blunt periodontal probe, hemorrhage of grades 1 and 2 occurs. This is a cardinal sign of gingivitis.

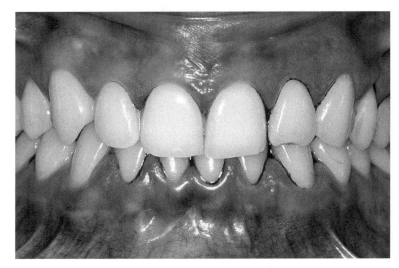

155 Stained Plaque
Around the necks of the teeth and in interdental areas, small plaque accumulations are visible.

Right: Gingival vascular plexus (**X**) in the region of the junctional epithelium in a case of mild gingivitis. Above the white arrows, one observes the most marginal vascular loops in the area of the adjacent oral sulcular epithelium (**OSE**; canine preparation).

Courtesy J. Egelberg

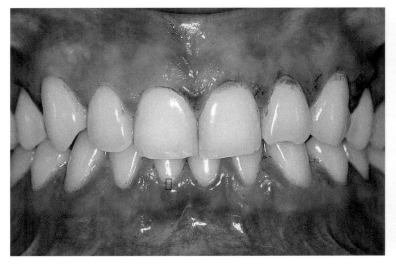
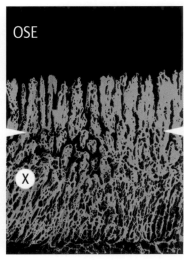

Moderate Gingivitis

A 28-year-old female presented with a chief complaint of gingival bleeding. She "brushes her teeth," but had never received any oral hygiene instruction from a dentist or hygienist. Calculus had been removed only infrequently, and a professional debridement had never been systematically performed. Generalized crowding of the teeth in both arches is evident, combined with an anterior open bite. These anomalies reduced any self-cleansing effects and made oral hygiene difficult. This also likely increased the severity of gingivitis.

Findings:
APERSPI: 50 %   PD: ca. 3 mm maxilla, ca. 4 mm mandible
PBI: maxilla 2.6, mandible 3.4. TM: 0 maxilla, 1 mandible
Diagnosis: Maxilla, moderate gingivitis; mandibular anterior region, severe gingivitis with pseudopockets.
Therapy: Motivation, oral hygiene, plaque and calculus removal; after re-evaluation, possible gingivoplasty.
Recall: Every six months initially.
Prognosis: With patient cooperation and compliance, very good.

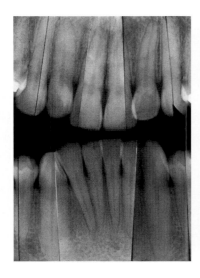
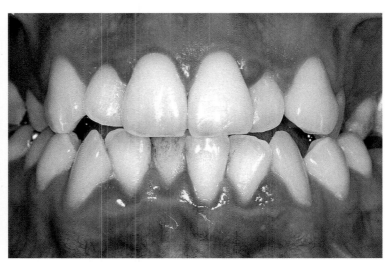

156 Moderate Gingivitis in Anterior Segments
Erythema and swelling of the gingiva. The symptoms are more pronounced in the mandible than in the maxilla.

Left: Radiographically there is no evidence of destruction (demineralization) of the interdental bony septa.

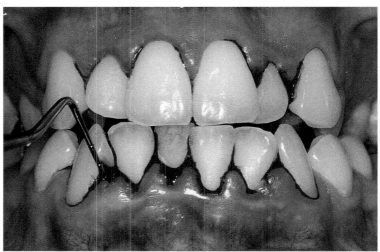

157 Papilla Bleeding Index (PBI)
The pronounced gingivitis that is particularly obvious in the mandibular anterior area is corroborated by the PBI. Bleeding scores of 2 and 3 are recorded after "sweeping" the sulcus with a periodontal probe in the papillary regions.

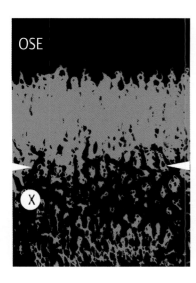
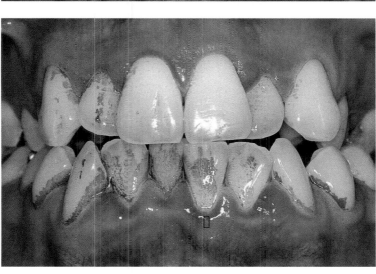

158 Stained Plaque
Moderate plaque accumulation in the maxilla. In the mandible, heavier plaque, especially at the gingival margins.

Left: Vascular plexus of the gingiva near the junctional epithelium in a case of severe gingivitis (Fig. 155, right)

Courtesy J. Egelberg

Severe Gingivitis

A 15-year-old male was referred for evaluation and treatment of suspected juvenile periodontitis (LJP/Type III A). The extremely pronounced gingivitis was, however, inconsistent with this diagnosis. Sulcus probing and radiographic examination revealed no attachment loss on anterior teeth or molars.

The patient practiced virtually no oral hygiene, stating that it was impossible to brush his teeth because the gingiva bled at the slightest touch. He had never received adequate motivation, nor any oral hygiene instruction, nor any treatment for his gingivitis.

Findings:

API: 88 %	PD: pseudopockets to 5 mm
PBI: 3.5	TM: 0

Diagnosis: Severe gingivitis with edematous hyperplastic enlargement of the facial aspect of the anterior area; mouth breathing as possible etiologic co-factor (?).

Therapy: Motivation, oral hygiene instruction, definitive debridement. After re-evaluation, possible gingivoplasty.

Recall: Initially every three months.

Prognosis: With patient cooperation and compliance, good.

159 Severe Gingivitis
The clinical symptoms of severe gingivitis including erythema, edema and hyperplastic enlargement, are observed. The anterior region is more severely affected (slight crowding, mouth breathing?). Probing reveals no attachment loss; the base of the pseudopockets are not apical to the cementoenamel junction.

Right: Radiographically, one observes no evidence of bone loss on the interdental septa.

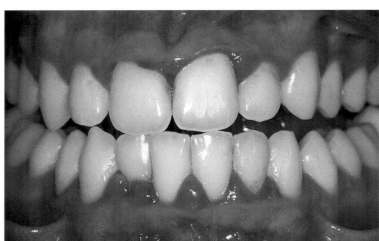
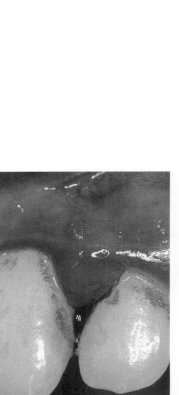

160 Papilla Bleeding Index (PBI)
Copious bleeding (PBI grade 4) occurs after sweeping the anterior sextant pseudopockets with a blunt periodontal probe. The inflammation is less pronounced in the premolar and molar regions.

If gingival hyperplasia is severe, the clinician must exclude other possible etiologic factors such as medicament-induced lesions and systemic disorders.

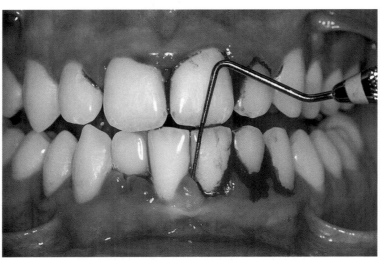

161 Stained Plaque
Moderately heavy accumulation of supragingival plaque. Not visible is the expanse of the subgingival plaque within pseudopockets. The pronounced inflammation, especially in the anterior region, anticipates significant plaque accumulation subgingivally.

Right: The papilla between 21 and 22 is grossly enlarged, erythematous and devoid of any stippling.

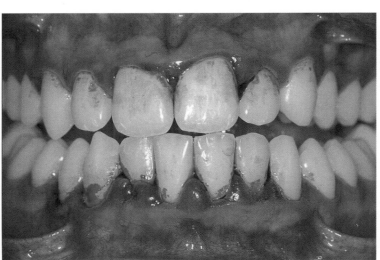

Ulcerative Gingivitis/Periodontitis

NUG/P = Necrotizing Ulcerative Gingivitis/Periodontitis, Types V A (NUG) and V B (NUP)

Ulcerative gingivitis is usually an acute, painful, rapidly progressing inflammation of the gingiva, which may enter a sub-acute or chronic stage. Without treatment, this disease usually develops quickly into localized ulcerative periodontitis. It seldom occurs as a generalized process, nor is its severity always identical. It may be quite advanced in anterior segments, while the premolars or molars are not affected at all, or only mildly so. The reasons for this remain unknown (oral hygiene? ischemia? locally predominating pathogenic bacteria? plaque-retentive areas? tooth type?). Probing depths are usually shallow because gingival tissue is lost to necrosis as attachment loss proceeds. Secondary ulceration of other oral mucosal surfaces is rarely observed, and only in severe cases (AAP 1996e). Caution: Ulceration can represent an early oral symptom in HIV-positive patients and AIDS victims (p. 151).

Ulcerative gingivitis/periodontitis has become less common in recent decades than earlier (exception: HIV-positive and AIDS patients). In the younger population, the *morbidity* has been variously reported between 0.1–1 %.

The *etiology* of NUG is not completely understood. In addition to plaque and a previously existing gingivitis, the following local and systemic predisposing factors are suspected:

Local Factors
- Poor oral hygiene
- Predominance of spirochetes, fusiforms and *P. intermedia*, and occasionally *Selenomonas* and *Porphyromoncs* in the plaque
- Smoking (local irritation by tar products)

Systemic Factors
- Poor general health, psychic stress, alcohol
- Smoking: nicotine as a sympatheticomimetic, and carbon monoxide (CO) as a chemotaxin (p. 216)
- Age (15–30 years)
- Season of the year (September/October and December/January; Skâch et al. 1970)

NUG/P patients usually exhibit similar *life styles and habits*: The teeth do not occupy a high position in the patient's consciousness. They are usually young adults, heavy smokers (tobacco: high content of tar and nicotine), exercise poor oral hygiene, and become interested in treatment only during acute, painful exacerbations.

The *clinical course* is acute, but fever occurs only seldom. Within only a few days, interdental papillae may be lost to ulceration. The acute phase may gravitate into a chronic interval stage if host resistance improves (see pre-disposing factors) or through self-treatment (rinsing with a disinfectant mouthwash). Untreated ulcerative gingivitis exhibits a high recurrence rate, and may develop rapidly into ulcerative periodontitis (attachment loss with shallow pockets!).

Therapy: In addition to local debridement, the early stages of treatment should be supported with medicaments. Topical application of ointments containing cortisone or antibiotics, or metronidazol may be effective. In severe cases, systemic metronidazol (e.g., Flagyl) may be prescribed (see Medicaments, p. 287). After reduction of the acute symptoms in advanced cases, surgery to correct gingival contours may be indicated.

Histopathology

The clinical and histopathologic pictures in NUG are correlated. The histopathology of NUG is, however, significantly different from that of simple gingivitis.

As a consequence of the acute reaction, an enormous number of PMNs transmigrate the junctional epithelium in the direction of the sulcus and the col. In contrast to the situation in simple gingivitis, PMNs also migrate toward the oral epithelium and the tips of papillae, which undergo necrotic destruction. The ulcerated wound is covered by a clinically visible, whitish pseudomembrane that consists of bacteria, dead leukocytes and epithelial cells as well as fibrin. The tissue subjacent to the ulcerated areas is edematous, hyperemic and heavily infiltrated by PMNs. In long-standing disease, the deeper tissue regions will also contain lymphocytes and plasma cells. Within the infiltrated area, collagen destruction progress rapidly.

Spirochetes and other bacteria often penetrate into the damaged tissues (Listgarten 1965, Listgarten & Lewis 1967).

162 Papilla Biopsy
Affected papilla excised from a patient with mild ulcerative gingivitis, resembling the clinical situation in Fig. 164. The tip of the papilla and the tissue approaching the col have been destroyed by ulceration (**U**).
The oral epithelium (**OE**, stained yellow) remains essentially intact. In the deeper layers of the biopsy, one observes the red-stained intact collagen, while beneath the decimated papilla tip the collagen is largely obliterated (van Gieson, x10).

The arrow indicates the section that is enlarged in Fig. 163.

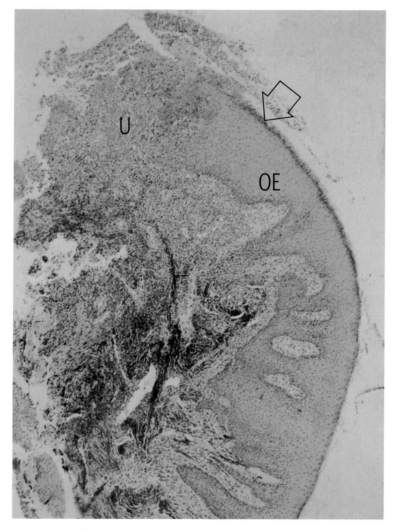

163 Surface of the Disintegrated Tissue
The upper portion of the figure exhibits thickly packed fusiform bacteria (**FUS**). Spirochetes present in the section are not visible with this staining technique, but the numerous **PMNs** are obvious. The brownish structures with weakly staining nuclei are dying epithelial cells (van Gieson, x1000).

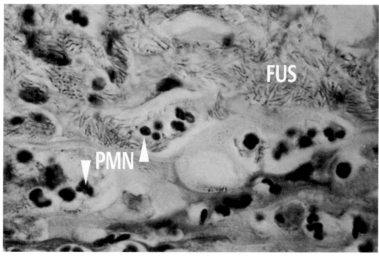

Clinical Symptoms—Bacteriology

- Necrotic destruction of the gingiva, ulceration
- Pain
- Halitosis
- Specific bacteria

Beginning in the tissues of the interdental col, there is *necrotic destruction* of papilla tips, followed by destruction of entire papillae and even portions of the marginal gingiva. It is not clear whether gingival destruction is caused primarily by vascular infarction or by invasion of bacteria into the tissues. In rare instances, depressed ulcerations may also be seen on the cheeks, lips or tongue. In the absence of treatment, the osseous portion of the periodontal supporting apparatus can also become involved. The earliest clinical symptom of ulcerative gingivitis is localized pain.

The patient with NUG is characterized by a typical, insipid, sweetish *halitosis*.

Generalized ulcerative gingivitis must be differentiated from acute *herpetic gingivostomatitis* (p. 131), which is generally accompanied by fever.

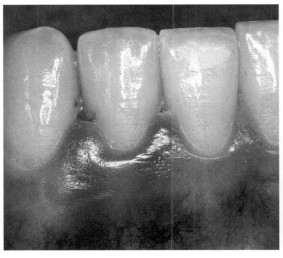
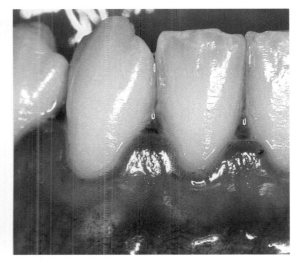

164 Earliest Symptom of NUG (left)
The most coronal portion of the papilla tip is destroyed by necrosis from the col outward. The defects are covered by a typical whitish pseudomembrane. The first pain may be experienced even before any ulcerations become visible clinically. NUG should be diagnosed and treated in this early, *reversible* stage!

165 Advanced Stage of Ulceration (right)

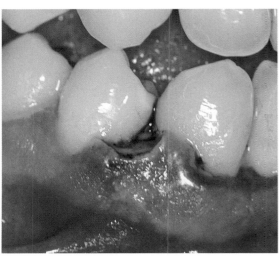
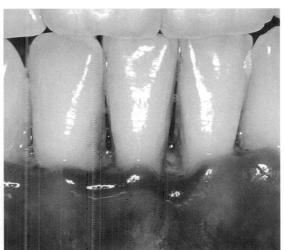

166 Complete Destruction of the Papilla (left)
Between the premolars there is no visible lesion, but areas of early necrosis can be seen on the mesial and marginal aspects of the canine. Note the complete destruction of the papilla between canine and first premolar.

167 Acute Recurrence (right)
The papillae have been completely destroyed. The previous acute stage has led to reverse architecture of the gingival margin. Beginning ulcerative periodontitis.

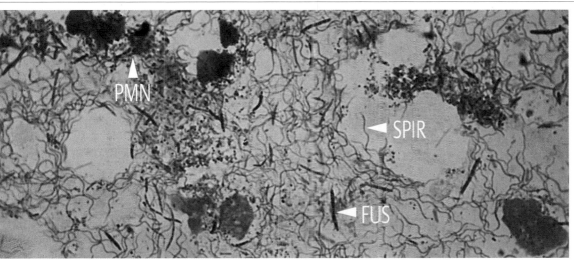
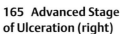

168 Bacteriology—Smear of the Pseudomembrane
In addition to dead cells, granulocytes (**PMN**) and fusiform bacteria (**FUS**), enormous numbers of spirochetes (**SPIR**) are visible (van Gieson, ×1000)

Ulcerative Gingivitis (NUG)

A 19-year-old female experienced gingival pain and hemorrhage for three days.

Findings:

- API: 70 %
- PBI: Anterior segments, 3.2
  Premolar and molar regions, 2.6
- PD: 2–3 mm proximal
- TM: 0–1

Diagnosis: Acute ulcerative gingivitis, early stage; NUG, Type V A.

Therapy: At the first appointment, careful mechanical debridement; topical medicaments: antibiotic or cortisone-containing ointment, metronidazol gel (e.g., Elyzol, p. 292). The patient may be instructed to rinse at home with mild hydrogen perborate solution.

Subsequent appointments: Motivation, repeated oral hygiene instruction, plaque and calculus removal.

Recall: Short-interval (information! plaque control!).

Prognosis: With treatment and *patient compliance*, good.

169 Initial Stage
Initial acute ulcerative destruction of several papilla tips (arrows). Other papillae exhibit signs of mild inflammation, but no destruction.

Right: Radiographically one observes no evidence of resorption of interdental septal bone.

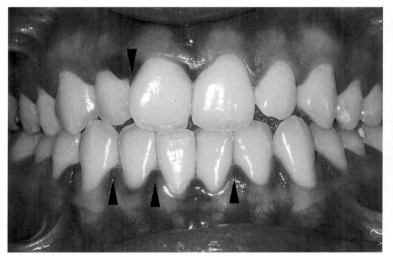 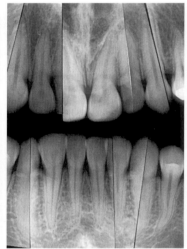

170 Initial Destruction of Papilla Tips in the Maxilla
Necrosis of the papilla tips between central and lateral incisors is apparent, with erythema and swelling. Note the initial necrosis of the papilla tips between the lateral incisor and canine. Between the central incisors, one notes erythema of the papilla, but not yet any signs of necrosis. If the patient experiences pain when this area is probed gently, it is evidence that the necrotic process has already begun in the col area.

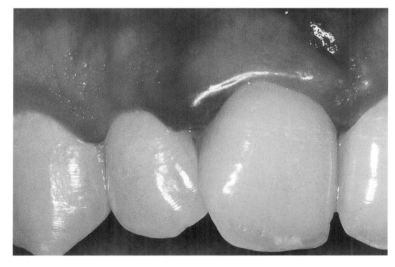

171 Destruction of Papilla Tips in the Mandible
Each papilla exhibits signs of incipient ulceration, and each is already covered by a pseudomembrane consisting of fibrin, dead tissue cells, leukocytes and bacteria.

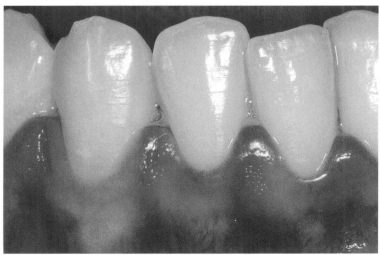

Ulcerative Periodontitis (NUP)

Ulcerative periodontitis always develops—often very rapidly—from a preexisting ulcerative gingivitis. Probing depths may be shallow because the destruction of tissue occurs simultaneously with the attachment loss. While the clinical signs associated with NUG can be eliminated by proper treatment, ulcerative periodontitis (NUP) always leads to irreversible damage (attachment loss, bone loss). Acute and subacute phases occur cyclically. Acute phases are always accompanied by pain, in contrast to simple gingivitis. Ulcerative periodontitis is seldom generalized.

Therapy: Similar to the case with ulcerative gingivitis, in the acute phase of NUP careful and complete plaque and calculus removal should be performed. This mechanical therapy can be supported by topical medicaments. After the pain subsides, systematic instrumentation (debridement) follows. In advanced cases, minor surgical procedures may be necessary after all acute symptoms subside: In mild cases, gingivoplasty; in advanced cases, contouring flap surgery. A strict recall program is absolutely necessary, because NUP has a tendency toward recurrence.

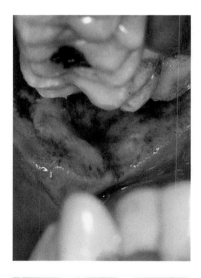
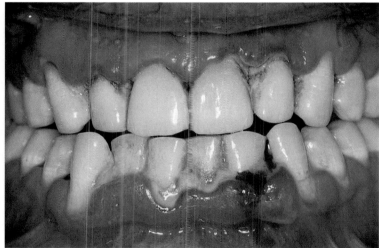

Acute Stage

172 Ulcerative Gingivoperiodontitis—Second Acute Episode
This 26-year-old male experienced a second, pronounced acute episode. In addition to gingivitis, in the maxillary anterior and molar segments attachment loss has occurred. (Treatment: p. 90)

Left: Expansive, painful mucosal ulcer adjacent to tooth 18. Extraction of tooth 18 is indicated following the acute episode.

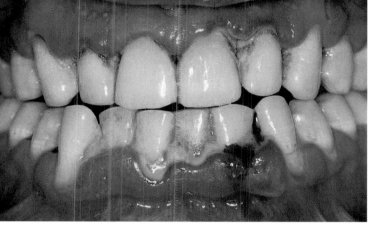
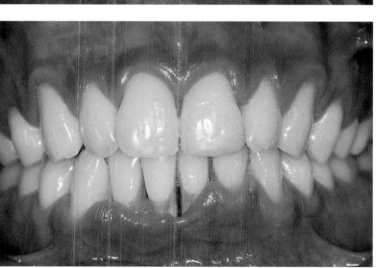

Interval Stage

173 Localized Ulcerative Periodontitis
This 22-year-old male had experienced two acute episodes, which were not treated professionally. In this *interval stage*, the patient is free of pain.

Left: Advanced but very localized attachment loss in the anterior segment of the mandible. The interdental crater presents a niche for plaque accumulation, which can lead to exacerbation if host response is compromised.

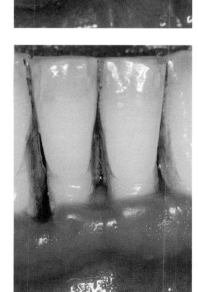
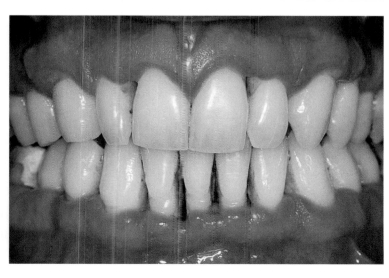

174 Expansive, Generalized Ulcerative Periodontitis
This 30-year-old male complained of gingival recession. He had experienced pain in recent years, but did not seek treatment. The now pain-free lesions have progressed to various degrees; *interval stage (HIV-patient)*.

Left: In the anterior region of the mandible, especially between teeth 41 and 42, the attachment loss has progressed significantly.

Puberty

178 Puberty Gingivitis
In this 13-year-old female, more or less severe hemorrhage occurred after gentle sulcus probing. Plaque and mouth breathing were causes of the gingival inflammation. The pubertal hormonal surge may have been a cofactor.

Right: Morbidity of gingivitis in 10,000 persons. A peak is observed during puberty (Stamm 1986).

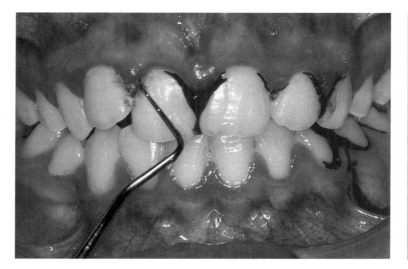

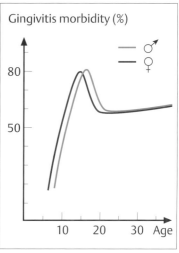

179 Puberty Gingivitis, Orthodontic Treatment
This 13-year-old male lost his maxillary central incisors due to an accident. Gingivitis, possibly puberty-related, was present before the accident.
Orthodontic means were used to move the lateral incisors mesially. In the absence of adequate plaque control, a severe inflammatory hyperplasia occurred between the maxillary lateral incisors.

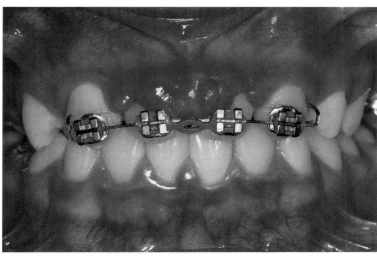

Pregnancy

180 Mild Pregnancy Gingivitis
In this 28-year-old female, who was in her seventh month of pregnancy, a cursory inspection did not reveal symptoms of gingivitis in the anterior region. In the premolar and molar areas, however, a moderate gingivitis was detected.

Right: Copious hemorrhage occurred immediately after probing in the area of a defective restoration (plaque niche).

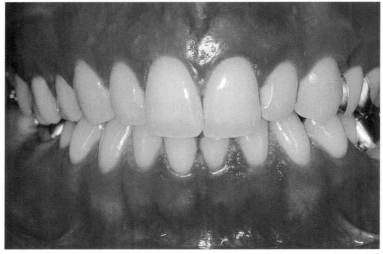

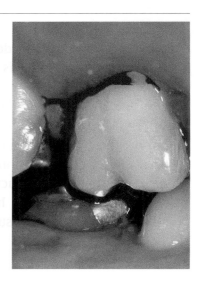

181 Severe Pregnancy Gingivitis
This 30-year-old patient exhibited moderate gingivitis even before her pregnancy. This photograph, taken during the eighth month, reveals severe inflammation and pronounced hyperplastic, epulis-like gingival alterations in the anterior segment.

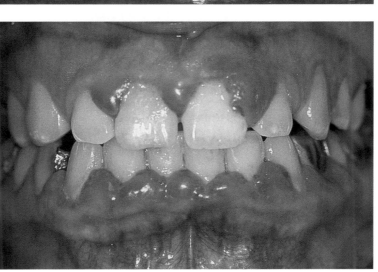

Severe Pregnancy Gingivitis—Gravid Epulis

This 24-year-old woman was eight months pregnant. She presented complaining that she "bites the swollen gums" on the left side of her mouth (gravid epulis). A severe, generalized gingivitis was also in evidence.

Findings:

API: 70%

PBI: 3.2

PD: 7 mm in the region of teeth 34 and 35 otherwise up to 4 mm (pseudopockets)

TM: 0–1

Diagnosis: Severe generalized pregnancy gingivitis with a large pyogenic granuloma (epulis) near teeth 34–35.

Therapy: During the pregnancy, repeated oral hygiene instruction, motivation, plaque and calculus removal; gingivoplasty (electrosurgery, laser) around teeth 34 and 35. After breast-feeding is terminated, re-evaluation and further treatment planning.

Recall: Frequency depends on patient compliance.

Prognosis: With treatment, good.

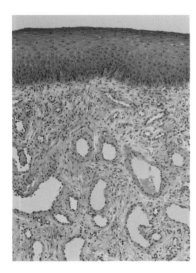
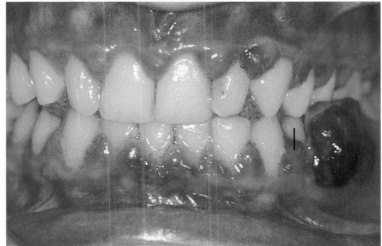

182 Severe Pregnancy Gingivitis
Due to poor oral hygiene, a pronounced gingivitis developed during the last half of the pregnancy. A large epulis is observed buccally and lingually around the mandibular premolars.

Left: The histologic section (of gingiva, not the epulis; see black line) exhibits normal oral epithelium, a relatively mild inflammatory infiltrate and widely dilated vessels (HE, x40)

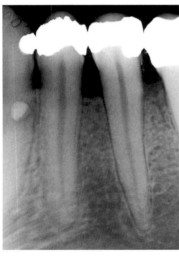
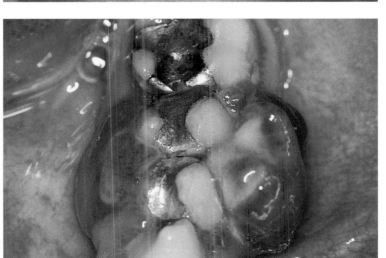

183 Gravid Epulis
The surface of the epulis is ulcerated because the patient's maxillary teeth bit into the tissue during mastication. For this reason, the redundant tissue had to be removed while the patient was still pregnant. Considerable hemorrhage may be expected during such surgery (laser, electrosurgery).

Left: The radiograph depicts some horizontal loss of the crestal compact bone of the interdental septa (demineralization).

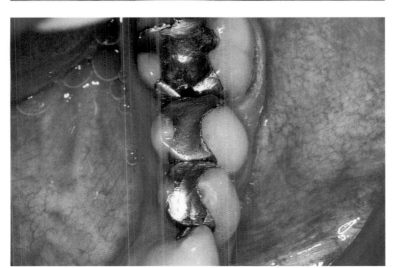

184 Three Months After Gingivoplasty; Two Months Post-Partum
Definitive periodontal therapy and treatment planning for restorative work that is sorely needed should begin at this time (e. g., replacement of the old amalgam restorations with inlays or composites).

Pathobiology—The Most Important Forms of Periodontitis

The pathobiological nomenclature for the various forms of periodontitis is not a rigid, definitive classification. Today, one differentiates between chronic and aggressive forms of the disease, which may be localized or generalized (pp. 327–330). The chronic form of the disease may transform into an aggressive form, e.g., in the elderly, where the immune system is less effective. Most types of periodontitis progress in a step-wise fashion (random burst theory). Stages of exacerbation alternate with stages of remission.

As science continually provides new knowledge concerning microbiology as well as pathogenesis—especially the host response to the infection—the diagnosis and the nomenclature can no longer simply be defined according to the clinical course of the disease; it is now possible to characterize periodontitis as an *Aa*- or a *Pg*-associated disease (etc.). In the future, it may become even more important to characterize the diverse parameters of the host immune response, the mediators and the risk factors; these are ultimately responsible for the existence of the disease and the speed of its progression.

Type II   (Chronic Periodontitis; formerly AP)

This most common form of periodontitis begins between the ages of 30 and 40 years, generally from a pre-existing gingivitis. The entire dentition may be equally affected (*generalized*, Type II B). More often, however, the distribution of the disease is irregular, with more severe destruction primarily in molar areas but secondarily also in anterior segments (*localized*; Type II A). The gingivae exhibit varying degrees of inflammation, with "shrinkage" in some areas and fibrotic manifestations elsewhere.

Exacerbations occur at rather lengthy intervals. Risk factors (e.g., heavy smoking, IL-1-positive genotype) can accentuate the clinical course. In the elderly, the disease can lead to tooth loss, which may also be due to a decrease in host immune response and more frequent acute stages.

Therapy: Chronic periodontitis can be successfully treated by means of purely mechanical therapy, even if the patient's cooperation/compliance is not optimum.

Type III B   (Aggressive Periodontitis; formerly EOP/RPP)

Aggressive forms of periodontitis are relatively rare (Page et al. 1983a, Miyazaki et al. 1993, Lindhe et al. 1997, Armitage 1999). They are usually diagnosed between the ages of 20 and 30 years. Females appear to be more frequently affected than males. The severity and distribution of attachment loss vary considerably. One observes infrequent acute stages, which may transition into chronic disease. The cause of the active stages is specific microorganisms (*Aa, Pg* etc.), which may actually invade the ulcerated tissues. Risk factors (smoking, systemic disease such as diabetes, conditions of psychic tension and stress) and pro-inflammatory mediators that reduce the immune response can amplify the disease picture.

Therapy: The majority of aggressive cases can be successfully treated by means of purely mechanical therapy. In severe cases, a supportive systemic antibiotic regimen may be indicated.

188 Characteristics of Type II—formerly AP

Clinical Symptoms

• Morbidity	ca. 85–95 % of all adults (?)
	ca. 95 % of all periodontal patients
• Initiation—Course	ca. 30th year of life
	slow, "chronic" course
• Periodontal Findings	– all teeth affected, localization to molars and incisors
	– gingival inflammation, gingival swelling, some recession
	– alveolar bone: uneven destruction
• Systemic Diseases	none

Blood Cell Defects

	neutrophilic granulocytes, monocytes
	– –

Bacterial Infection

	mixed flora; in *active pockets*, frequently *P. gingivalis, P. intermedia, Fusobacterium nucleatum, A. actinomycetemcomitans*

Heredity

	none (possible polymorphisms, e.g., IL-1)

189 Characteristics of Type III B—formerly EOP/RPP

Clinical Symptoms

• Morbidity	ca. 5–15 % of all periodontitis patients
• Initiation—Course	possible in all ages, young individuals predominate rapid cyclic course
• Periodontal Findings	– many to all teeth affected
	– gingiva more or less inflamed
	– rapid bone loss
	– frequent symptoms of activity
• Systemic Diseases	?, possible genetic determination

Blood Cell Defects

	neutrophilic granulocytes, monocytes	
Chemotaxis reduced	++	++
Increased migration	++	++

Bacterial Infection

	mixed flora and specific *P. gingivalis, T. forsythia, F. nucleatum, A. actinomycetemcomitans* (invasion?), *P. intermedia*, spirochetes

Heredity

	sex-linked dominant (?)

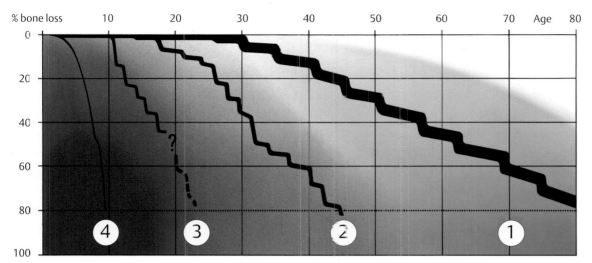

1 Chronic, slowly progressive periodontitis in adults—Type II

2 Aggressive, rapidly progressing periodontitis—Type III B

3 Aggressive, localized (juvenile) periodontitis—Type III A

4 Aggressive, generalized, pre-pubertal, rapidly progressing periodontitis—Type IV B

Type III A   (Aggressive Periodontitis, formerly EOP/LJP)

This rare disorder occurs early and attacks the permanent dentition. It begins in puberty, but is usually not diagnosed until several years later, often when lesions are discovered serendipitously (e.g., on bitewing radiographs taken for caries assessment). In the initial stages, incisors and/or first molars are affected in both maxilla and mandible; later, other teeth may also be affected. Hereditary factors (genetics, ethnic origin) have been demonstrated. Girls are affected more frequently than boys. In the early stages of aggressive periodontitis, one seldom observes pronounced gingivitis. The gingival pockets almost always (90 %) harbor *Aa*. The patient's serum contains immunoglobulins against *Aa* leukotoxins, which damage PMNs.

Therapy: With early diagnosis and therapy consisting of vigorous mechanical debridement and supportive systemic administration of medicaments, the destructive process can be halted rather easily. Osseous defects may eventually regenerate.

Type IV B   (Aggressive Periodontitis; formerly EOP/PP)

This extraordinarily rare form of periodontitis may be detected even upon eruption of the deciduous teeth and is usually associated with genetic aberrations and systemic disorders (Page et al. 1983b, Tonetti & Mombelli 1999, Armitage 1999; cf. p. 118). The disease progresses rapidly and is usually generalized:

• A localized form begins at ca. age 4 and exhibits only mild gingival inflammation with relatively little plaque.
• The generalized form (Type IV B) begins immediately after eruption of the deciduous teeth. It is associated with severe gingivitis and gingival shrinkage. The microbiology remains unclear.

Therapy: The localized form can be halted by a combination of mechanical therapy and systemic antibiotics. The generalized form appears to be refractory to therapy.

191 Characteristics of Type III A (formerly EOP/LJP)		
Clinical Symptoms		
• Morbidity	0.1 % in young Caucasians, > 1 % in young Blacks	
• Initiation—Course	ca. age 13, at the beginning of puberty often rapid "burst-like" course	
• Periodontal Findings	– primarily only in first molar and/or incisor teeth – gingiva often appear normal – crater-like bone loss	
• Systemic Diseases	none, genetically determined	
Blood Cell Defects	*neutrophilic granulocytes, monocytes*	
Chemotaxis reduced	++	+
Phagocytosis reduced	+	-
Receptor defect	+	?
Bacterial Infection	mixed flora and specifically *A. actinomycetemcomitans* (serotypes a, b), *Capnocytophaga* sp. (?)	
Heredity	autosomal recessive (sex-linked dominant?)	

192 Characteristics of Type IV B (formerly EOP/PP)		
Clinical Symptoms		
• Morbidity	very rare (few cases reported)	
• Initiation—Course	immediately after eruption of deciduous teeth clinical course is almost continuous and destructive	
• Periodontal Symptoms		
– generalized form	– all teeth affected – gingiva inflamed and hyperplastic	
– localized form	– individual teeth affected, very rare	
• Systemic Diseases	Hypophosphatasia, susceptibility to respiratory tract infections, otitis media, skin infections	
Blood Cell Defects	*neutrophilic granulocytes, monocytes*	
Adherence (vessel wall) disturbed	++	+
Chemotaxis reduced	++	++
Receptor deficiency	+	+
Bacterial Infection	mixed flora, specific bacteria are unknown	
Heredity	autosomal recessive	

(Figs. 188–192 modified from *Page et al. 1983a/b, 1986; Schroeder 1987b*)

Pathomorphology—Clinical Degree of Severity

Periodontitis is a general term. As already described, it sub-sumes *pathobiologically dynamic forms of disease progressing at varying rates*, and exhibits differing microbial etiologies and varying influences by the host immune response (p. 21). It may sound trite, but one must understand that all forms of periodontitis *begin* at some point in time. They develop at various times during a patient's life, usually from a pre-existing plaque-elicited gingivitis. In the absence of treatment, the disease progresses, albeit at varying rates. It is therefore clear that during clinical data collection, which leads to the diagnosis for an individual case, not only must the type of disease be ascertained, it is also necessary to determine in what pathomorphologic stage the disease process currently exists or, in other words, how far attachment loss has pro-gressed. From these diagnostic criteria, clinical course, ex-panse (*localized*, e.g., less than 30% of all sites, or *general-ized*) and clinical degree of severity, the practitioner can derive a prognosis and estimate the degree of difficulty of the necessary treatment, which will naturally be higher for aggressive periodontitis (Type III) than for a similarly ad-vanced chronic periodontitis (Type II).

Case Diagnosis—Single-Tooth Diagnosis—"Sites"

While it is usually possible to diagnosis the type of peri-odontitis for the entire dentition, it is rather a more difficult matter to precisely define the clinical degree of severity. Periodontitis almost always progresses at different rates in different areas of the mouth, on different teeth, and even at different sites on individual teeth. Therefore, any statement about "average" disease severity is usually meaningless.

The following pathomorphologic classification (degree of severity) cannot be understood as pertinent to the indivi-dual case (patient); it relates more to *single tooth diagnosis* as well as *single tooth prognosis*. The reasons for the often quite irregular localized destruction are not always clear (oral hygiene, plaque-retentive niches, localized specific bacteria, tooth type, function?). In addition to describing gingivitis, practitioners will continue to use the terms mild, moderate and severe to differentiate the stages of periodon-titis. It is perhaps important to remember that different au-thors, "schools," and periodontologic societies use various synonyms for these different clinical manifestations of di-sease.

Clinical Degrees of Severity

• mild/slight	... *levis*	... *superficialis*
• moderate	... *media*	... *media*
• severe/advanced	... *gravis*	... *profunda*

Most recently, the AAP (1996c) has defined the degree of severity of periodontitis not exclusively according to prob-ing depths and terms such as mild, moderate or severe; rather, more consideration is given also to gingival inflam-mation, bone loss, attachment loss, furcation invasion and tooth mobility.

Clinical Degrees of Severity		Gingival Inflammation, Bleeding (BOP)	Probing Depths (PD)	Clinical Attachment Loss (AL)	Bone Loss	Furcation Invasion	Tooth Mobility (TM)
Class	Form						
Class 1	Gingivitis	+ to +++	1–3 mm	–	–	–	– ?
Class 2	Slight Periodontitis	+ to +++	4–5 mm	1–2 mm	+	–	– ?
Class 3	Moderate Periodontitis	+ to +++	6–7 mm	3–4 mm	horizontal ++ individual vertical	~ F1	+
Class 4	Severe Periodontitis	+ to +++	>7 mm	≥5 mm	multiple vertical ++	F2, F3	++

Conclusions

All of the pathomorphologic classifications of periodontitis presented on this page (cf. AAP Glossary 2001) attempt to describe the severity of the disease *as it exists immediately after clinical examination*; these descriptors say very little about the pathobiology, the *dynamics* or the speed of pro-gression of periodontitis (prognosis).

Pockets and Loss of Attachment

Pocket formation without any loss of connective tissue attachment is seen in gingivitis in the form of the *gingival pocket* and the *pseudopocket* (p.79). A *true* periodontal pocket will exhibit attachment loss, apical migration of the junctional epithelium, and transformation of the junctional epithelium into a pocket epithelium (Müller-Gauser & Schroeder 1982). The *true* periodontal pocket may assume two forms (Papapanou & Tonetti 2000):

- *Suprabony* pockets, resulting from horizontal loss of bone

- *Infrabony* pockets, resulting from vertical, angular bone loss. In such cases the deepest portion of the pocket is located apical to the alveolar crest.

Whether pocket development is horizontal or vertical appears to be due to the thickness of the interdental septum or the facial and oral bony plates.

True loss of attachment results from microbial plaque and the metabolic products of plaque microorganisms. The range and effective radius of destruction is ca. 1.5–2.5 mm (Tal 1984; Fig. 195).

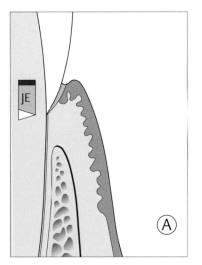
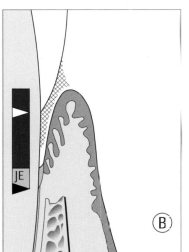
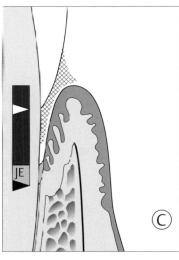

193 Types of Periodontal Pockets

A Normal Sulcus
The apical termination of the junctional epithelium (JE) is at the cementoenamel junction (open arrow).

B Suprabony Pocket (red)
Attachment loss; proliferation of pocket epithelium. A remnant of junctional epithelium (pink) persists at the base of the pocket.

C Infrabony Pocket
Bony pocket

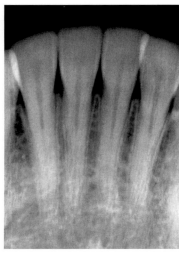
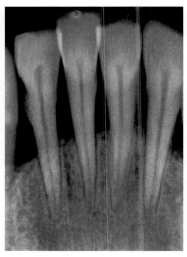
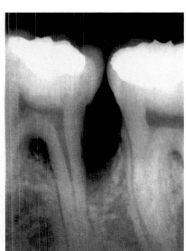

194 Types of Bone Loss

No Attachment Loss (left)
Normal alveolar septa. Lamina dura and alveolar crest remain intact.

Horizontal Bone Loss (middle)
Up to 50 % loss of interdental septal bone.

Vertical Bone Loss, Furcation Involvement (right)
Severe bone loss distal to the first molar. The furcation of this tooth is also involved.

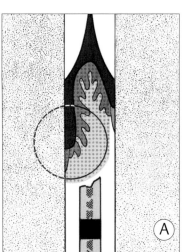
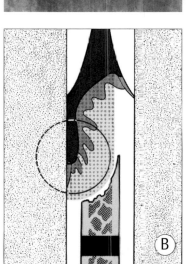
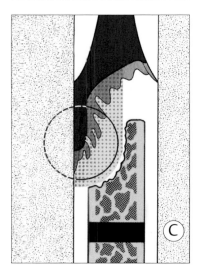

195 "Range" of Destruction = Contour of Bone Resorption
The destructive process radiating from the plaque measures ca. 1.5–2.5 mm (red circle). The *expanse (width) of the interdental septa* therefore determines for the most part the type (morphology) of bone loss.

A Narrow: horizontal resorption
B Average: horizontal resorption, incipient vertical resorption
C Wide: vertical resorption, bony pocket

Intra-alveolar Defects, Infrabony Pockets

The infrabony pocket (infra-alveolar vertical bone loss) may exhibit various forms in relation to the affected teeth (Goldman & Cohen1980, Papapanou & Tonetti 2000).

Classification of Bony Pockets

- *Three-wall bony pockets* are bordered by one tooth surface and three osseous surfaces
- *Two-wall bony pockets* (*interdental craters*) are bordered by two tooth surfaces and two osseous surfaces (one facial and one oral)
- *One-wall bony pockets* are bordered by two tooth surfaces, one osseous surface (facial or oral) and soft tissue
- *Combined bony pockets (cup-shaped defects)* may be bordered by several surfaces of a tooth and several of bone. The defect surrounds the tooth.

The causes for this wide variation in pocket morphology and resorption of bone are myriad and cannot always be wholly elucidated in each individual case.

196 Schematic Representation of Pocket Morphology

A **Three-Wall** bony defect
B **Two-Wall** bony defect
C **One-Wall** bony defect
D **Combined** bony defect, crater-like resorption ("cup")

The walls of each pocket are shown in red (1–3).

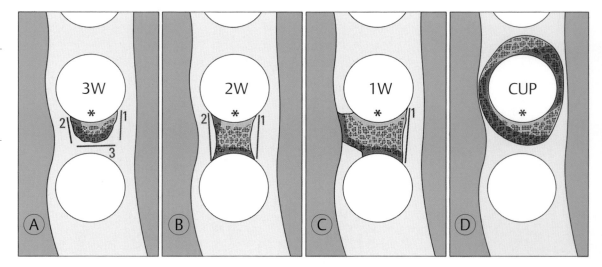

197 Small Three-Wall Defect
Early pocket formation on the mesial aspect of the second premolar. The color-coded probe (CP12) measures a depth of ca. 3 mm. If gingiva were present, the total probing depth would be ca. 5 mm.

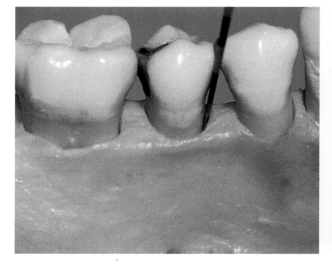
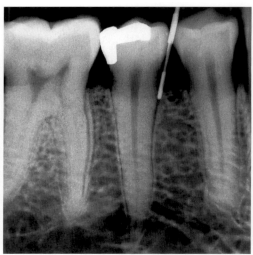

198 Deep Three-Wall Bony Pocket
The periodontal probe descends almost 6 mm (measured from the alveolar crest) to the base of this three-wall defect.

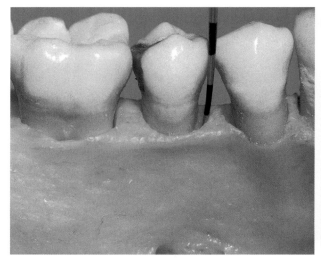
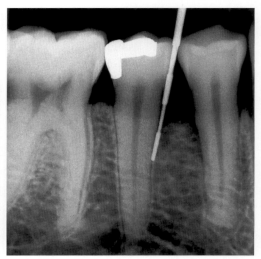

Mention was already made of the significance of bone thickness (Fig. 195). Since the bony septa between the roots become thinner coronally, the initial stage of periodontitis generally presents as horizontal resorption. The greater the distance between the roots of two teeth, the thicker will be the intervening septum, and the development of a vertical defect is more likely.

In addition to such simple osseous morphology, other factors almost certainly play some role in the type of resorption:

- local acute exacerbation elicited by specific bacteria in the pocket
- local inadequate oral hygiene (plaque)
- crowding and tipping of teeth (plaque-retentive areas)
- tooth morphology (root irregularities, furcations)
- improper loading due to functional disturbances (?).

The morphology of the bony pocket is of importance in both prognosis and treatment planning (defect selection). The amount of bone remaining will affect the chances of osseous regeneration after treatment.

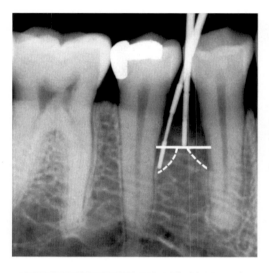
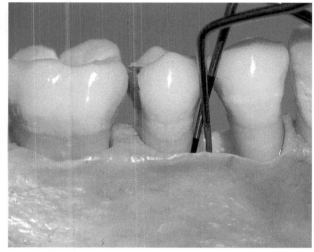

199 Two-Wall Bony Pocket, Interdental Crater
The coronal portion of this defect is bordered by only two bony walls (and two tooth surfaces). In the apical areas the two-wall defect becomes a three-wall defect (see left probe tip in the radiograph, left).

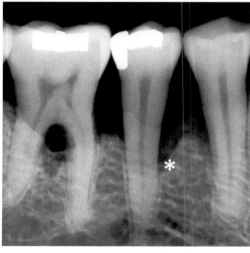
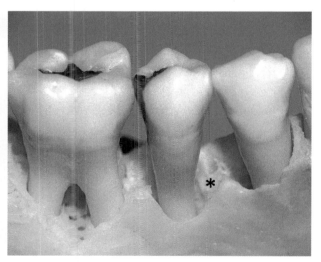

200 One-Wall Bony Pocket on the Mesial of Tooth 45
Advanced bone loss in premolar/molar area. On tooth 45, the facial wall of bone is reduced almost to the level of the mesial pocket (✳). A portion of the lingual plate of bone remains intact. The facial root surface and the interdental spaces could be covered with soft tissue to the cementoenamel junction, masking the defect clinically.

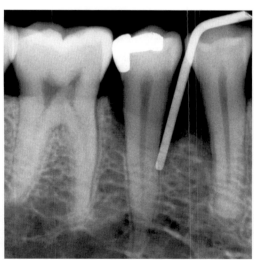
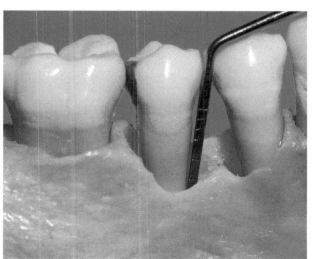

201 Combined Pocket, Cup-shaped Defect
In the region of tooth 45, the apical portion of the osseous defect courses around the tooth, creating a "moat" or "cup" (Goldman probe in situ). The bony pocket is therefore bordered by several osseous and several tooth surface walls.

Furcation Involvement

Periodontal bone loss around multirooted teeth presents a special problem when bi- or trifurcations are involved. Partially or completely open furcations tend to accumulate plaque (Schroeder & Scherle 1987). Exacerbations, abscesses, progressive loss of attachment and rapid deepening of periodontal pockets occur frequently, especially with through-and-through furcation involvement. In addition, open furcations are particularly susceptible to the development of dental caries.

Modified from Hamp et al. (1975), three classes of *horizontally* measured furcation invasion are acknowledged:

Classes—Horizontal

Class F1: The furcation can be probed in the horizontal direction up to 3 mm.
Class F2: The furcation can be probed to a depth of more than 3 mm, but is not through-and-through.
Class F3: The furcation is through-and-through and can be probed completely.

202 Classification of Furcation Involvement—
Horizontal Measurement
Furcation involvement may be combined with infrabony pockets.

A **F0:** Pocket on the mesial root, but without furcation involvement.
B **F1:** Furcation can be probed 3 mm horizontally.
C **F2:** Furcation can be probed deeper than 3 mm.
D **F3:** Through-and-through furcation involvement.

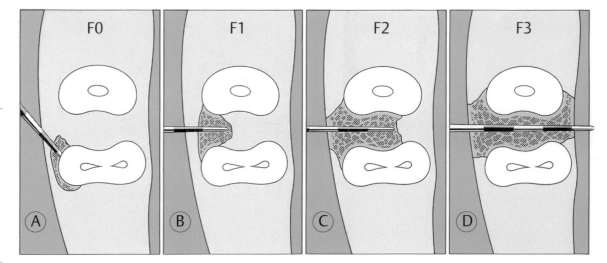

203 No Furcation Involvement—F0
In a clinical situation, in the region of the buccal furcation entrance, a ca. 5 mm deep *suprabony pocket* would be detectable.

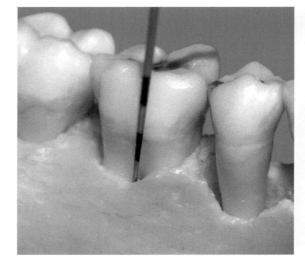

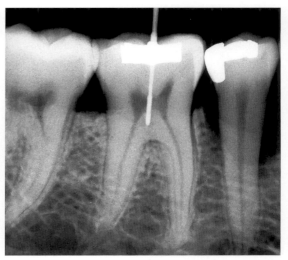

204 Furcation Involvement—F1
Using a curved, pointed explorer (CH3; Hu-Friedy) the buccal furcation can be probed to a depth of less than 3 mm. Probing is performed from both buccal and lingual aspects. Special furcation probes are available on the market today. They are rounded and have millimeter indications; e.g. Nabers-2 (Hu-Friedy).

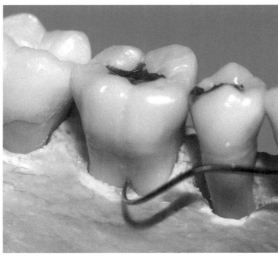

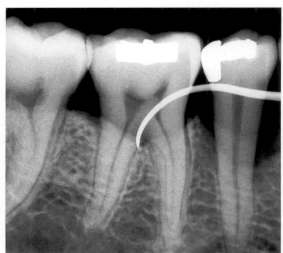

This classification of bifurcation involvement in the mandible is also applicable to the maxilla, where trifurcation involvement is virtually impossible to diagnosis on the radiograph. In the case of maxillary trifurcations, it is imperative to differentiate between which roots the invasion exists and the extent of the horizontal bone loss. For a complete diagnosis, probing most be performed not only from the buccal, but also from distopalatal and mesiopalatal aspects.

Vertical bone loss in a furcation can also be classified (subclasses A-C, Tarnow & Fletcher 1984). It is measured in millimeters from the roof of the furcation (see also pp. 172, 306):

Subclasses—Vertical

Subclass A:	1–3 mm
Subclass B:	4–6 mm
Subclass C:	>7 mm

Therapy: Class F1 and F2 furcation involvement may be successfully treated by root planing alone or by flap procedures (conventional and regenerative). Class F3 furcations are usually treated by means of hemisection or by amputation of one root (p. 305).

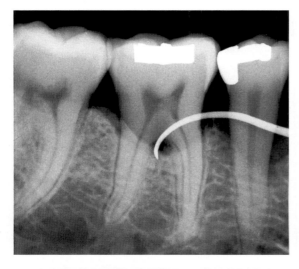

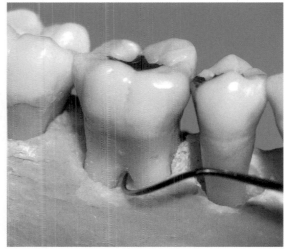

205 Furcation Involvement—F2
The explorer can probe more than 3 mm into the furcation, which is not yet through-and-through.

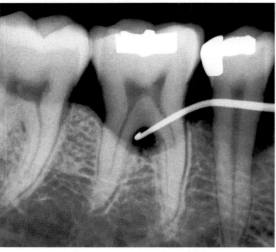

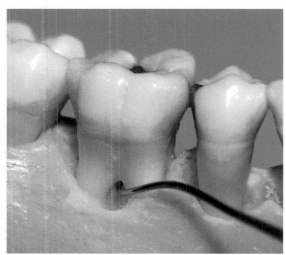

206 Furcation Involvement—F3, Mild, Subclass A
Narrow, through-and-through bifurcation involvement in the face of relatively minor bone loss (Nabers-2 probe).
Less than 3 mm of bone loss in the vertical dimension; this corresponds to subclass A.

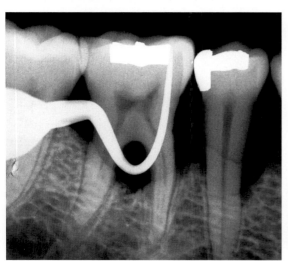

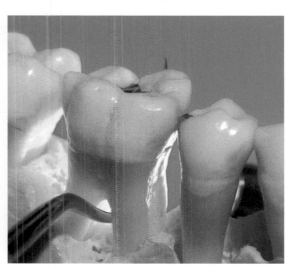

207 Furcation Involvement—F3, Severe, Subclass C
Wide, through-and-through bifurcation in a case exhibiting severe horizontal and vertical bone loss (Cowhorn explorer). The vertical extent of the furcation exceeds 6 mm: Subclass C.

Histopathology

The primary symptoms of periodontitis are attachment loss and pocket formation. *Pocket epithelium* exhibits the following features (modified from Müller-Glauser & Schroeder 1982):

- irregular boundary with the subjacent connective tissue, exhibiting rete pegs; toward the periodontal pocket, epithelium is often very thin and partially ulcerated
- in the apicalmost region, the pocket epithelium becomes a very narrow and short junctional epithelium

- transmigration of PMNs through the pocket epithelium
- defective basal lamina complex on the connective tissue aspect.

Within the *subepithelial connective tissue,* collagen is lost and numerous inflammatory cells invade. In acute stages, pus formation and microabscesses occur. Bone is resorbed, and deeper osseous marrow is transformed into fibrous connective tissue.

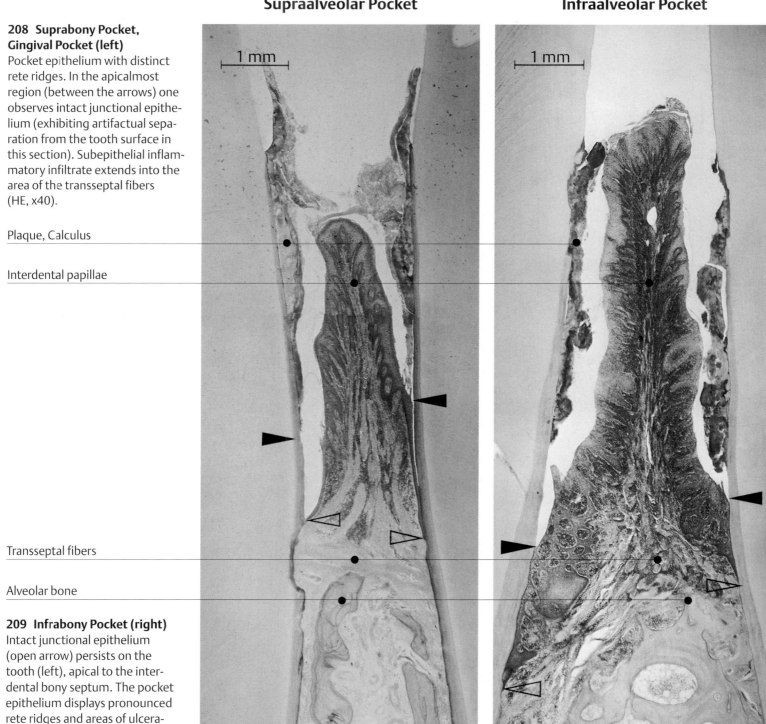

Supraalveolar Pocket **Infraalveolar Pocket**

208 Suprabony Pocket, Gingival Pocket (left)
Pocket epithelium with distinct rete ridges. In the apicalmost region (between the arrows) one observes intact junctional epithelium (exhibiting artifactual separation from the tooth surface in this section). Subepithelial inflammatory infiltrate extends into the area of the transseptal fibers (HE, x40).

Plaque, Calculus

Interdental papillae

Transseptal fibers

Alveolar bone

209 Infrabony Pocket (right)
Intact junctional epithelium (open arrow) persists on the tooth (left), apical to the interdental bony septum. The pocket epithelium displays pronounced rete ridges and areas of ulceration. Inflammatory infiltrate extends into the periodontal ligament and marrow (HE, x40).

Additional Clinical and Radiographic Symptoms

Primary Symptoms

- Inflammation (gingivitis)
- True periodontal pockets
- Bone resorption
} Attachment Loss

These *obligate* primary symptoms of periodontitis must be present simultaneously for a diagnosis of "periodontitis" (= inflammation-induced attachment loss); they can occur in different forms and in measurable degrees of severity.

Additional Symptoms

The additional symptoms, listed below, are *not obligate* in every case of periodontitis, but they may modify or complicate the disease picture:

- Gingival shrinkage
- Gingival swelling
- Pocket activity: bleeding, exudate, pus
- Pocket abscess, furcation abscess
- Fistula
- Tooth migration, tipping, extrusion
- Tooth mobility
- Tooth loss

Gingival Shrinkage

During the course of periodontitis, especially the slowly progressive, chronic type in adults, gingival shrinkage may occur with time. Gingival shrinkage can also occur after spontaneous transition of an acute exacerbation into a chronic, quiescent stage, or following comprehensive periodontal therapy or after draining of abscesses. Whatever the cause, shrinkage leads to exposure of root surfaces.

This type of shrinkage must not be confused with true gingival *recession*, which can occur in the *absence* of clinical inflammation. True recession occurs without the formation of periodontal pockets and is most often observed on the facial aspect of roots. On the other hand, gingival shrinkage due to periodontitis may also be quite pronounced in the papillary regions.

If, as a result of shrinkage, the gingival margin is located apical to the cementoenamel junction, clinical probing of any pockets will underestimate the actual loss of attachment. True attachment loss must be measured from the cementoenamel junction to the base of the pocket.

Gingival Swelling

Enlargement of the gingiva is a symptom of gingivitis that may remain if progression to periodontitis occurs.

If the gingivae are edematous or hyperplastically enlarged beyond the cementoenamel junction, pocket depth (probing depth) may be overestimated, while true attachment loss may be underestimated (Fig. 212).

Pocket Activity

The activity of a pocket and the frequency of active episodes are of more importance than absolute pocket depth in mm, especially in regard to treatment planning and prognosis.

Bleeding on probing, presence of exudate, and suppuration after application of finger pressure are all signs that an *active phase of periodontitis* is in progress (Davenport et al. 1982). Such signs are often observed in the aggressive forms of periodontitis, but may also be seen in older patients with chronic periodontitis and reduced host immune response.

Pocket and Furcation Abscess

An additional symptom of active periodontitis is the pocket or furcation abscess. This develops *during an acute exacerbation* if necrotic tissue cannot be either resorbed or expelled (for example, due to closure of the coronal gingiva above deep pockets, furcations and retentive areas). An abscess (macronecrosis) may also be the consequence of *injury*, for example biting upon hard, sharp foodstuffs, improper oral hygiene efforts (e. g., a broken toothpick), or iatrogenic trauma. In rare instances a periodontal abscess can develop into a submucosal abscess (parulis).

An abscess is one of the few manifestations of periodontitis that may elicit *pain*. If an abscess is expansive, extending to the apical region, the tooth may become sensitive to percussion. A painful abscess must be drained on an emergency basis, either by way of the pocket orifice itself or via incision through the lateral wall. An abscess may release spontaneously through a fistulous tract or via the gingival margin.

Fistula

A fistula may be the result of spontaneous opening of an abscess if the gingival margin is sealed. If the underlying cause (active pocket) is not eliminated, the fistula may persist for an extended period of time without any pain. The orifice of the fistula is not always located directly above the acute process; this can lead to improper diagnosis of the location of an abscess (probe the fistulous tract with a blunt probe!). Pulpal *vitality* of the tooth in question, and its neighbors, must also be checked, to ascertain possible endodontic complications.

Shrinkage—Swelling

In advanced periodontitis, additional clinical symptoms include shrinkage (gingival recession) or swelling of the gingiva; tooth migration and tipping of individual teeth or groups of teeth can occur. The result of such tooth movements is the creation of diastemata, which can present an esthetic problem. There are many factors that could be responsible for tooth migration and it is not possible in every case to determine the specific cause. It is nevertheless clear that compromised tooth-supporting apparatus is a prerequisite for tooth migration, tipping etc. Numerous other factors may also play a role: missing antagonists, functional occlusal disturbances, oral parafunctions (lip biting, cheek biting, tongue thrust etc.).

A tooth exhibiting a deep pocket on one side and intact periodontal fiber structure on the other side may migrate not so much as a result of pressure exerted by granulation tissue in the pocket, as by forces deriving from the still intact collagenous supracrestal fiber bundles in the healthy tissues. The fact that migrated teeth usually exhibit their unilateral pocket on the side opposite the direction of wandering would appear to support this hypothesis.

The figures below present typical *clinical* measurements (probing depth, recession of the marginal gingiva, *clinical attachment loss*; see also p. 171).

Clinical Attachment Loss

210 Pocket Measurement: Probing Depth (PD) = Attachment Loss (AL)

The measurement (8 mm) is made from the gingival margin, which in this case is still in its normal position near the cementoenamel junction; only in such cases does probing depth correspond identically to attachment loss.

Right: The schematic clearly depicts that the pocket depth corresponds to the attachment loss.

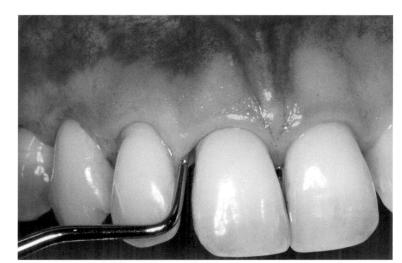 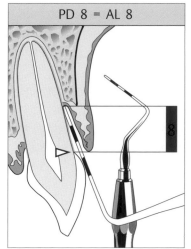

211 Pocket Measurement: Probing Depth Underestimates Attachment Loss

The measurement (7 mm) is made from the gingival margin, which is 3 mm apical to the cementoenamel junction. Thus, the true attachment loss is 10 mm.

Right: The schematic diagram reveals that the probing depth underestimates the attachment loss because of the recession (**RE**) of the gingival tissues.

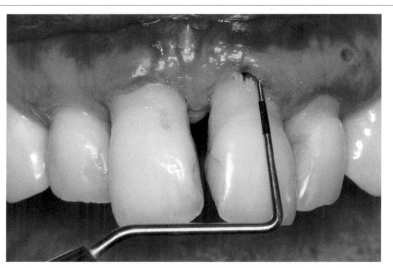 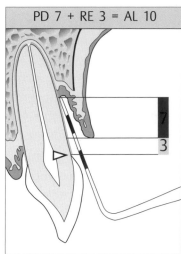

212 Pocket Measurement: Probing Depth Overestimates Attachment Loss

The measurement (7 mm) is made from the gingival margin, but the hyperplastic gingivae (**HY**) extend beyond the CEJ, creating a pseudopocket. The clinical attachment loss (**AL**) is 4 mm less than probing depth.

Right: The schematic diagram reveals that the attachment loss is overestimated as a result of the gingival swelling.

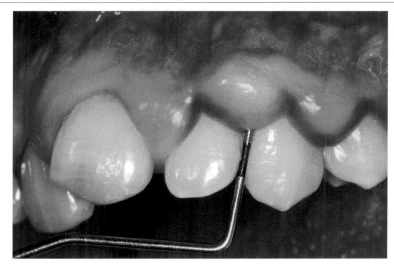 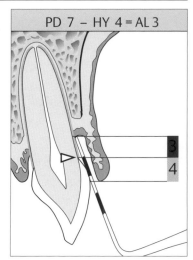

Pocket Activity, Tooth Migration and Tooth Mobility

Pocket activity and tooth mobility are symptoms of severe, advanced periodontitis. Elevated tooth mobility must, however, be interpreted carefully because it can be influenced by numerous factors.

Even in a healthy periodontium, the teeth exhibit physiologic differences in mobility depending on number of roots, root morphology and root length.

Even in a healthy periodontium, occlusal trauma can lead to an increase in tooth mobility (p. 174). In cases of periodontitis, it is the quantitative loss of bone that is the primary de-terminant of tooth mobility, but superimposed occlusal trauma can increase tooth mobility still further. In such cases, one may observe a continuously increasing (progressive) tooth mobility, which is very unfavorable in terms of single tooth prognosis.

Tooth Loss

The final "symptom" of periodontitis, the one which ultimately stops the disease process, is tooth loss. It seldom occurs spontaneously because extremely mobile teeth that are no longer functional are usually extracted prior to spontaneous exfoliation.

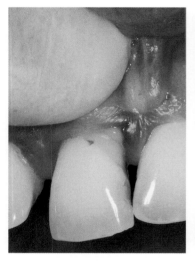

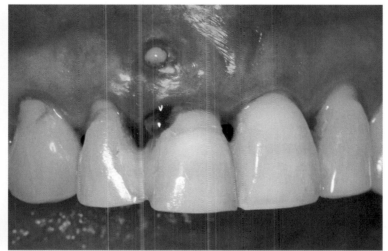

213 Periodontal Fistula—Pus
13 mm pocket on the distal of tooth 11, which is a candidate for extraction. After probing, pus escapes from both the fistulous tract and the gingival margin.

Left: Pus exudes from an active pocket on tooth 11 after finger pressure is applied.

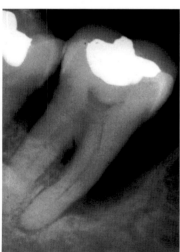

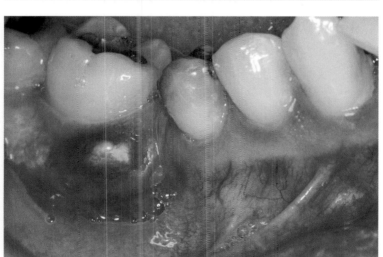

214 Periodontal Abscess
Originating from a 12 mm pocket on the mesial aspect of the tipped, vital tooth 47, an abscess has developed, which is just about to open spontaneously.

Left: The radiograph reveals a severe vertical bony defect on the mesial of tooth 47.

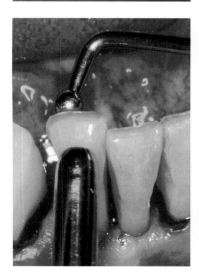

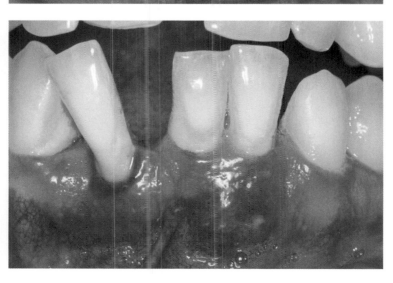

215 Tooth Migration and Tipping
Creation of a diastema by severe tipping of tooth 41 after loss of 42. Patient exhibits a heavy tongue thrust when swallowing.

Left: Tooth mobility. Increased tooth mobility can be caused by functional disturbances and/or by periodontal attachment loss. Mobility is measured clinically by using two instruments or one instrument and a fingernail (degrees of mobility, see p. 174).

Chronic Periodontitis—Mild to Moderate

This 51-year-old male had received restorative dental care at irregular intervals. The dentist had never performed any periodontal diagnostic procedures, nor any therapy. The patient himself complained of occasional gingival bleeding and calculus that bothered him. He was unaware of any periodontal disease and felt that he was completely functional in mastication.

Findings: See charting and radiographic survey (p. 109).

Diagnosis: Slowly progressing, mild to moderate chronic periodontitis (Type II B; p. 329).

Therapy: Motivation, oral hygiene instruction and follow-up initial therapy. Closed scaling and root planing. After *re-evaluation*, modified Widman procedure at several sites. No systemic therapy. Possible bridgework in mandibular posterior segments.

Recall: Every 4–6 months.

Prognosis: Even if the patient's compliance is only average, the prognosis is good. In cases such as this, the dentist or hygienist is always "very successful."

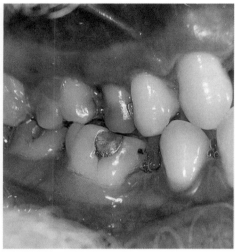
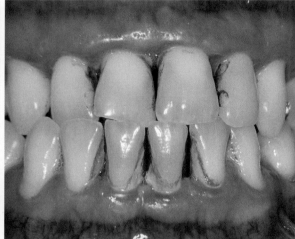
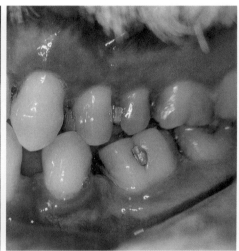

216 Clinical Overview (above)
A cursory inspection reveals only gingivitis and the absence of interdental papillae. The mandibular first molars were extracted 30 years previously, with resultant slow tooth migration, tipping and diastemata. Occlusion is poor.

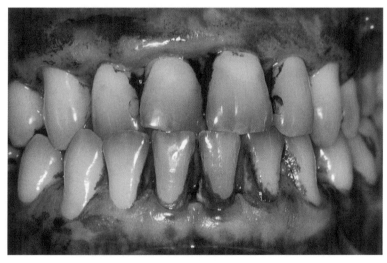

217 Plaque Disclosure, Oral Hygiene (right)
The labial surfaces exhibit almost no plaque accumulation, while the interproximal areas are filled with plaque and calculus.

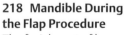

218 Mandible During the Flap Procedure
The facial crest of bone is somewhat bulbous but shows no signs of active destruction. Interdental 3 mm craters were detected.

Treatment consisted solely of root planing, minor recontouring of the bulbous bony margin (osteoplasty) and repositioning of the flaps at their origin position (no apical repositioning).

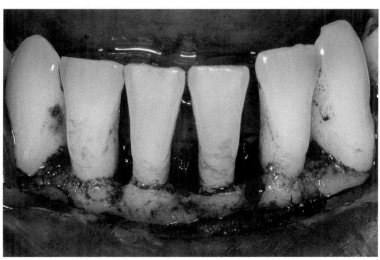

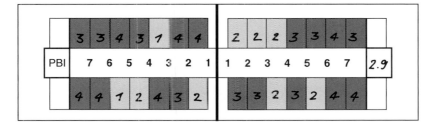

API

API	7	6	5	4	3	2	1	1	2	3	4	5	6	7	
	+	+	+	+	−	+	+	+	+	+	+	+	+	+	93%
	+	+	+	−	+	+	+	+	+	+	+	+	+	+	

219 Aproximal Plaque Index (API) and Papilla Bleeding Index (PBI)

API 93 %. Oral hygiene is poor. Almost all of the interdental spaces harbor plaque.

PBI

PBI	7	6	5	4	3	2	1	1	2	3	4	5	6	7	
	3	3	4	3	1	4	4	2	2	2	3	3	4	3	2.9
	4	4	1	2	4	3	2	3	3	2	3	2	4	4	

PBI 2.9. The index is very high. All papillae bled during performance of the PBI.

The procedure for performing this index is described on pp. 68–70.

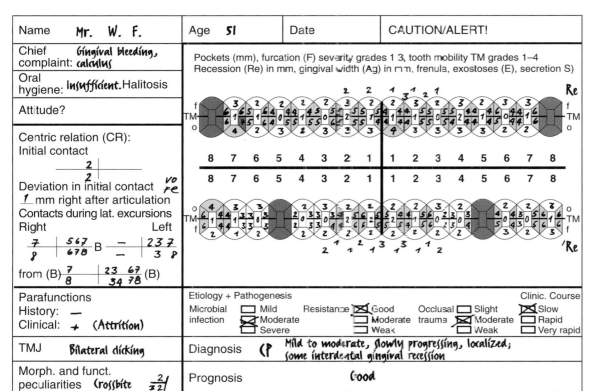

Name	Mr. W. F.	Age	51	Date		CAUTION/ALERT!

Chief complaint: Gingival bleeding, calculus

Oral hygiene: Insufficient. Halitosis

Attitude?

Centric relation (CR):
Initial contact
$\frac{2}{2}$
Deviation in initial contact vo/re
1 mm right after articulation
Contacts during lat. excursions
Right   Left
$\frac{7}{8}$ | $\frac{567}{678}$ B — | $\frac{237}{3}$ P
from (B) $\frac{7}{8}$ | $\frac{23\ 67}{34\ 78}$ (B)

Parafunctions
History: —
Clinical: + (Attrition)

TMJ   Bilateral clicking

Morph. and funct. peculiarities   Crossbite $\frac{2}{32}$

Pockets (mm), furcation (F) severity grades 1 3, tooth mobility TM grades 1–4
Recession (Re) in mm, gingival width (Ag) in mm, frenula, exostoses (E), secretion S)

Etiology + Pathogenesis

Microbial infection	☐ Mild	Resistance	☒ Good	Occlusal trauma	☐ Slight	Clinic. Course	☒ Slow
	☒ Moderate		☐ Moderate		☒ Moderate		☐ Rapid
	☐ Severe		☐ Weak		☐ Weak		☐ Very rapid

Diagnosis   CP   Mild to moderate, slowly progressing, localized; some interdental gingival recession

Prognosis   Good

220 Periodontal Charting—I
This periodontal chart (description p. 194, Fig 439) is used in many dental offices, and has convenient places for recording probing depth, recession, furcation involvement and tooth mobility using numerical scores.
This case exhibits uniform probing depths throughout, especially in the interdental areas. For an assessment of the true attachment loss, the millimeter measurements entered by "Re" (recession) must be considered; these indicate the amount of gingival shrinkage.
Tooth mobility is low (grade 0–2). Functional analysis revealed premature contact between the upper and lower right lateral incisors (cross bite, increased mobility). Disturbances in lateral excursion and protrusion.

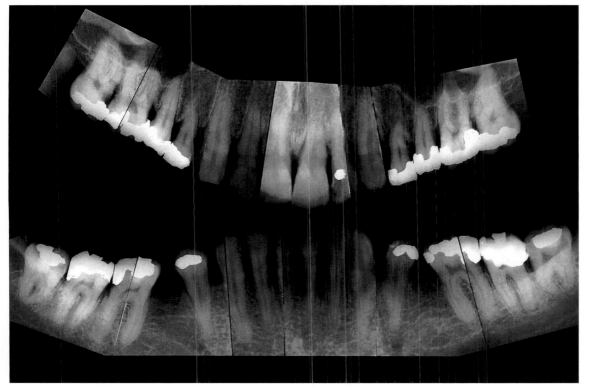

221 Radiographic Survey
The radiographs confirm the clinical observations: localized, mild to moderate, mainly horizontal bone loss.
Note migration and tipping of several teeth in the mandible. Some of the restorative work is inadequate.
Most important is that the "strategically" important canines and molars will be easy to restore (no furcation involvement).

(Note: This is not a "panoramic radiograph" in the usual sense of that term. Rather this survey was prepared by cutting and fitting individual periapical radiographs into a unified whole. This practice provides a more detailed overview of each individual segment of the dentition than any available panoramic film.)

Chronic Periodontitis—Severe

For decades, this 61-year-old male patient had "scrubbed" his maxillary anterior teeth using a horizontal motion. He had never received oral hygiene instructions, and virtually all of other areas of his dentition were completely neglected. Restorations were inadequate.

Findings: See chart and radiographic survey (p. 111).

Diagnosis: Moderate to severe generalized chronic periodontitis (Type II B; cf. p. 329). The pronounced gingival shrinkage in the maxillary anterior sextant should not be confused with classical gingival *recession*!

Therapy:

- Immediate: Extraction of teeth 18, 17, 28 and 46 and the root of 41. The crown will be used as a temporary pontic by attaching it to the adjacent teeth (acid etch).
- Definitive treatment: Motivation, modification of oral hygiene, extraction of 26 and 31. Initial periodontal therapy (definitive debridement) and possible subsequent surgical procedures and a cast framework partial denture.

Recall: Every 4–6 months.

Prognosis: For the teeth to be maintained and treated periodontally, the prognosis is good.

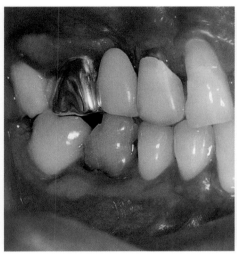 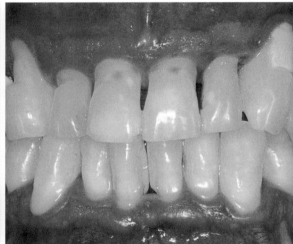 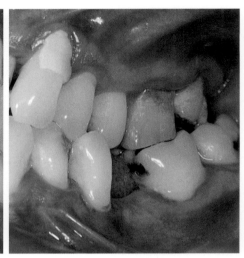

222 Clinical Overview (above)
Noticeable in maxillary anterior region are the severe gingival shrinkage and the wedge-shaped defects (hard-bristle toothbrush, abrasive dentifrice). Periodontal pockets were "brushed away" by the patient!

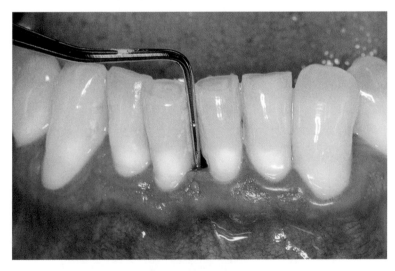

223 Mandibular Anterior Probing Depths (right)
Probing of a 9 mm pocket on the mesial aspect of 41 provoked only slight bleeding. The cervical areas of the mandibular anterior teeth also exhibit abrasion.

224 Retained Root (Tooth 41)
Tooth 41 was no longer functional and had to be extracted. Its root, which had virtually no bony support remaining, was amputated and the natural crown was used as a *temporary pontic* during periodontal treatment, by bonding it to the adjacent teeth using the acid etch technique.

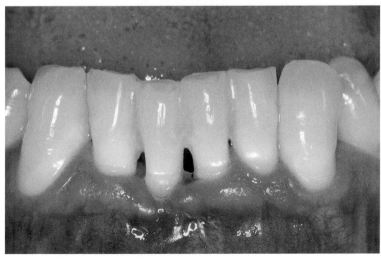

PI

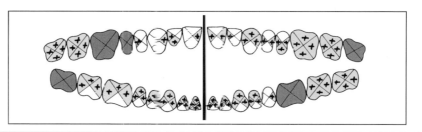

BOP

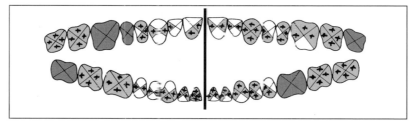

225 Plaque Index (PI) and Bleeding Index (BOP)
PI 69 %. With the exception of the maxillary anterior and some facial surfaces in the mandibular anterior regions, plaque was present on almost all tooth surfaces.

BOP 75 % of the pockets examined bled after gentle probing.

All teeth present were probed at all four surfaces (mesial, distal, facial and oral; pp. 68–69).

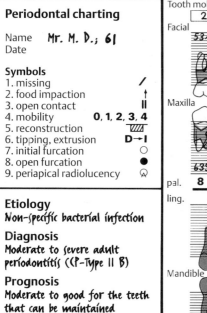

Periodontal charting

Name Mr. M. D.; 61
Date

Symbols
1. missing /
2. food impaction ↑
3. open contact ‖
4. mobility 0, 1, 2, 3, 4
5. reconstruction ▨
6. tipping, extrusion D→I
7. initial furcation ○
8. open furcation ●
9. periapical radiolucency Ⓡ

Etiology
Non-specific bacterial infection

Diagnosis
Moderate to severe adult periodontitis (CP-Type II B)

Prognosis
Moderate to good for the teeth that can be maintained

Systemic diseases:
None

226 Periodontal Charting—II
Using this modified "Michigan Chart," gingival contour, probing depths and attachment loss are represented visually.
Probing depths around each tooth are measured first from the facial aspect at mesial, mid-buccal and distal sites, then from the lingual aspect at 3 similar sites. Because of the pronounced gingival recession, the pockets in the anterior area are not very deep, despite great attachment loss. All anterior teeth were highly mobile.

Complete information concerning the periodontal chart II and its use is presented on page 194 (Fig. 440).

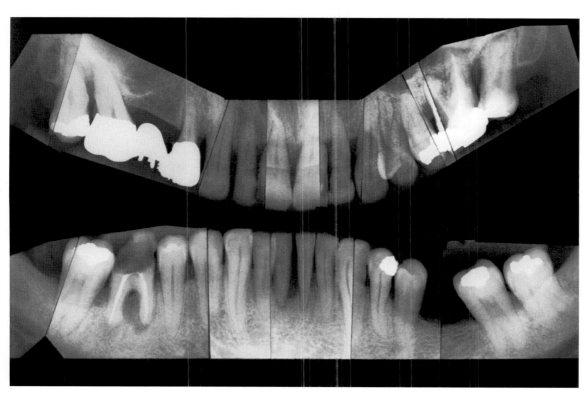

227 Radiographic Survey
The radiographs reveal a very typical, irregular distribution of bone resorption; this is commonly observed in older patients. While some teeth and/or some tooth surfaces have already lost all attachment, hardly any bone resorption is observed on the mandibular canines and the premolars.
At tooth 46, the apical and periodontal lesions appear to communicate.

Aggressive Periodontitis—Ethnic Contributions?

This 31-year-old female immigrated to Switzerland from Ethiopia ten years previously. She complained of loose teeth and the formation of a diastema between her maxillary central incisors. Hemorrhage occurred during tooth brushing. She had never undergone any periodontal treatment.

Findings: See microbiology (Fig. 229), charting and radiographs (p. 113).

Diagnosis: Aggressive, moderate periodontitis, generalized: Type III B; an ethnic component must be considered.

Therapy: Motivation, oral hygiene instruction and follow-up initial therapy. Systemic administration of metronidazol and amoxicillin (van Winkelhoff et al. 1989). After re-evaluation, flap surgery in quadrants 1, 2 and 4 (excluding the maxillary anterior). Extraction of teeth 18 and 28.

Supportive Therapy: Recall at 3-month intervals.

Prognosis: With good patient compliance, the prognosis is good.

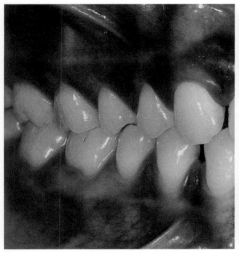
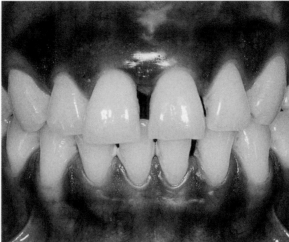
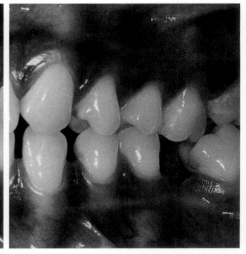

228 Clinical Overview (above)
Pigmented gingiva; very little sign of inflammation. Interdental plaque and bleeding on probing. Calculus on the mandibular anterior teeth. The diastema between the maxillary central incisors had developed in the previous two years; tooth 11 is slightly supererupted.

229 Bacterial Cultures (right)
In deep pockets, high levels of *Aa*, *Pg*, *Ec*.
Right: Classification of the bacterial counts (Socransky et al. 1991).

Bacterial type		Relative percentage	Number of bacteria
Black pigmenting bacteria		50%	
Aa	*Actinobacillus actinomycetemcomitans*	+ + + +	$\geq 10^6$
Pg	*Porphyromonas gingivalis*	+ + + +	$\geq 10^6$
Tf	*Tannerella forsythia*	+ + +	$\sim 10^4$
Pi	*Prevotella intermedia*	+ +	$\sim 10^3$
Ec	*Eikenella corrodens*	+ + + +	$\geq 10^6$
Fn	*Fusobacterium nucleatum*	–	–

Bacterial Cultures	
Bacterial counts Classes 0 – 5	
0	non-detectable
1	below 10^5
2	$\approx$ 10^5
3	10^5 to 10^6
4	$\approx$ 10^6
5	above 10^6

230 Flap Surgery
Clinical view during flap surgery on teeth 25, 26 and 27, following amputation of the distal roots of teeth 26 and 27.

Right: Tooth 27 as viewed from the distal aspect (mirror image).

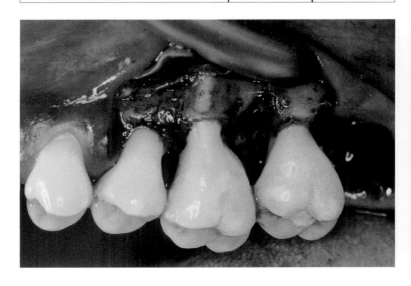
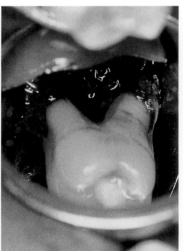

Courtesy J-P. Ebner

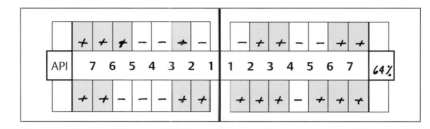

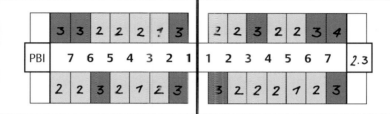

231 Approximal Plaque Index (API) and Papilla Bleeding Index (PBI)

API 64 %. Interdental hygiene is inadequate; smooth surfaces are relatively clean.

PBI Bleeding was more or less pronounced from all interdental papillae. The papilla bleeding index is very high at 2.3.

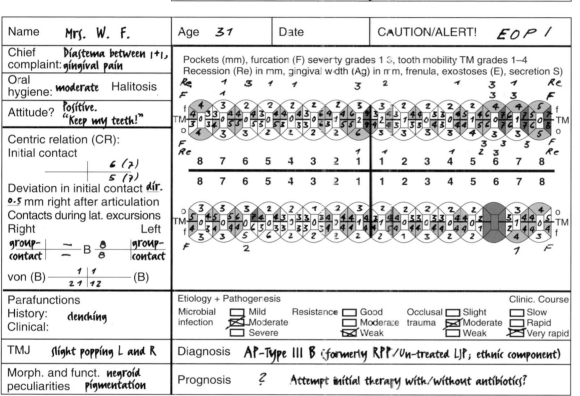

232 Periodontal Charting—I
Probing revealed a very irregular distribution of attachment loss. Remarkable are the deep pockets on teeth 11, 26, 27 and 46. Teeth 26 and 27 exhibit Class III furcation involvement. The furcations are through-and-through from buccal to distal.
Tests of function revealed premature contacts between teeth 26 and 35, with a mild deviating slide of the mandible forward and to the right. This led to trauma on tooth 11. With the exceptions of teeth 11 and 21, the teeth are not mobile. The history revealed that the patient occasionally clenches during the day.

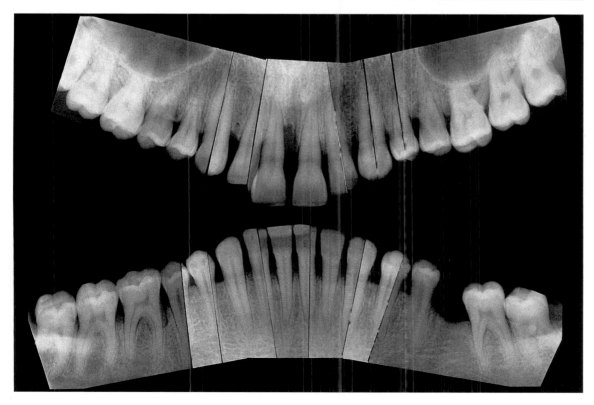

233 Radiographic Survey
The pronounced attachment loss revealed in the periodontal charting is corroborated in the radiographs. The distobuccal roots of teeth 26 and 27 exhibit almost no bony support.
The slightly elongated and distally migrated tooth 11 exhibits a deep pocket on the mesial surface. A typical situation: The most severe attachment loss on a tooth that has migrated is usually on the side opposite the direction of migration.

Aggressive Periodontitis—Acute Phase

This 32-year-old female was referred by her general dentist because of multiple periodontal abscesses. She complained for years about ever-recurring pain and "pus discharge" from her gingiva.

Findings: See charting and radiographs (p. 115) and microbiologic DNA test (IAI Padotest 4.5; Fig. 235 and p. 184).

Diagnosis: Aggressive, moderate, localized profound and acute periodontitis (Type III B, active stage).

Therapy: Incision of the abscess; motivation, oral hygiene instructions and check-up, immediate extraction of teeth 25, 37, 32, 31, 41 and 42. Temporary replacement for mandibular anterior teeth. Supra- and subgingival scaling. Systemic antibiotic supportive therapy (metronidazol), and topical application of metronidazol (p. 289) at recall appointments. At Phase 1 evaluation, decision concerning additional procedures, depending upon patient compliance (radical, maintenance or regenerative/GTR).

Supportive Therapy: Initially, very short-interval recall.

Prognosis: With the exception of teeth 15, 24 and 37, and with good patient compliance, the prognosis is average.

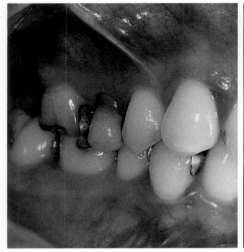
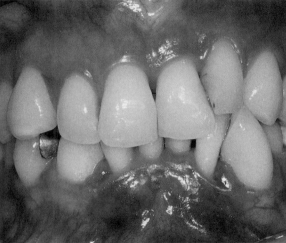
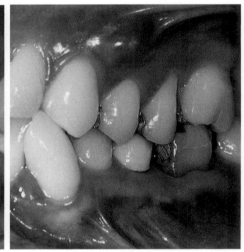

234 Clinical Overview (above)
Acute stage of periodontitis. Localized severe gingival inflammation, abscess formation and pus release from several pockets. Awkward occlusion and severe crowding in the area of the left incisors and canines.

**235 DNA Test Results—
IAI Padotest 4.5 (p. 184)**
Results from the two maxillary teeth that were tested (teeth 16 and 26). Noteworthy is an elevated proportion of *Pg* with a high bacterial load (TBL).

Tooth 16, mesiopalatal; PD 8 mm

Marker	n	ML	Status
Aa	–		
Tf	7.84	6.3%	★★★
Pg	8.2	6.6%	★
Td	7	4.0%	★★
TBL	125.0	–	★★★
TML		17%	Type 5

Tooth 26, distobuccal; PD 6 mm

Marker	n	ML	Status
Aa	–		
Tf	2.41	1.7%	★
Pg	6.2	4.5%	★
Td	7	3.8%	★★
TBL	140.9	–	★★★
TML		10%	Type 5

Microbial Test Results

- *Aa:* not detected
- *Pg:* present in Red Complex (cf. pp. 37, 191)

- *TML:* Total marker load, i. e., pathogenic marker bacteria with 17% and 10% very high

- Finding: Pocket type 5 (p. 185)

- Treatment recommendation: Mechanical pocket therapy plus Metronidazol

**236 Abscess Formation
and Pus Release**
Finger pressure applied to the gingiva elicited release of pus from the deep pocket between teeth 32 and 33.

Right: Clearly visible is the abscess between teeth 23 and 24, which emanated from the 10 mm pocket between these two teeth. The abscess will soon break through the muscosa.

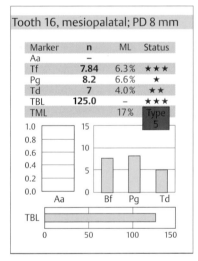
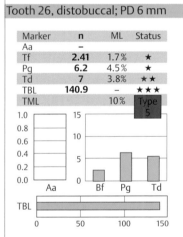
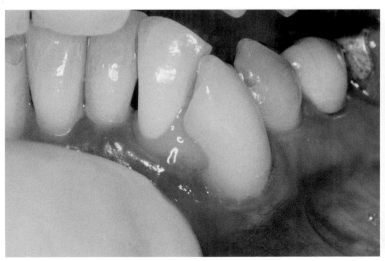
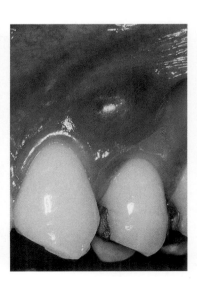

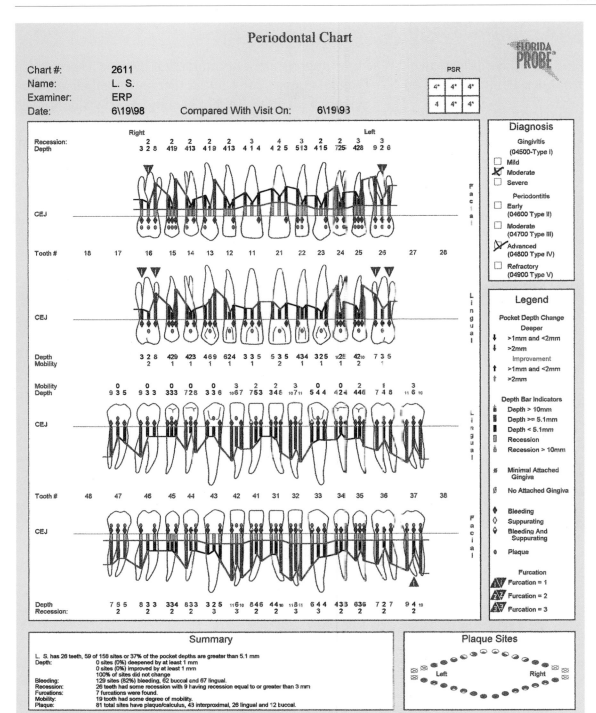

Periodontal Chart

FLORIDA PROBE

Chart #:	2611
Name:	L. S.
Examiner:	ERP
Date:	6\19\98 Compared With Visit On: 6\19\93

PSR

4*	4*	4*
4	4*	4*

Right   Left

Recession:
Depth
    2   2 2   2   2   3   4   3 2   2 3 3
   3 2 8 419 413 419 413 4 1 4 4 2 5 513 415 725 428 9 2 6

CEJ

Tooth # 18   17   16   15   14   13   12   11   21   22   23   24   25   26   27   28

Facial

CEJ

Depth
Mobility
    3 2 8 429 423 469 624 3 3 5 5 3 5 434 325 12E 42₁₀ 7 3 5
    2   1   1   1   1   1   2   1   1   1   2   1

Lingual

Mobility
Depth
  0   0   0   0   0   3   2   2   3   0   0   2   1   3
  9 3 5 9 3 3 333 728 336 ₁₀67 753 348 ₁₀7₁₁ 5 4 4 424 446 7 4 8 ₁₁ 6 ₁₀

CEJ

Lingual

Tooth # 48   47   46   45   44   43   42   41   31   32   33   34   35   36   37   38

CEJ

Facial

Depth
Recession:
  7 5 5 8 3 3 334 833 325 ₁₁6₁₀ 846 44₁₀ ₁₁8₁₁ 6 4 4 433 636 7 2 7 9 4 ₁₀
  2   2   2   2   3   3   2   2   3   2   2   2   2

Diagnosis

Gingivitis
(04500-Type I)
☐ Mild
☒ Moderate
☐ Severe

Periodontitis
☐ Early (04600 Type II)
☐ Moderate (04700 Type III)
☒ Advanced (04800 Type IV)
☐ Refractory (04900 Type V)

Legend

Pocket Depth Change
Deeper
↓ >1mm and <2mm
↓ >2mm
Improvement
↑ >1mm and <2mm
↑ >2mm

Depth Bar Indicators
▮ Depth > 10mm
▮ Depth >= 5.1mm
▮ Depth < 5.1mm
▮ Recession
▮ Recession > 10mm

✗ Minimal Attached Gingiva
∅ No Attached Gingiva

♦ Bleeding
◇ Suppurating
♦ Bleeding And Suppurating
● Plaque

Furcation
◭ Furcation = 1
◭ Furcation = 2
◭ Furcation = 3

Summary

L. S. has 26 teeth, 59 of 156 sites or 37% of the pocket depths are greater than 5.1 mm

Depth:
  0 sites (0%) deepened by at least 1 mm
  0 sites (0%) improved by at least 1 mm
  100% of sites did not change
Bleeding: 129 sites (82%) bleeding, 62 buccal and 67 lingual.
Recession: 26 teeth had some recession with 9 having recession equal to or greater than 3 mm
Furcations: 7 furcations were found.
Mobility: 19 tooth had some degree of mobility.
Plaque: 81 total sites have plaque/calculus, 43 interproximal, 26 lingual and 12 buccal.

Plaque Sites

Left   Right

237 Periodontal Charting III—Florida Probe Charting

In the cases previously described, and in those which follow, probing depths were determined using a manual periodontal probe (e. g., CP-12 or CP-15 UNC; Hu-Friedy), and the data entered by hand into prepared charts.

With progressive computerization of the dental practice, electronic devices such as the Florida Probe are being used more and more often for clinical data collection (description p. 195).

The Florida Probe (Gibbs et al. 1988) functions with a standardized pressure (0.25 N). The measured values for recession, probing depth etc. are stored by means of a foot pedal. The findings can be seen on the monitor (information, motivation) and can be expressed in color.

In addition to recession, probing depths and attachment level, other parameters such as furcation involvement, tooth mobility, plaque accumulation, bleeding and suppuration can be noted tooth-by-tooth. At recall appointments, new software in this system (FP 32) permits a long-term comparison of the findings: "progression" or "improvement" are depicted graphically.

The present case is one of generalized, aggressive periodontitis (III B). Probing depths up to 5 mm are shown by black bars, deeper pockets by red bars.

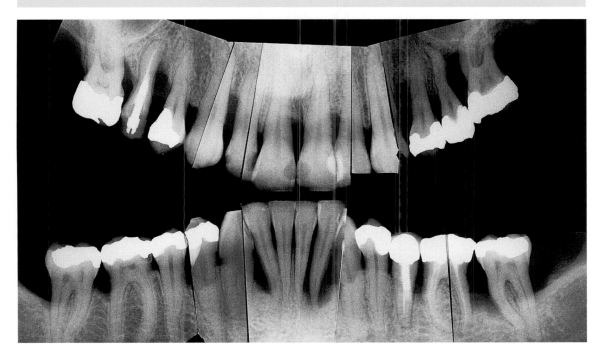

238 Radiographic Survey

The radiographic picture corroborates the clinical examinations. Pronounced bone loss, almost to the apex of the roots, is clearly visible on those teeth that were determined to be non-salvageable from the very beginning: teeth 25, 37, 32, 31, 41 and 42.

Aggressive Periodontitis—Initial Stage

This 15-year-old female was referred from her private dentist because of "suddenly occurring" periodontal defects on all first permanent molars.

Bitewing radiographs had been taken periodically to check for dental caries, and gingival findings were noted. Thus, the localized osseous defects were not "serendipitous findings."

Findings: See charting and radiographs (p. 117).

Diagnosis: Incipient LJP (Type III A). Typical involvement of first molars, with as yet no pocket formation around incisors: Localized Juvenile Periodontitis (LJP).

Therapy: Improvement of interdental hygiene, especially in the molar areas. After initial therapy, modified Widman surgery with intensive root planing (direct vision!) on all involved molars.

Microbiologic DNA test (e.g., PadoTest): *Aa* present, pocket type 4 (p. 185).

Systemic medicinal support with *tetracycline* (p. 289).

Possible filling of osseous defects.

Recall: Repeated professional plaque control during the wound healing phase; subsequent 6-month recall.

Prognosis: Good.

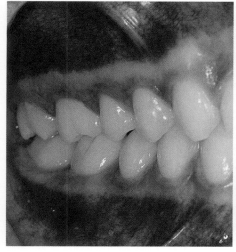
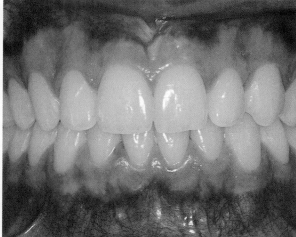
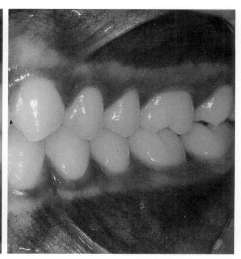

239 Clinical Overview—15-year-old Female (above)
Caries-free dentition.
Upon cursory inspection, the gingivae also appear healthy; however, numerous sites bled after gentle probing.

240 Bitewing Radiograph; Healthy 13-year-old (right)
The radiograph reveals healthy interdental septa of compact bone around the first permanent molars (empty arrows).

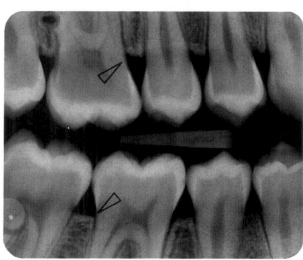

241 Bitewing Radiograph; 15-year-old with LJP (Type III A)
Two years later, obvious bony defects are visible mesial to tooth 16 and distal of 46 (red arrows), with identical defects on the opposite side: early diagnosis—**LJP**!
The significance of regular clinical and radiographic examination of young adults is clear.

Right: Osseous crater distolingual to tooth 46 during surgery.

Radiographs courtesy
U. Hersberger

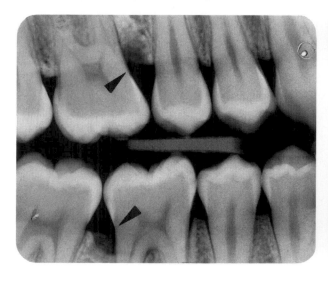
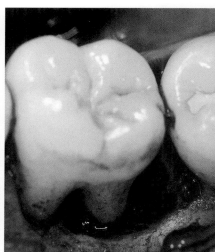

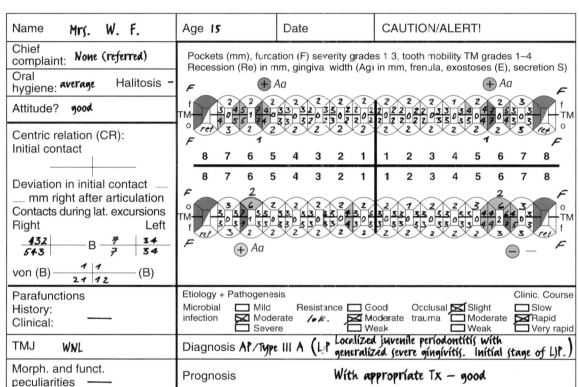

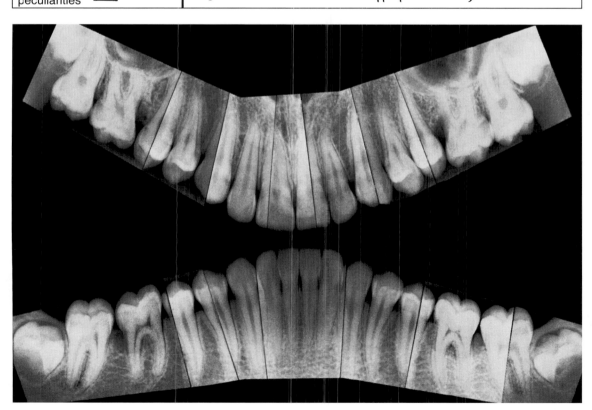

API

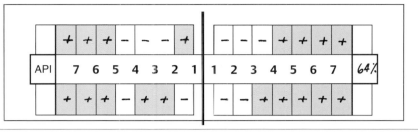

PBI

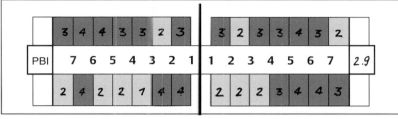

242 API and Papilla Bleeding Index (PBI)

API 64 %. Only ten of the 28 interdental spaces examined were free of plaque (-), despite the fact that the dentition appeared relatively clean (Fig. 239).

PBI 2.9; number of bleeding sites, 80!
Upon cursory inspection, the gingiva appeared to be inflammation-free. Only after recording the PBI was the massive gingivitis identified.

243 Periodontal Charting—I

All four first permanent molars have probing depths up to 7 mm, which corresponds to about 5 mm of true attachment loss (see bitewing radiograph, Fig. 241). The two maxillary first molars exhibit Class F1 furcation involvement from the mesiopalatal aspect. There is no evidence at this time of pocket formation around the incisors, an area that is often affected in such patients.

The occlusion is normal, without parafunctions or occlusal trauma! The mobility of tooth 36 is slightly elevated.

Caution: In three of the four 7 mm pockets, *Aa* was identified (color circles).

| Name | Mrs. W. F. | Age 15 | Date | CAUTION/ALERT! |

Chief complaint: **None (referred)**

Oral hygiene: **average** Halitosis —

Attitude? **good**

Centric relation (CR): Initial contact

Deviation in initial contact — mm right after articulation
Contacts during lat. excursions
Right — Left

$\frac{132}{543}$ — B $\frac{7}{7}$ — $\frac{34}{34}$

von (B) — $\frac{1|1}{21|12}$ — (B)

Parafunctions History: Clinical: —

TMJ **WNL**

Morph. and funct. peculiarities —

Pockets (mm), furcation (F) severity grades 1–3, tooth mobility TM grades 1–4
Recession (Re) in mm, gingiva width (Ag) in mm, frenula, exostoses (E), secretion S)

Etiology + Pathogenesis

Microbial infection	Resistance	Occlusal trauma	Clinic. Course
☐ Mild	☐ Good	☒ Slight	☐ Slow
☒ Moderate /o.k.	☒ Moderate	☐ Moderate	☒ Rapid
☐ Severe	☐ Weak	☐ Weak	☐ Very rapid

Diagnosis AP/Type III A (LP Localized juvenile periodontitis with generalized severe gingivitis. Initial stage of LJP.)

Prognosis **With appropriate Tx — good**

244 Radiographic Survey

Routine periapical radiographs do not portray the osseous craters—especially on the mandibular first molars—as well as the bitewings (x-ray projection angle). No bone loss is apparent on any teeth other than the first permanent molars, especially the maxillary and mandibular incisors exhibit no bone loss.

Prepubertal Periodontitis—PP (Aggressive Periodontitis)

This 2$\frac{1}{2}$-year-old boy was referred from his private dentist. The medical history, gathered from his parents (Japanese mother, Swiss father) revealed that the mandibular deciduous incisors and the maxillary right deciduous incisor had "fallen out" in the previous few months. The left deciduous incisor and also the lateral incisor and canines in the maxilla were highly mobile, but their roots exhibited no resorption. This case is difficult to classify in the absence of an identification of possible hematologic defects. Even though most of the teeth are affected, the relatively mild gingival inflammation and the absence of gingival hyperplasia speak against the generalized form of PP (Type IV B). Laboratory studies should be performed to rule out hypophosphatasia.

Findings: See charting and radiographs.
Diagnosis: Localized, pre-pubertal periodontitis
(PP, Type IV B).
Therapy: Palliative or extraction (Page et al. 1983b). Intensive periodontal preventive maintenance upon eruption of the permanent teeth.
Prognosis: Poor for the deciduous dentition, questionable for permanent teeth.

245 Clinical Picture—2$\frac{1}{2}$-year-old boy
Maxillary anterior tooth 51 and all mandibular anterior teeth, as well as the canines, exfoliated spontaneously.
The gingiva is unimpressive. Aphthous-like lesion near 73.

Right: The radiograph clearly depicts the pronounced attachment loss on the anterior teeth, in the presence of complete roots.
The pulp chambers appear to be above average in size (hypophosphatasia?).

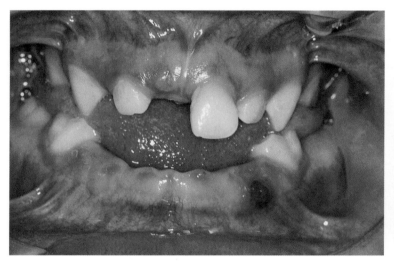 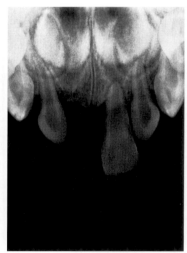

246 Probing Depths and Tooth Mobility
Pocket probing was only possible at four sites around tooth 61 (upper left central incisor), because the 2$\frac{1}{2}$-year-old boy was very sensitive and understandably impatient.
All deciduous teeth exhibited elevated mobility. Teeth 52, 54, 61, 62 and 63* were highly mobile
* (Roman numbers in this graph for deciduous teeth).

*FDI-International tooth numbering of deciduous teeth cf. bookmark.

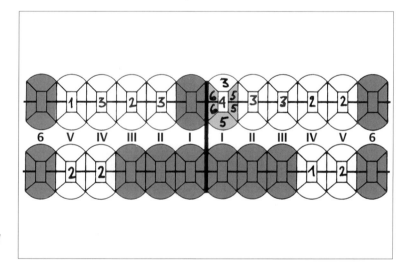

247 Panoramic Radiograph
Irregular and in some areas extreme attachment loss is revealed on all maxillary deciduous teeth. The mandibular deciduous molars appear to be only slightly involved at this time.
Tooth 61, which was present in the clinical picture above (Fig. 245) was spontaneously exfoliated before the panoramic radiograph was taken, some two weeks after the initial clinical visit.

Panorex courtesy *B. Widmer*

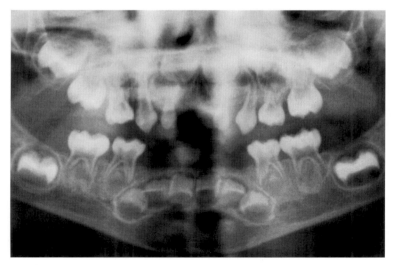

Oral Pathologic Alterations of Gingiva and Periodontium *

As they traverse their clinical course, plaque-induced inflammatory gingival and periodontal diseases may be enhanced or co-initiated by hormonal disturbances and the side effects of systemic medications. Additional oral pathologic alterations accompanying systemic diseases are frequently observed on the gingiva and in the periodontium. In this milieu, clinical differentiation between gingivitis and periodontitis on the one hand and diseases of the oral mucosa on the other may become blurred.

It is impossible in this book to depict and describe each and every oral pathologic alteration that also manifests on the *gingiva* or in the *periodontium*. A comprehensive review of *all* such oral lesions can be found in the *Color Atlas of Oral Pathology* (Reichart & Philipsen 1999).

In the pages that follow, several of the relatively frequently occurring diseases or alterations will be described:

Primarily Gingival Alterations

- Hormonal complications (p. 91)
- Hyperplasia caused by medicaments
- Gingival overgrowth, tumors
- Autoimmune diseases, desquamative and bullous gingival alterations, anomalies of keratinization, dermatologic diseases
- Specific infections
- Allergies
- Toxic manifestations
- Injuries, chemical injuries

Gingival and Periodontal Disorders

- Metabolic disturbances
- Nutritional deficiencies
- Genetically-related systemic syndromes
- Blood cell disorders
- Immune deficiency, AIDS

---

* In the new AAP Classification (Armitage 1999, see Appendix pp. 327–330), a portion of the oral pathologic alterations on the *gingiva* are classified under Type I A and B, and in the *periodontium* under Type IV, "periodontitis as a manifestation of systemic diseases."

Primarily Gingival Alterations (Type I B)

In the following pages, the disorders shown below with a black dot are described and depicted.

Hormonal Complications
- Pregnancy gingivitis (p. 92)
○ Gingivitis due to the "pill"
- Puberty gingivitis (p. 92)
○ Gingivitis menstrualis and intermenstrualis
○ Gingivitis climacterica

Medicament-Elicited Hyperplasia
- Phenytoin gingival overgrowth (p. 121)
- Dihydropyridine-induced gingival overgrowth (p. 122)
- Cyclosporine-induced gingival overgrowth (p. 123)
- Medicament combinations
  (cyclosporine/nifidepine, p. 124)

Gingival Overgrowth, Tumors
- Epulis (p. 125)
- Idiopathic and hereditary fibrosis (p. 126)
- Neoplasms
  – benign tumors (p. 126)
  – malignant tumors (p. 127)

Autoimmune Diseases, Desquamative and Bullous Gingival Alterations, Anomalies of Keratinization, Dermatologic Diseases
- Gingivosis (p. 128)
- Pemphigoid (p. 128)
- Pemphigus vulgaris (p. 128)
○ Epidermolysis bullosa

○ Exudative erythema multiforme
- Lichen (p. 129)
- Leukoplakia—precancerous lesions (p. 130)
- Oral granulomatosis (p. 130)
○ Dermatomyositis, scleroderma, psoriasis etc.

Specific Infections
- Herpes (p. 131)
- Aphthae ? (p. 131)
○ Toxoplasmosis
○ Actinomycosis, candidiasis
○ Gonorrhea, syphilis etc.

Allergies
○ To medicaments
○ To metals, mercury

Toxic Reactions
These may occur locally in the oral cavity through release of metal ions possessing high toxic potential, from dental materials (nickel, cadmium, bismuth, beryllium, vanadium etc; Wirz et al. 1997 a, b):
○ Dental materials of varying composition
○ Lead and other metals

Injuries, Chemical Injuries

Gingival and Periodontal Alterations (Type IV A/B)

Metabolic Disturbances
- Diabetes (p. 132)
○ Acatalasemia (Takahara's Disease)
○ Eosinophilic granuloma
○ Pre-leukemic syndrome

Nutritional Deficiency
Nutritional deficiency as a cause or co-factor in gingivitis or periodontitis is practically no longer observed in the western/northern hemispheres. In extreme conditions (e.g., in the Third World) one may observe:
○ Ascorbic acid deficiency (scurvy)
○ Kwashiorkor (protein deficiency) etc.

Genetically-Elicited Systemic Syndromes
It is not uncommon that rare, partially inherited systemic syndromes are characterized by severe periodontitis:
- Down syndrome (p. 134)
- Papillon-Lefèvre syndrome (p. 136)

○ Chediak-Higashi Syndrome
○ Hypophosphatasia (Rathbun Syndrome)
○ Pelger-Huet nucleus anomaly
○ Ehlers-Danlos syndrome etc.

Blood Cell Diseases
Every blood cell disorder reduces the immune response and, therewith, local defense reactions.
○ Leukemia
○ Panmyelopathy—Fanconi anemia
○ Cyclic neutropenia
○ Agranulocytosis
○ Erythroblastic anemia etc.

Immune Deficiencies
Any weakening of the immune system may elicit or enhance periodontitis. Perhaps most important today is infection by the human immunodeficiency virus HIV.
- HIV infection, AIDS (p. 139)

Phenytoin-induced Gingival Overgrowth

Phenytoin (hydantoin) prevents or reduces the incidence or severity of seizures associated with most types of epilepsy (grand mal), with the exception of petit mal. Phenytoin is also often prescribed following neurosurgical operations or cranial trauma. The anticonvulsive effect is probably due to the inhibition of the spread of nerve potentials in the brain cortex (Hassell 1981).

Systemic side effects of phenytoin are relatively minor. Some bone pathology may be observed after long-term therapy. The patient's mental capacity and reaction time may be negatively influenced (thus, no driver's license!).

The most important *oral side effect* is an often pronounced and secondarily inflamed gingival overgrowth.

Therapy: Motivation, repeated oral hygiene instructions, professional plaque and calculus removal. Once inflammation subsides, fibrous tissue can be excised. Lesions frequently recur.

In collaboration with the patient's physician, in some cases it may be possible to change to a different medication, e.g., valproic acid, benzodiazepine, barbituric acid derivatives, etc.

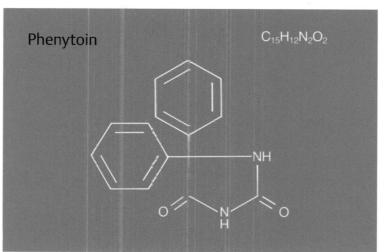

248 Mild Phenytoin-induced Gingival Overgrowth
Fibrous form of phenytoin induced overgrowth in a 19-year-old female with epilepsy.
Following initial periodontal therapy, a gingivoplasty was performed. The oral hygiene of this patient was relatively good, and this made it possible to eliminate secondary inflammation for the most part.

Phenytoin—Trade Names

– Dilantin
– Antisacer
– Danten
– Diphantoin
– Diphenin
– Diphenylan Sodium
– Epanutin
– Minetoin
– Solantyl
– Tacosal

The Merck Index no. 7475
(12th ed. 1996, p. 1259)

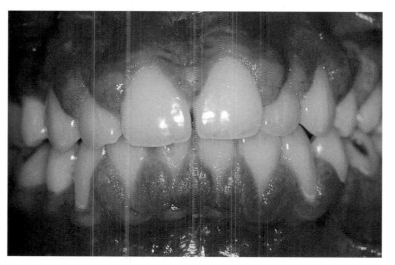

Phenytoin $C_{15}H_{12}N_2O_2$

249 Phenytoin—Structural and Chemical Formula
The medicament phenytoin (diphenylhydantoin) is a 5,5-diphenyl-2,4-imidazolodine-dione.
The overgrowth occurs in only approximately 50 % of patients, usually young individuals (pharmacogenetic factor; Hassell 1981). Participating in the etiology are probably macrophages and fibroblasts that stimulate catabolic mediators, growth factors and collagen (Type IV; Sinha Morton & Dongari-Bagtzoglon 1999).

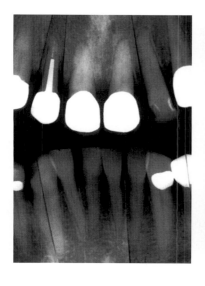

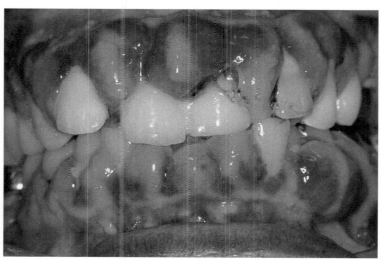

250 Severe Phenytoin Overgrowth—Severe Secondary Inflammation
This 44-year-old female had taken phenytoin on a chronic regimen for six years, since a neurosurgical procedure. She was mildly debilitated and therefore unable to perform adequate oral hygiene. Following initial periodontal therapy, gingivoplasty was performed.

Left: There is radiographic evidence of bone resorption at the interdental septa.

Dihydropyridine-induced Gingival Overgrowth

The substituted dihydropyridines (nifedipine, nitrendipine etc.) are calcium antagonists that reduce the influx of calcium ions into heart muscle and thereby reduce the strength of contraction as well as the vascular resistance. This reduces oxygen consumption by the heart while simultaneously increasing cardiac circulation. Thus, dihydropyridines exert both anti-anginal and anti-hypertensive effects. Some general side effects as well as interactions with other drugs are observed. In contrast to phenytoin, dihydropyridines are taken by primarily by *older* cardiac patients, who often have a pre-existing periodontitis.

The most important *oral* side effect is an often pronounced, secondarily inflamed gingival overgrowth. The pathogenesis of the overgrowth is suspected to be similar to that observed in phenytoin-treated individuals (connective tissue accumulation), but an increase in acid mucopolysaccharides (ground substance) also appears to occur (Lucas et al. 1985, Barak et al. 1987).

Therapy: Following patient motivation, repeated oral hygiene instruction and initial periodontal therapy, severe lesions may be eliminated surgically (gingivoplasty).

251 Mild to Moderate Nifedipine-induced Gingival Overgrowth
This 55-year-old male exhibited lesions of varying severity, with evidence of secondary inflammation. He had been taking "Adalat" (nifedipine) for two years because of his high blood pressure. The physician changed his medication to a different drug.

Right: The radiograph clearly shows that the gingival alterations were superimposed upon an existing periodontitis; the latter is *not* due to the drug.

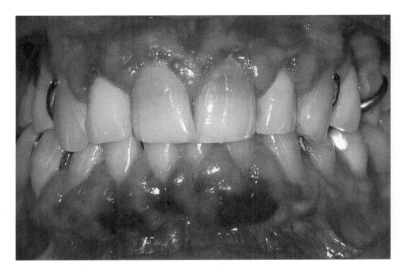
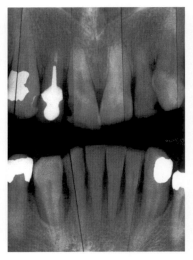

252 Nifedipine—Structure and Chemical Formula
This drug is a 1,4-dihydro-2,6-di-methyl-4-(2-nitrophenyl)-3,5-pyridine-dicarbonic acid dimethyl ester.

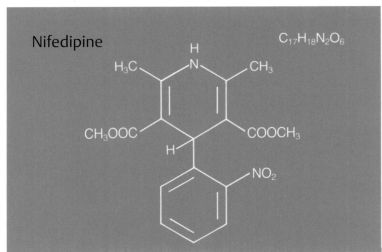

Nifedipine

$C_{17}H_{18}N_2O_6$

Nifedipine—Trade names (from 31 available preparations)

– Procardia
– Adalat
– Adapress
– Aldipin
– Alfadat
– Anifed
– Bonacid
– Hexadilat
– Nifelan
– Zenusin

Merck Index no. 6617

253 Severe Nifedipine-induced Gingival Overgrowth
This 58-year-old Black female presented with severe, secondarily highly inflamed gingival overgrowth. The patient had taken "Procardia" (nifedipine) for four years. Note also the mild gingival pigmentation.

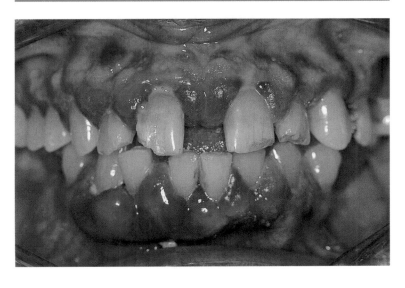

Cyclosporine-induced Gingival Overgrowth

The immunosuppressive effect of cyclosporine-A ("Sand-immune," Novartis Co.) derives from the suppression of antibody formation against *T cell*-dependent antigens, the suppression of cell-mediated immunity, and interference with the production of cytokines (IL-2 etc).

Systemic side effects occur frequently: increased blood pressure, increase in body hair (hirsutism), formation of lymphoma, as well as *nephro-* and *hepatotoxicity*.

The oral manifestation of cyclosporine is the side effect of gingival overgrowth, which is usually secondarily inflamed.

The incidence and severity of the gingival lesions are strictly dose-dependent and correlated to blood levels of the drug. New medicines (e.g., Prograf, Cellcept etc.) are reported to have fewer side effects.

Therapy: Good oral hygiene coupled with initial periodontal therapy can reduce both the inflammation and the overgrowth. If instituted early, such measures may actually prevent development. In severe cases, surgical gingivoplasty may be indicated. Organ transplant patients should receive comprehensive dental care *before* organ transplant (Rateitschak-Plüss et al. 1983a, b).

Cyclosporine-A—Trade names

– Cyclosporine-A
– Sandimmune
– Neoral

Merck Index no. 2821

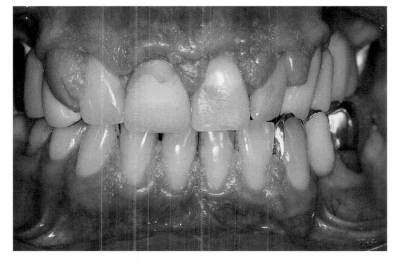

254 Mild to Moderate Cyclosporine-induced Gingival Overgrowth
This 45-year-old female began taking cyclosporine-A two years previously, following kidney transplantation. The gingival overgrowth is pronounced only in the maxilla; secondary inflammation is in evidence.
In order to avoid excessive doses of cyclosporine-A, this medicament is often combined today with azathioprine and/or cortisone.

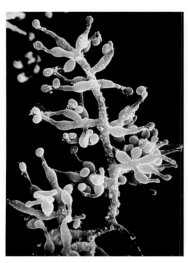

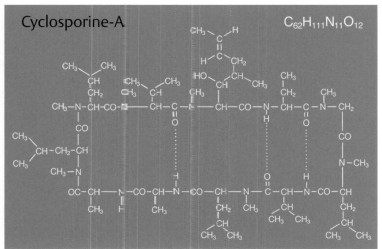

255 Cyclosporine-A—Structure and Chemical Formula
The drug is a cyclic peptide (undecapeptide) consisting of eleven amino acids. It is used to prevent rejection reactions following solid organ and bone marrow transplantation.

Left: Tolypocladium inflatum is the fungus from which cyclosporine was originally isolated during research on antibiotics.

SEM courtesy *R. Guggenheim*

Cyclosporine-A $C_{62}H_{111}N_{11}O_{12}$

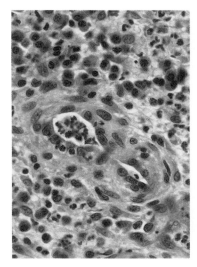

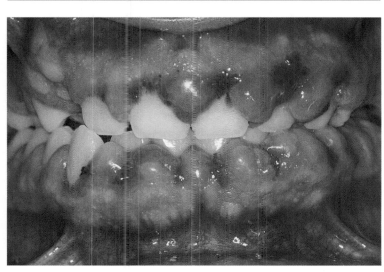

256 Severe Cyclosporine A-induced Gingival Overgrowth: Overdose
Dramatic enlargements such as in this 51-year-old female are infrequently observed today. This patient had received approximately three times the dosage of cyclosporine-A that is common today. In addition, the patient exhibited poor oral hygiene.

Left: PMN granulocytes and plasma cells are observed histologically in the infiltrated subepithelial connective tissue.

Gingival Hyperplasia Following Combined Drug Therapies

Dihydropyridine and Cyclosporine

When systemic medications are prescribed, every effort should be made to reduce adverse side effects by setting the dose as low as possible. In certain cases, the use of a *combination of medications* can also serve to reduce the dosage. For example, today, following organ transplantation (kidney, heart etc.), cyclosporine is often combined with azathioprine and prednisone.

On the other hand, the necessary combination of two medications that may *both* possess the same side effect (e.g., gingival overgrowth) may massively increase the adverse effect.

Therapy: In the case presented here, a 30-year-old male (kidney transplant), cyclosporine was prescribed. This medicament can increase blood pressure, so she was also treated with the calcium-antagonist nifedipine (p. 122). Very severe gingival overgrowth was the consequence of this co-medication. In such cases, alternative antihypertensive medications should be employed.

257 Severe Gingival Overgrowth
Simultaneous use of Sandimmune (cyclosporine-A) and Adalat (nifedipine), in conjunction with inadequate oral hygiene, led to severe and secondarily inflamed gingival overgrowth (with formation of pseudopockets) throughout the entire dentition.

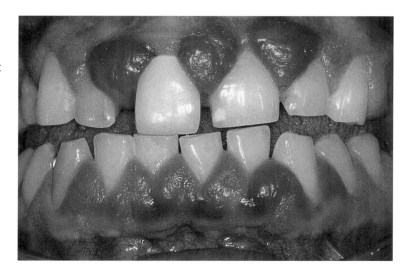

258 Following Gingivoplasty in the Maxilla
The "contouring" gingivectomy shown here in the maxillary anterior and canine regions was subsequently performed throughout the entire dentition.
Unfortunately, no particular efforts were expended to improve the patient's oral hygiene.

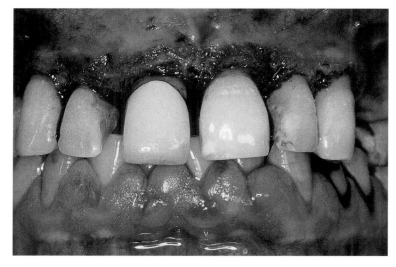

259 Recurrence in the Maxilla
Eight months after the surgery, a recurrence of the tissue overgrowth was obvious in the maxilla. This occurred despite changing the patient's antihypertensive medication to a different class of drugs (beta blocker). The patient's oral hygiene remains less than optimum.
Patients who have undergone a serious medical procedure such as organ transplantation have more important "problems" to deal with than the achievement of "maximal" oral hygiene!

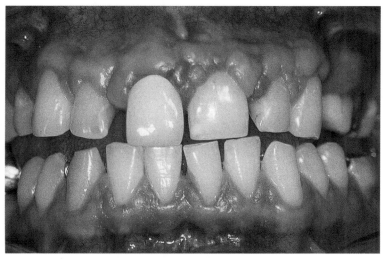

Benign Tumors—Epulis

Gingival epulis represents a family of benign tumors. The classification includes:

- Granulomatous epulis, pyogenic granuloma
- Giant cell epulis
- Fibrous epulis

Giant cell epulis and granulomatous epulis may develop relatively quickly; fibrous epulis grows slowly. The etiology of such tumors is not completely understood, but marginal irritation is one likely cause. Some pathologists contend that

giant cell epulis is the *only true epulis.* It is a fact that no histologic differences exist between fibrous epulis and fibromas in other areas of the oral cavity.

Therapy: Pyogenic granuloma and fibrous epulis can be removed by simple excision.

The giant cell epulis has a tendency to recur; following excision of such tumors, a gingival flap should be reflected, the tooth (and root) surfaces thoroughly cleaned and planed, and the bone filed.

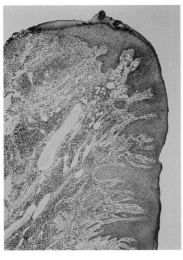

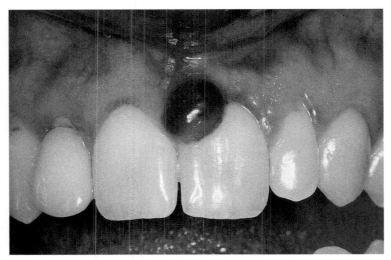

260 Pyogenic Granuloma, Granulomatous Epulis
Localized, tumor-like bright red, soft mass on the labial gingival margin in a 34-year-old female. Epulis is usually seen in the papillary region, and less frequently, as in the present case, on the gingival margin. When probed or injured, the lesion exudes a copious mixture of blood and pus.

Left: The histologic view exhibits a loose granulation tissue that is highly vascularized (HE, x40).

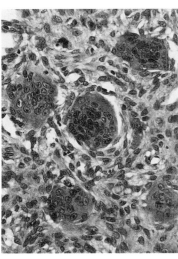

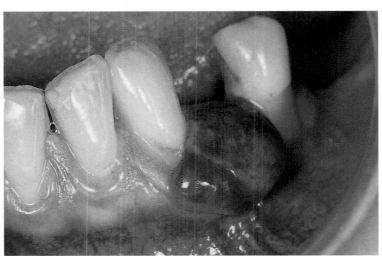

261 Giant Cell Epulis— "True" Epulis
Clinically resembling the granulomatous epulis, the giant cell epulis can only be differentiated and diagnosed histologically. Such lesions can become very large and, as in this 50-year-old female, can cause displacement of adjacent teeth.

Left: The histologic section reveals an inflammatory infiltrate including *multinucleated giant cells* in the subepithelial connective tissue (HE, x 400).

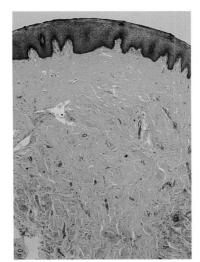

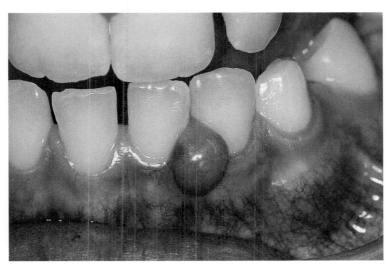

262 Fibrous Epulis
This 45-year-old female exhibited a localized, fibrous, firm mass upon the gingiva between the central and lateral incisors. The etiology of such lesions can only seldom be ascertained.

Left: Histologically one observes an accumulation of fibrous connective tissue. If the mass becomes secondarily inflamed, a typical inflammatory infiltrate can be expected.

Courtesy B. Maeglin

Benign Tumors—Fibrosis, Exostosis

The list of benign tumors of the oral cavity is long (Pindborg 1987, Reichart & Philipsen 1998). Mention will be made here of only *gingival* tumors, as well as gingival and osseous lesions that must be distinguished from the plaque-elicited, inflammatory swellings (gingivitis) and epulis:

- Fibrosis
- Exostosis
  - Verrucous hyperplasia, papilloma, hemangioma, gingival cysts, peripheral ameloblastoma, nevi

Fibrosis and exostosis may be localized or generalized on the gingiva. Their causes are for the most part unknown. Hassell & Jacoway (1981a, b) described a genetically determined (autosomal dominant) form of gingival hyperplasia (Elephantiasis gingivae).

Therapy: True gingival hyperplasia (histologically determined) is treated by simple gingivoplasty. Osseous thickening can be reduced by osteoplasty following flap reflection. These procedures may also be combined (Fig. 264, right). Recurrence is, however, frequent.

263 Hereditary Gingival Overgrowth

This 28-year-old male exhibited generalized gingival overgrowth with regionally varying severity. His family history revealed that similar gingival alterations had been observed in his father (who today wears a complete denture). The tissue overgrowth occasioned pseudopocket formation; these act as niches for plaque accumulation and therefore can lead to secondary inflammation. Following surgical resection, such overgrowth often recurs.

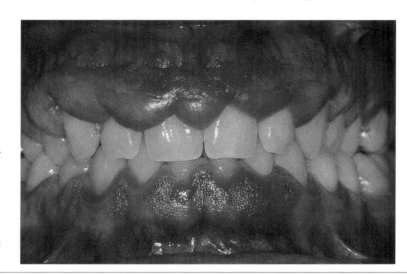

264 Idiopathic Gingival and Osseous Thickening

This 26-year-old female exhibited pronounced gingival overgrowth *and* osseous thickening. The latter could be diagnosed by passing a sterile injection needle through the soft tissue ("sounding").

Right: The treatment consisted of a combined procedure including gingivoplasty and osteoplasty following flap reflection. Depicted is the suture closure of the flap, which was previously thinned by external gingivectomy.

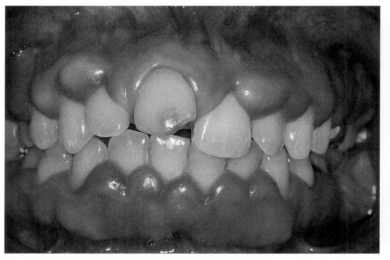
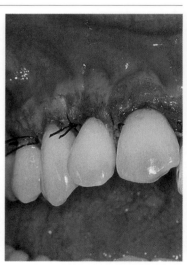

265 Exostosis

Exostosis is a harmless "idiopathic" thickening of bony tissue, whose cause is unknown (bruxism?). Such osseous lesions can be left untreated if they do not negatively influence function, well-being or periodontal health (niches?).
The maxillary right segment exhibits a particularly pronounced idiopathic osseous thickening, which could render oral hygiene more difficult.

Courtesy B. Maeglin

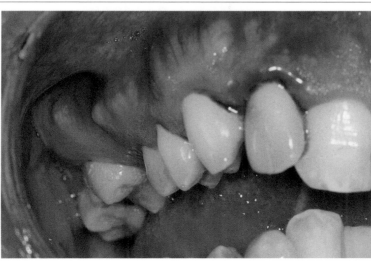

Malignant Tumors

- Carcinoma
- Melanoma
- Sarcoma (chondrosarcoma, fibrosarcoma, rhabdomyosarcoma, lymphoma etc.)

Malignant epithelial and mesenchymal tumors are frequently observed on the mucosa of the oral cavity. In the Western world, oral carcinoma accounts for 1–5 % of all carcinomas (Pindborg 1987). Malignant tumors are, however, seldom observed on the *gingiva*.

In addition to *primary tumors*, the gingiva may also be the recipient site for metastases, from the kidneys, lungs, prostrate, breast or other organs.

Therapy: If there exists even the slightest suspicion of malignancy, the patient should be referred immediately to the oral surgeon, who may perform diagnosis, biopsy and frozen-section diagnosis, as well as radical surgical removal, radiotherapy and/or chemotherapy. The dentist should avoid manipulation of the tumor mass, and should never attempt a biopsy!

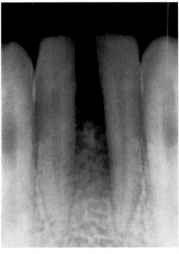
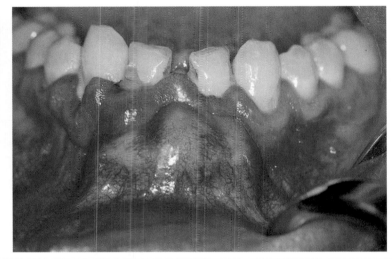

266 Chondrosarcoma
This 25-year-old female complained of a large swelling in the mandibular anterior area. The tumor extended from the gingiva into the oral mucosa and was ca. 2 cm wide. Histopathologic diagnosis: Highly differentiated chondrosarcoma. Metastases had not been detected up to this time.

Left: The radiograph reveals resorption of bone between the mandibular central incisors.

All photos courtesy *B. Maeglin*

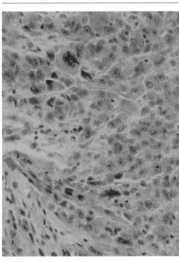
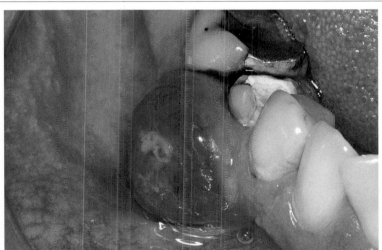

267 Rhabdomyosacroma
A large, epulis-like swelling in a 38-year-old female was diagnosed by the pathologist as the rare malignant rhabdomyosacroma. The tumor grows by invading the alveolar bone. Metastasis to other skeletal sites occurs rapidly.

Left: The histologic picture is one of growth of "strands" of the malignant tissue. Note the dramatic number of mitotic figures (HE, x400).

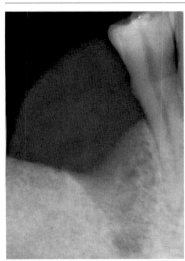
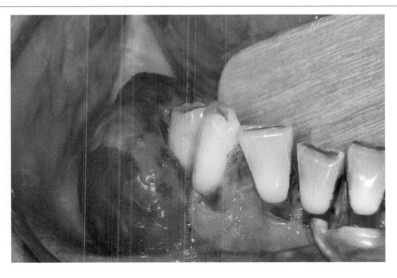

**268 Adenocarcinoma—
Metastasis**
Poor wound healing occurred in this 63-year-old male following extraction of tooth 45. A large swelling developed one month later on the right side of the mandible. Histopathologic diagnosis: Poorly differentiated, clear cell adenocarcinoma. (Metastasis from prostate carcinoma!)

Left: The radiograph depicts the non-healing alveolus of tooth 45.

Gingivosis / Pemphigoid

Mild forms of gingivosis (desquamative gingivitis) are characterized by spotty gingival erythema. In more severe cases, epithelial desquamation occurs. If blister formation is also in evidence, the clinical descriptor is pemphigoid.

Therapy: True "causal" therapy is not possible. Therapy therefore is polypragmatic and symptomatic (pain medications and vitamin-A containing ointments). In severe cases (pemphigoid) topical (and systemic) corticosteroid preparations may be indicated.

Pemphigus vulgaris

Pemphigus vulgaris may affect the skin, as well as all mucosal surfaces and the gingiva. With or without blister formation, the epithelial layer sloughs, leaving behind expansive and painful erosions. The histologic diagnosis may be substantiated by immunofluorescence serology and by identification of "Tzanck cells."

Therapy: Immunosuppressive drugs and systemic corticosteroids. The painful lesions can be treated topically and symptomatically with ointments containing cortisone and antibiotics. The prognosis is relatively poor.

269 Gingivosis/Desquamative Gingivitis
Severe, spotty erythema of the attached gingiva in this 62-year-old female. Epithelium can be easily separated from subepithelial connective tissues. Secondary gingivitis is elicited by plaque.

Right: Histology exhibits a thin oral epithelium (**OE**) devoid of rete ridges and not keratinized. The epithelium has separated (carbol fuchsin, x100).

Courtesy *H. Mühlemann*

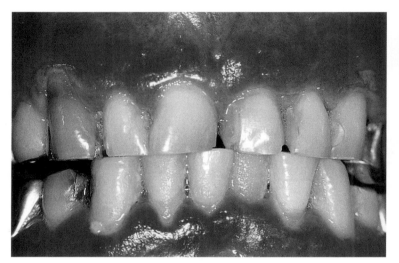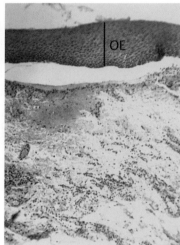

270 Pemphigoid
There are no strict criteria for clinical differentiation between gingivosis and pemphigoid. In this 54-year-old female, one observes a severe, marginally localized erythema of the gingiva. The patient reported recurring blister formation, especially on the lingual aspect.

Right: Blister formation and sloughing of the epithelium in another patient with pemphigoid.

Courtesy *U. Saxer*

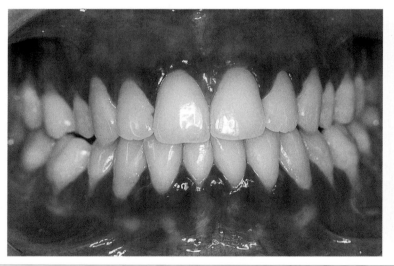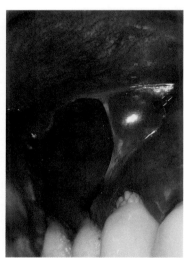

271 Pemphigus vulgaris
Fiery red gingiva with secondary effluorescences (burst vesicles). This 50-year-old female also manifested pronounced symptoms on her skin and on other areas of the oral mucosa.
Right: It is obvious that vesicle formation and sloughing of the superficial layer of gingiva occurs intra-epithelially. The basal cell layer remains attached to the connective tissue.
OE = oral epithelium (HE, x250).

Courtesy *B. Maeglin*

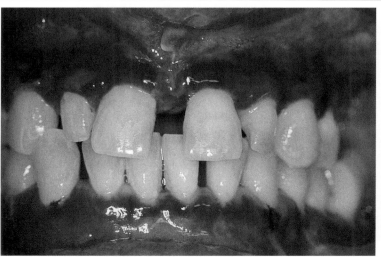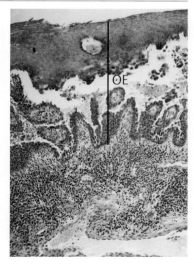

Lichen planus: Reticular and Erosive

Lichen (intertwined) is a general term for a family of similar-appearing yet differentiable skin (lichen ruber) and mucosal alterations (lichen planus *reticularis, erosivus, nitidus, pilaris, acutus, verrucosis* etc.). Lichen occurs relatively frequently; morbidity figures of 0.2–1.9 % of the adult populations have been reported (Axéll 1976).

The symptoms of reticular lichen planus are milky-white, pebbly, hyperkeratotic effluorescences and/or net-like coatings, the so-called "Wickham's striae." The white lesions may also be expansive (plaque-forming type) and resemble a leukoplakia. The affected mucosa may atrophy (atrophic form), and may subsequently erode (erosive lichen planus; pre-malignant?).

Therapy: There is no true causal therapy. The lesions should be monitored closely. Treatment for erosive forms include systemic administration of corticosteroids, often combined with retinoids.

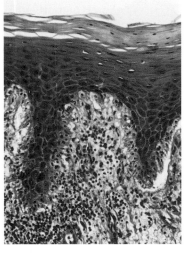
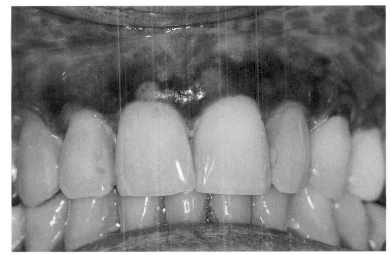

272 Lichen Planus
This 42-year-old male presented with generalized erythema as well as a whitish, hyperkeratotic, net-like coating (Wickham's striae) on the gingiva and oral mucosa, as well as secondary gingivitis.

Left: Histologically the epithelium exhibits rete ridges and appears to be hyperkeratinized. A subepithelial inflammatory infiltrate is visible (HE, x400).

Courtesy B. Maeglin

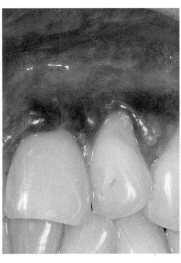
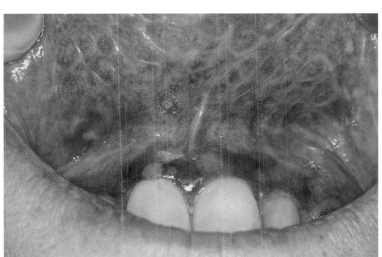

273 Reticular Lichen Planus (Wickham's Striae)
In addition to the red and whitish gingival lesions, the pronounced striae of this lesion are impressive, extending from the vestibular fold and covering the entire mucosa of the internal surface of the lip.

Courtesy B. Maeglin

Left: Bullous lichen with secondary gingivitis.

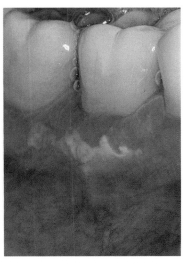
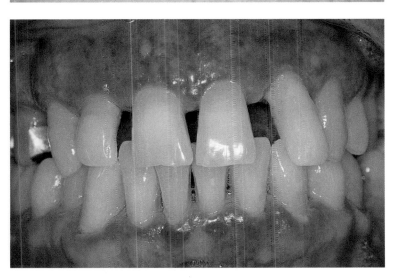

274 Erosive Lichen
Red-whitish spots, some of which show initial, quite painful erosions (rendering oral hygiene difficult!). Secondary plaque-induced gingivitis.

Left: The lesions extend over the entire gingiva into the molar region.

Periodontitis with Systemic Diseases (Type IV)—Diabetes Type I and Type II

Numerous investigations of the relationships between Diabetes mellitus and gingivitis/periodontitis have been published. Most investigators found correlations between uncontrolled or poorly controlled diabetes and gingivitis/periodontitis (Firatli 1997; Salvi et al. 1997; Tervonen & Karjalainen1997; Katz 2001). Today, diabetes is an established risk factor.

One explanation for this could be the defects of polymorphonuclear granulocytes (PMNs) that are regularly observed in diabetes patients (Manouchehr-Pour et al. 1981a,

b). Furthermore, the hyperglycemia increases the presence of AGE (advanced glycated end-product), which stimulates the macrophage receptor (RAGE) toward increased synthesis of TNFα, IL-1β and IL-6. Both the form and function of extracellular matrix components, such as collagen, become altered.

It is possible that the vascular pathology associated with diabetes (cf. retinopathy, Fig. 285) may also play a role in terms of periodontal blood supply, but this has yet to be proven (Rylander et al. 1987).

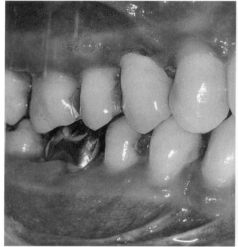
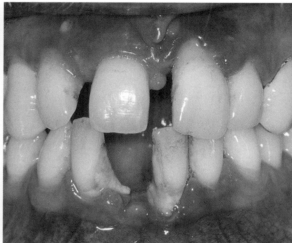
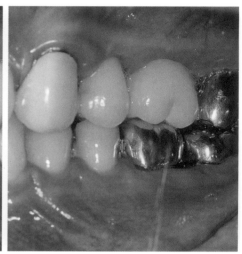

281 Clinical Overview (above)
Localized acute inflammation of the gingivae, which exhibit some edematous swelling as well as areas of shrinkage. Plaque and calculus are abundant. Almost all of the deeper pockets exhibit signs of activity (pus).

282 Probing Depths, Gingival Recession (Re) and Tooth Mobility (TM, right)
Immediately apparent is the extraordinarily irregular attachment loss. Probing depths in the interproximal areas ranged from 4 to 12 mm. Some teeth exhibited extreme mobility (cf. radiographic survey).

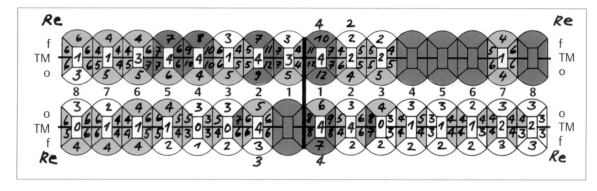

283 Radiographic Survey
The radiographs confirm the clinical findings. Teeth 15, 14, 12, 21 and 32 had to be extracted on an emergency basis.

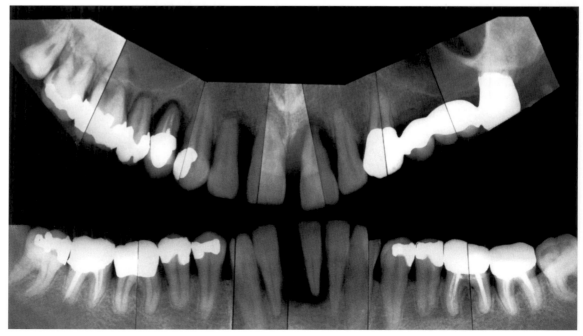

A 28-year-old male had developed severe, *insulin-dependent juvenile diabetes* at age 15. The associated periodontitis had never been treated.

Findings :
API: 69%   PBI: 3.2
Probing depth, gingival recession and tooth mobility: see Fig. 281.

Diagnosis: Rapidly progressing, advanced periodontitis in conjunction with juvenile diabetes.

Therapy: The treatment plan for patients with juvenile diabetes is usually rather radical.
– Maxilla: Extraction of all teeth with the exception of teeth 13 and 23 (periodontal treatment); temporary partial denture.
– Mandible: Extraction of the remaining anterior teeth and the third molars. Periodontal treatment of the remaining teeth, cast framework partial denture. Dental implants are not indicated in diabetes patients.

Recall: Initially, every 3 months.

Prognosis for the abutment teeth: "Guarded" at best, in view of the proposed radical therapy.

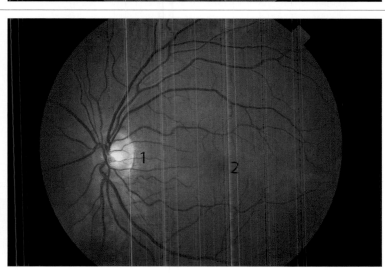

284 Maxillary Anterior Area—Initial Findings
Diastemata had formed over the course of the previous years. Tooth 21 appears elongated, exhibits no bony support, is highly mobile and painful (see radiographic survey, Fig. 283). It was extracted along with the other teeth after a temporary removable partial denture was constructed.

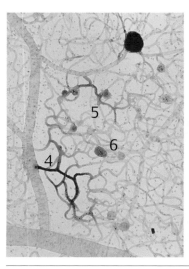
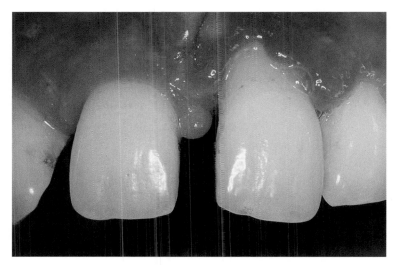

285 Retinoscopy in Diabetic Retinopathy
1 Yellow lipid bodies in the retina
2 Disseminated hemorrhage and microaneurysms
3 Neovascularization bundle due to ischemia

Left: Histologic view of diabetic retinal microangiopathy
4 Closure of a precapillary
5 Atrophic capillaries, cell-free zone
6 Microaneurysms

(Trypsin digestion, x25)

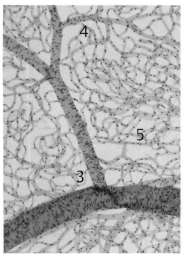
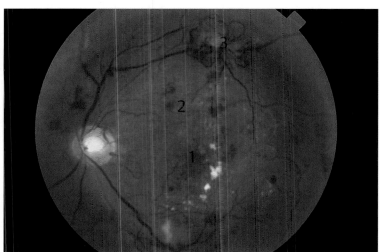

286 Normal Retinoscopy, Healthy Eye
1 Optic nerve papilla with exiting retinal vessels
2 Macula free of vasculature

Left: Normal histology of the retina
3 Retinal arterioles
4 Precapillaries
5 Capillaries

(Trypsin digestion, HE, x25)

Courtesy *B. Daicker*

Periodontitis Associated with Systemic Diseases (Type IV B)
Down Syndrome, Trisomy 21, "Mongolism"

Trisomy 21 (previously: Mongolism) carries the name of John Langdon Down who first described the condition in detail in 1866 (Rett 1983; literature review by Reuland-Bosme and Van Dijk 1986). The basis for this condition is a chromosomal aberration: During meiosis, which is the cell division process for reproductive cells, the separation of the paired chromosome 21 does not occur during nuclear division. Two homologues fail to disjoin at the first meiotic division, and therefore two of the resulting gametes carry a "double dose" of the chromosome. Thus, instead of a zygote containing one chromosome 21 from the male and one chromosome 21 from the female, the genotype of the zygote contains three chromosomes at position 21 (trisomy 21; see karyotype, Fig. 290).

Mongolism occurs at a rate of one in about every 700 live births. It is likely, however, that the prevalence of mongolism will diminish significantly in the future as a result of increased use of ultrasound prenatal analysis and amniocentesis, as well as more liberal abortion laws (Schmid 1988).

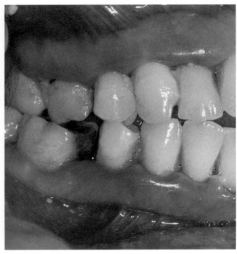
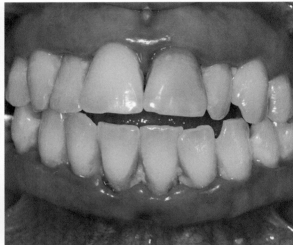
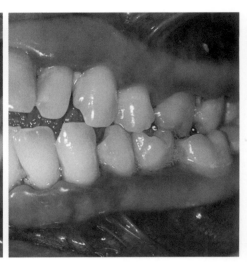

287 Clinical Overview (above)
Poor plaque control, severe gingivitis, anterior open bite, crossbite and end-to-end occlusion in molar segments.

288 Probing Depths and Tooth Mobility (TM, right)
The deeper pockets exhibit signs of activity. As a result of the massive attachment loss, all teeth exhibit varying degrees of mobility.

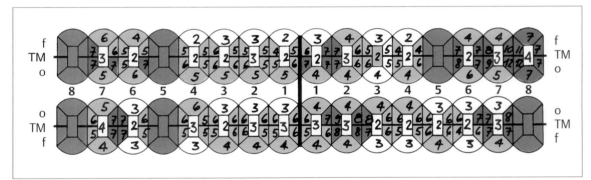

289 Radiographic Survey
The radiographs corroborate the generalized and profound attachment loss: Horizontal and in some areas vertical bone loss of up to two-thirds of the root length. The widened periodontal ligament space anticipates the elevated tooth mobility.
Tooth 21 is non-vital and exhibits an apical radiolucency.

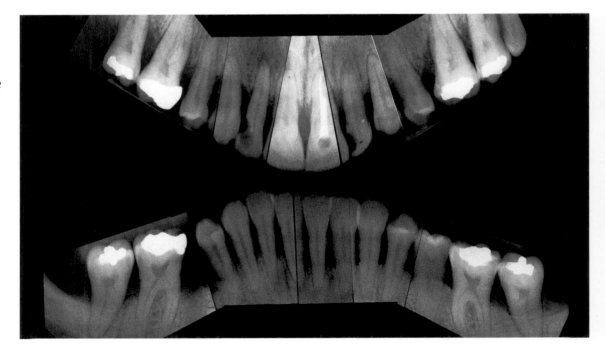

This 27-year-old female (without cardiac complications) has the mental development of a 6-year-old. She was raised in her parent's home, is well cared for and can converse readily. For these reasons every attempt was made to maintain as many teeth as possible.

Findings:
    API: 100%   PBI: 3.8
    Probing depths and tooth mobility: See Fig. 288.
Diagnosis: Advanced, rapidly progressive periodontitis in this patient with Down Syndrome.

Therapy: Professional debridement and oral hygiene instruction. (Tooth brushing by the patient, interdental cleaning by her mother).
    Modified Widman surgical procedures in all quadrants; extraction of teeth 17, 27, 28, 37 and 47.
Recall: Frequent but brief appointments.
Prognosis: Patient compliance will always be poor. Plaque control will depend for the most part on her caretakers. The prognosis is therefore guarded.

Thanks to today's modern medical treatments, the life expectancy for Trisomy 21 patients has increased dramatically in the past few decades.

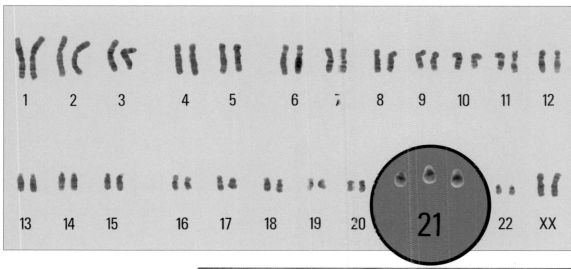

290 Karyotype in Trisomy 21
The abnormal chromosomal picture results from triplication of the small autosome 21. This "Trisomy 21" occurs in about 94% of all "mongoloid" patients.

Modified from *H. Müller*

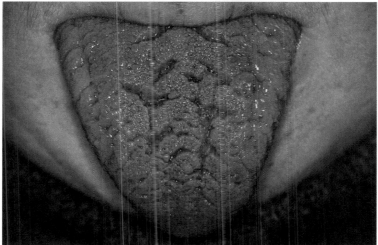

291 Symptoms of Down Syndrome—
Scrotal (Fissured) Tongue
The deeply fissured tongue is one of the typical symptoms in Down Syndrome.

Symptoms of Down Syndrome:
– Scrotal tongue
– Ocular peculiarity
– Small head
– Stocky physique
– Short, soft hands
– Cardiac defects (one-third have a short life expectancy)

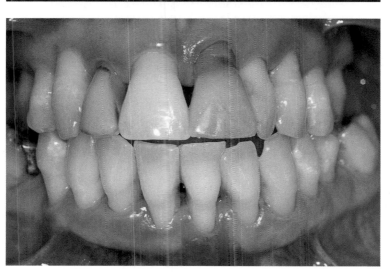

292 7 Years After Treatment
Following initial therapy, the entire dentition was treated by means of modified Widman surgical procedures. The end result, 7 years after the final surgery, was an acceptable result in comparison to the initial situation. A short-interval recall is recommended, and possibly also the use of a custom tray for daily application of chlorhexidine gel.

Pre-pubertal Periodontitis Associated with Systemic Disease
Papillon-Lefèvre Syndrome (Type IV B)

Papillon-Lefèvre Syndrome (PLS) is a rare, inherited, *autosomal recessive*, "dermatologic" disease (Haneke 1979). Obligate symptoms include severe periodontitis and hyperkeratoses, usually localized to the palms and soles of the feet, as well as other skin areas that commonly absorb minor trauma (HPP = *Hyperkeratosis palmaris* and *plantaris*).
The deciduous teeth are lost prematurely in most cases. The permanent teeth are always periodontally involved.
The primary etiologic factors include a mutation of the cathepsin-C gene (chromosome 11q14-q21; Hart et al.

1998), which regulates epithelial cells and immune cells, as well as a particularly aggressive pocket flora (gram-negative anaerobes).
Earlier therapeutic attempts were without success. During the 1980's, however, Preus & Gjermo (1987) as well as Tinanoff et al. (1986) reported that extraction of the deciduous teeth as well as the already present permanent teeth in a 9-year-old patient led to maintenance of the subsequently erupting permanent teeth.

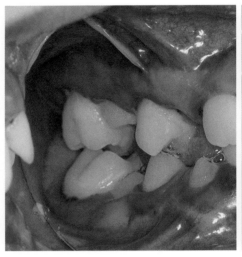
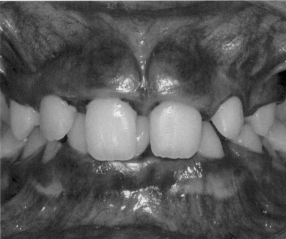
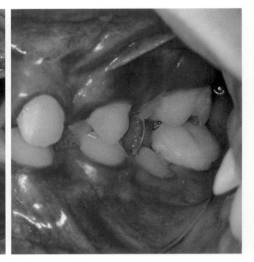

293 Clinical Overview (above)
Extremely severe gingivitis and periodontitis, plaque, spontaneous hemorrhage, exudate and suppuration from the pockets. Initial abscess formation on the facial of 11 and 21. Poor occlusion, severe overbite.

294 Probing Depths and Tooth Mobility (right)
All of the deeper pockets exhibit signs of advanced activity (pus).

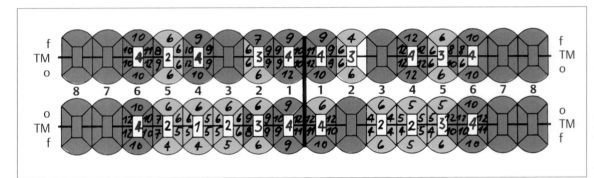

295 Radiographic Survey
The marked (∗) teeth

· ·	6	·	4	·	·	1	1	·	·	4	·	6	· ·
· ·	6	·	·	·	·	1	1	·	·	·	·	6	· ·

are all in the process of being spontaneously exfoliated, and will be immediately extracted (plaque-retentive niches). Periodontal destruction appears to begin after eruption of the teeth, and subsequently progresses rapidly. Vertical defects (infrabony pockets) predominate. Class F3 furcation involvements.

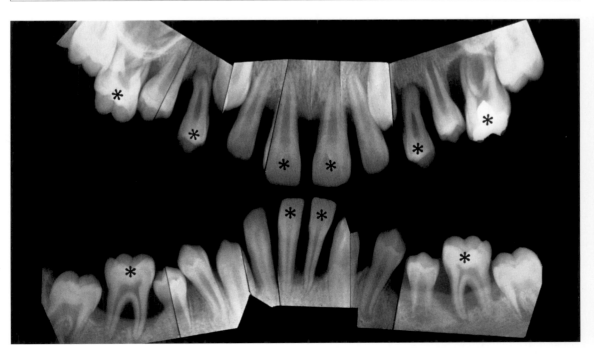

A 9-year-old boy was referred from his pediatrician because of severe halitosis and extreme tooth mobility.

Findings:
API: 100% PBI: 3.9
Probing depths, radiographic survey, tooth mobility and skin lesions: See figures below.
Special findings: PMN defects, specific pocket flora (*Porphyromonas* and spirochetes).
Diagnosis: Acute, severe pre-pubertal periodontitis associated with Papillon-Lefèvre Syndrome.

Therapy: Extraction of the hopeless teeth (Fig. 295; note asterisks on teeth to be extracted).
Mechanical periodontal debridement and simultaneous topical (chlorhexidine) and systemic (metronidazol/tetracycline) treatment; temporary removable partial denture (hygiene).
Recall: Very short interval.
Prognosis: Teeth that can be "saved" beyond puberty may be maintained over the long term (see next case, p. 138).

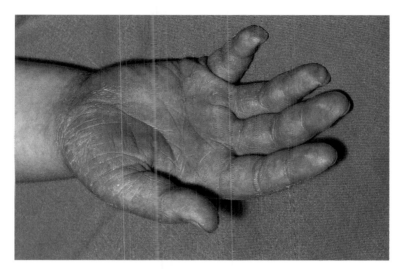

Papillon-Lefèvre Syndrome PLS with Palmar and Plantar Hyperkeratosis

296 Hyperkeratosis on the Palm of the Hand
The hyperkeratotic area exhibits cracks and fissures, which are actually wounds that have occurred due to normal function. These heal poorly and slowly. The patient suffers from these palmar lesions especially in winter.

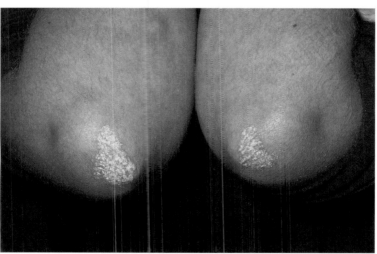

297 Hyperkeratosis on the Elbows

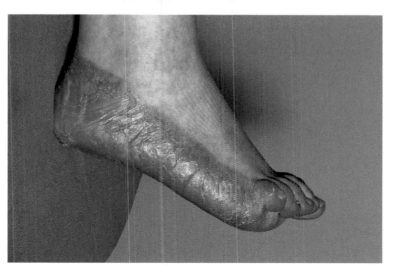

298 Hyperkeratosis on the Foot
The sharp line of demarcation between hyperkeratotic areas and normal-appearing skin on the lateral border of the foot correspond to the outline of the shoe worn by this patient.

Minor trauma to the skin elicits this type of severe hyperkeratotic response. Even dermatologists treat this disease only symptomatically and polypragmatically.

Papillon-Lefèvre Syndrome—"An Exception for Every Rule"

A 7-year-old girl was referred to the dental clinic because of severe mobility of her recently erupted permanent incisors and first molars. The patient remained under dental care for 24 years thereafter.

As a teenager, the patient was reconciled to wearing a cast framework partial denture. At age 18, she underwent surgery to correct her mandibular prognathism (note osteosynthesis wires in the radiograph, Fig. 301). At age 25, the remaining dentition was treated with splinted total reconstructions in both mandible and maxilla, which were cemented temporarily.

Diagnosis: Acute, severe periodontitis in a case of Papillon-Lefèvre Syndrome (PLS).

Course of the disease, and treatment: In this exceptional case, it was possible to retain a large number of permanent teeth as a result of timely extractions, intensive periodontitis therapy, frequent recall and the excellent cooperation of the patient (Fig. 301).

It is worthy of note that the treatment rendered 24 years ago was purely mechanical and did not include any systemic or topical supportive medicinal therapy.

299 Radiographic and Dental Survey of the 7-year-old Female

Erupted permanent teeth:

```
· · 6 · · · 2 1  1 2 · · · 6 · ·
· · 6 · · · 2 1 │1 2 · · · 6 · ·
```

The first permanent molars were exfoliated one year after eruption. The mandibular anterior teeth exhibit severe periodontitis. All permanent teeth are present (as yet unerupted).
The primary teeth were lost prematurely.

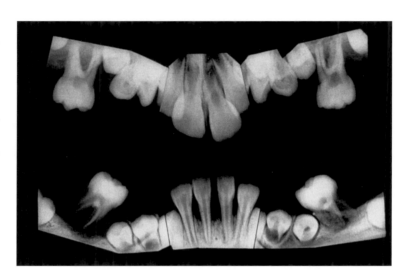

300 Same Patient, Age 31
The patient smiles with (many of) her own teeth, which were deemed to be "hopeless" due to her Papillon-Lefèvre syndrome. She displays advanced hyperkeratosis on both palms, and painful cracks and chapping on her heel. The skin on the back of her hands is paper thin, hyperkeratotic, dry and visibly erythematous.

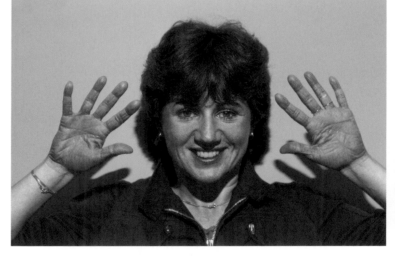
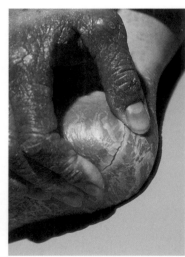

301 Radiographic Survey of the 31-year-old Female
Destructive periodontitis came to a halt after the patient traversed puberty. The remaining teeth served as abutments for fixed bridgework:

```
8 7 · · · 3 · · │· · 3 · 5 · · 8
8 7 · 5 4 · · · │· · · 4 5 · 7 8
```

This bridgework is seated only temporarily (Temp-Bond), and is periodically removed, cleaned and re-cemented.

Radiographs courtesy *U. Saxer*

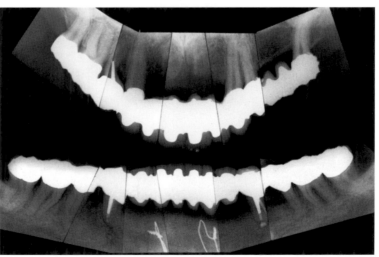

HIV Infection—AIDS

The immune deficiency disease AIDS (Acquired Immunodeficiency Syndrome) is caused by the HIV virus 1, a retrovirus. It is a complex virus, whose RNA genome (8,700 bases) contains at least nine genes. The three most important of these nine are *env* (virus capsule protein), *gag* (group-specific antigen) and *pol* (polymerase, enzyme-coding portion in the retrovirus genome; Fig. 302).

The virus exhibits the following structural characteristics: an RNA genome at the center of which the reverse transcriptase (RT, p66 *pol*-gene product) is bound; *gag*-coded proteins determine the virion structure; the phospholipid membrane (PL) provided by the host; two *env* gene products; a membrane-penetrating (gp 41) glycoprotein and an externally localized glycoprotein (knobs, gp 120) anchored to it. Three genes (*tat, rev, nef*) have regulatory functions. The specific functions of the remaining genes have not yet been completely elucidated.

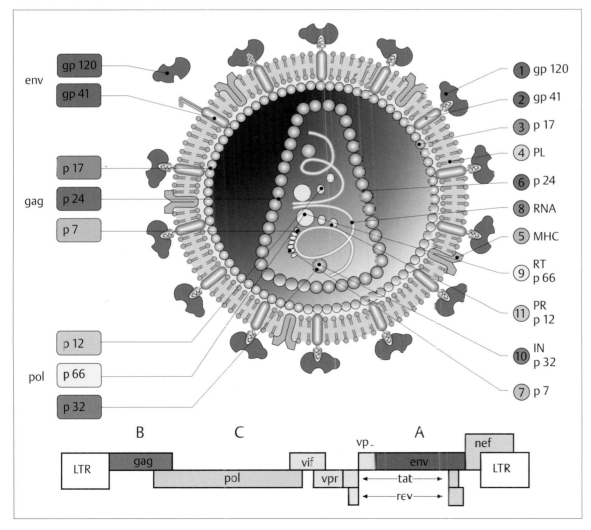

302 HI Virus
The *env*-, *gag*- and *pol*-coded proteins (**p**) and glycoproteins (**gp**) are shown at the left, and all other structures (**1–11**) on the right.

HIV Envelope
– *Virus-coded*

1	Knob bodies	gp120
2	Transmembrane portion	gp41
3	Capsule matrix	p17

– *Host-coded*

4	Phospholipid bilayer	
5	MHC-proteins (receptors, p. 46)	

Capsid/Core

6	Capsomere proteins	p24
7	RNA capsule protein	p7

Genome/Enzymes

8	HIV-RNA, 2 single strands	
9	**RT** reverse transcriptase	p66
10	**IN** integrase	p32
11	**PR** protease	p12

HIV Genome (below)

A *env*-coded viral surface proteins (binding sites for CD4 and membrane fusion)

B *gag*-coded nucleocapsid and nuclear membrane

C *pol*-coded for the enzymes RT, IN, PR and ribonucleases

HIV Disease—Epidemiology

The world wide dissemination of the HIV disease continues to increase. At the end of 2002, over 41,000,000 persons were infected with the HI virus. There are grave differences between the industrialized nations on the one hand and the developing countries on the other: While in the USA, Western Europe, Japan, Australia and New Zealand the new infections of adults have generally stabilized, the rates for the African countries south of the Sahara Desert, and in Russia continue to increase. At the present time, two thirds of all the HIV-infected adults are found in sub-Saharan Africa and Russia, and 90% of all infected children!

Unprotected heterosexual intercourse, the dissemination of uncontrolled blood products and above all the lack of prevention (information), as well as the enormous costs of treatment may be responsible for the current situation. Even more perplexing is the fact that the HI virus appears in various types and subtypes (Reichart & Gelderblom 1998, Reichart & Philipsen 1999), which makes efforts toward treatment or even immunization infinitely more complex. The battle against the AIDS pandemic must also be waged against the socioeconomic backdrop.

Ninety percent of all HIV-infected individuals world wide live in developing countries, but 90% of all monies spent for information, prevention and treatment are expended in the industrialized countries—ca. $10,000 per infected person per year.

Epidemiologic research has shown that we must differentiate not only between countries and their various stages of economic development. Even within the industrialized nations, there are clear differences between persons of different socioeconomic classes. For example, in the USA the infection rate for Blacks is almost five times higher than for white males. The difference between Afro-American and Caucasian females in the USA is even more dramatic (Fig. 304, right).

Because it is extremely unlikely that the differences between industrialized and developing nations, as well as between different socioeconomic standards will ever be reconciled, the highest priority must be given to the development of effective and inexpensive medicines, and above all an effective vaccine (Mann and Tarantola 1998).

303 World Wide Distribution of HIV-infected Individuals, 1997
By far the majority of HIV-infected person live in sub-Saharan Africa (20,800,000), as well as in south and southeast Asia (6,000,000), followed by Latin America (1,800,000).
Various HIV subtypes (A–G) can be differentiated.
Type B predominates (80%) in Europe and North America.

By the end of 2002, over 41,000,000 persons world wide were infected with HIV.

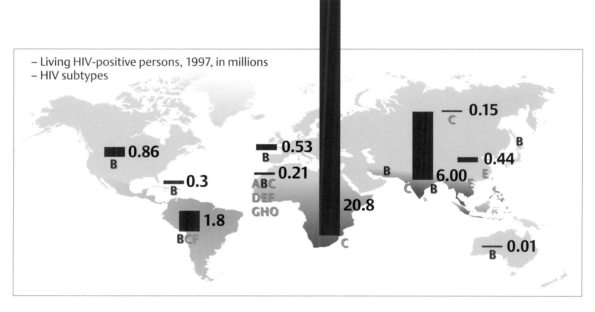

304 Increase in HIV-infected Adults, 1980–1998

Left: In the industrialized countries, the number of infected adults has decreased somewhat, following the initial increase. South of the Sahara Desert—but also in south and southeast Asia—a dramatic increase occurred.

Right: New infections per 100,000 adults and adolescents in the USA, 1996; the numbers are higher in individuals in lower socioeconomic groups.

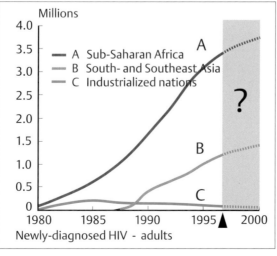

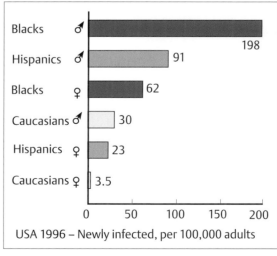

Classification and Clinical Course of HIV Disease

With ever-increasing knowledge, the classification of the HIV disease has already been modified many times, and additional variations will surely be implemented in the future. The classification derives from data from the USA *Centers for Disease Control and Prevention* (CDCP). This classification is based on the number of CD4 cells (stages 1–3) in relation to clinical symptoms (stages A-C) (Fig. 305).

Besides this classification, today the most significant parameter of the clinical course of disease is the number of free virus copies per milliliter of blood plasma, the so-called "viral load." This is determined using the polymerase chain reaction (PCR).

HIV disease develops very rapidly following the initial infection. Billions of HIV particles destroy millions of CD4 lymphocytes. This bitter "war of attrition" between HI viruses and host cells goes on continually for years. During the further (average) course of the disease—about 6 months after infection—the number of freely circulating viruses decreases dramatically and the number of immune cells again increases. A balance between attack and defense can remain constant for ca. 10 years, until the number of viruses again increases dramatically and the host defense breaks down (Fig. 306).

Even from patient to patient, the disease can assume extraordinarily different clinical courses. "Long survivors" are those individuals who live longer than 10 years after infection, while others with the disease have only a short post-infection life span. A prognosis concerning the course of the disease is possible by measuring the viral load. Mellors (1998) measured the viral load in 1,600 untreated HIV-infected males, and reported that 70 % of his study population who exhibited more than 30,000 virus copies per milliliter of blood plasma died within six years (mean lifespan: 4.4 years). In contrast, less than 1 % of the untreated patients died within six years if their viral load was below 500 copies/ml. In the latter group, the mean life expectancy was more than 10 years.

It is now clear that the determination of viral load provides important information concerning prognosis and therapy. Using today's anti-retroviral medicinal polytherapy (p. 149), the number of virus particles can be held below the level of detection.

Clinic. symptomatic ▶ Grade – CD4+-cell no. ▼	**A** Asymptomatic or acute HIV infection	**B** ARC syncrome, e g, oral candidiasis	**C** AIDS indicator diseases
1 >500	A1	B1	C1
2 200–500	A2	B2	C2
3 <200	A3	B3	C3

305 CDCP Classification
Close scrutiny of the CDCP classification clearly reveals that patients with a relatively high number of CD4 cells may already exhibit AIDS symptoms (**C2**), while, on the other hand, infected individuals with only low levels of CD4-cells may remain asymptomatic (**A2**).

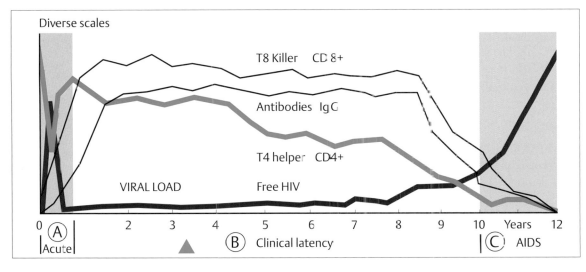

306 "Average" Clinical Course of HIV Disease
Immediately following HIV infection, there follows a ca. 6-month acute phase (bouts of fever, lymphadenitis etc), followed by a years-long asymptomatic period. This is characterized by a low *viral load* and a positive immune response (T-helper and T-killer cells, antibodies etc.). On average, 8–12 years later, the viral load increases and host defense collapses. The "average" clinical course depicted here varies significantly from patient to patient.

Oral Manifestations of HIV Disease

In addition to numerous somatic symptoms, the HIV disease can also be characterized by pronounced oral manifestations. The progress in systemic medical therapy has fortunately reduced many oral symptoms, e. g., bacterial and fungal infections, viral infections, neoplasms and other pathology of unknown etiology (Fig. 307).

The oral lesions are often painful and can compromise the patient's quality of life. The time of appearance of oral manifestations will be determined by the CD4 cell count and the viral load (Fig. 308). Occasionally, however, oral alterations—especially linear gingival erythema (LGE) and necrotizing periodontitis (NUP)—occur at unpredictable times during the course of the HIV disease.

The dentist must be fully aware of the oral manifestations of HIV disease; in numerous cases, a dentist has diagnosed oral alterations that lead to suspicion of HIV infection, only to have those suspicions subsequently corroborated after medical examination by the physician.

307 Some Oral Manifestations of HIV Disease
Most of the alterations (listed to the right) can be diagnosed by the dentist. LGE, NUG and NUP can only be treated in the dental practice (p. 151). All other disease manifestations must be treated in collaboration with the physician.

Non-specific Bacterial Infections	Fungal Infections	Neoplasms
• Linear gingival erythema (LGE) • Necrotizing ulcerative gingivitis (NUG) and periodontitis (NUP) • Exacerbation of periapical processes	• Candidiasis • Histoplasmosis	• Kaposi sarcoma • Non-Hodgkin lymphoma • Spinal cell carcinoma
	Viral Infections	**Unknown Etiology**
Specific Bacterial infections	• Human herpes viruses (HHV) • Herpetic stomatitis • Human papilloma virus (HPV) (Details, see pp. 131, 145)	• Delayed wound healing • Aphthae • Ulcerations • Pigmentations • Idiopathic thrombocytopenia (hemorrhage) • Xerostomia • Salivary gland disorders
• MAI (Intracellular *Mycobacterium avium*) • *Enterobacter cloacae*		

308 Occurrence of Disease in Correlation with the CD4 Cell Number ("Marker" Diseases)
While *candidiasis* can occur relatively early, the severe systemic diseases such as *Pneumocystis carinii pneumonia* (PcP), *Toxoplasmosis, infections with intracellular Mycobacterium avium* (MAI), *Cytomegalovirus (CMV) pneumonia* etc. occur only when the CD4 cell count drops.

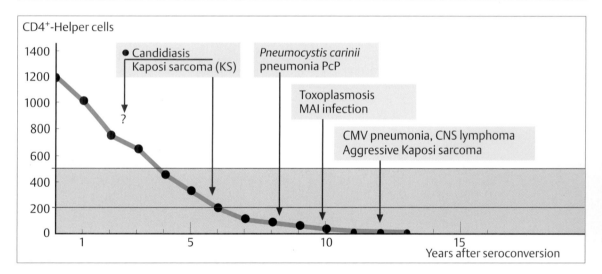

309 Association Between Certain Oral Symptoms and HIV Disease
The frequency of occurrence of these opportunistic diseases is also dependent on the stage of the HIV disease (Weinert et al. 1996).

Most Frequent Occurrence +++	Occasionally Occurring ++	Seldom Occurring +
• **Candidiasis** • **Hairy Leukoplakia** • **LGE** • **NUG/NUP** • **Kaposi Sarcoma** • **Non-Hodgkin Lymphoma**	• Bacterial infections such as tuberculosis (frequent in S. Africa) • MAI • Viral infections (Herpes simplex virus, Varicella-zoster virus, Papilloma virus) • Atypical ulcerations • Thrombocytopenic purpura • Salivary gland alterations • Pigmentations	• Fungal infections (except Candida) • Other poorly understood infections • Neurologic disturbances, viral infections (cytomegalovirus etc.) • Recurring aphthous stomatitis • Reactions to medicaments

Bacterial Infections in HIV

- Linear gingival erythema (LGE)
- Necrotizing gingivitis/periodontitis (NUG/NUP)

The disease states marked with a solid bullet (•) on this page and the pages that follow are depicted and described.

LGE is clearly differentiable from simple plaque-elicited gingivitis. It is characterized by a clearly demarcated band of reddening in the marginal gingiva. Classic periodontitis—both "chronic" and "aggressive" forms—do not occur in HIV-disease patients any more frequently than in other individuals; on the other hand, *NUP* occurs much more frequently, often exhibiting an extremely rapid clinical course of attachment loss.

Th significance of certain microorganisms in the etiology of LGE and NUP remains unclear. One finds periodontopathic microorganisms as seen in aggressive forms of periodontitis (p. 96), but often also significant increases in *Candida albicans* (*Ca*). The spotty erythema on the attached gingiva, and the frequent observation of this fungus in niches and pockets can be attributed to *Ca*. In those not responding to mechanical therapy, the cytomegalovirus is often detected.

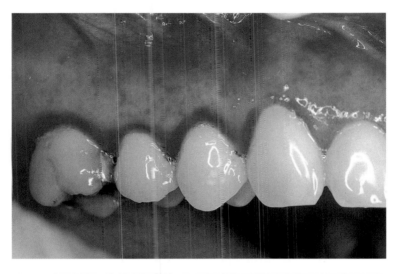

310 Linear Gingival Erythema (LGE)
Note the even band of erythema along the gingival margin and papillae. It is unclear whether such LGE (in the absence of treatment) can develop into NUP. The latter appears to be much more closely associated with ulcerative gingivitis (Fig. 311). Treatment consists of mechanical cleaning with betadine irrigation, motivation to improve oral hygiene and, in severe cases, CHX rinses.

Courtesy J. Winkler

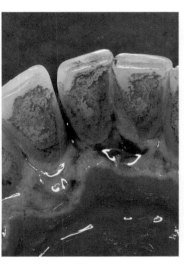

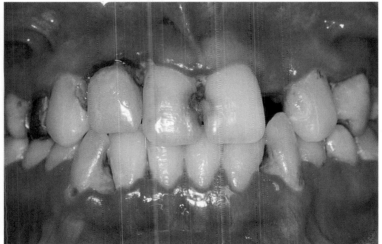

311 Ulcerative Gingivitis—NUP, Initial Stage
23-year-old female drug addict. The inflammation and ulcerations are similar to those observed in classic ulcerative gingivoperiodontitis. In the absence of treatment, the destruction of gingival tissue can progress rapidly.

Left: Severe, painful, ulcerative gingivitis in a 28-year-old female drug addict. The case was treated successfully (Figs. 329–335); she returns for regular recall and is recurrence-free for 7 years.

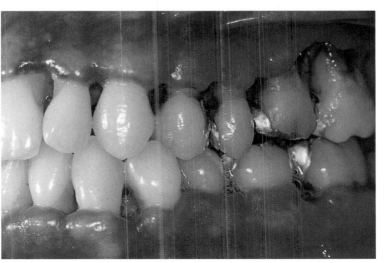

312 Very Advanced NUP
45-year-old homosexual male with extremely severe and painful NUP. Exposed bone could be probed in the interdental areas. In such severe cases, osseous sequesters may form. This patient was in the end stage of AIDS, and died 3 months later.

The standard NUP therapy used here is described on pages 151–154.

Fungal Infections

- Candidiasis
  - Atrophic/Erythematous
  - Angular cheilitis
  - Pseudomembranous
  - Hyperplastic

○ Histoplasmosis

The most common and earliest appearing fungal infection in HIV disease is candidiasis in its many and varied forms. Approximately 95 % of all fungal diseases are caused by *Candida albicans*; other fungi have only minor medical significance. *Candida albicans* is also found in a high percentage of healthy individuals, without causing any clinical symptoms. If host defense mechanisms are reduced, as is the case in HIV disease, proliferation of the fungi can occur by growth of hyphae and the formation of mycelia. The latter can invade the mucosa and lead to clinical manifestations of the types listed above. Oral Candida infections have a tendency to recur. Spread into the respiratory tract or the gastrointestinal tract is an indication of progression of the HIV disease, and is a complication to be taken very seriously by the patient and the physician.

313 Pseudomembranous Candidiasis
The whitish, painless layer on the gingiva and mucosa of this 27-year-old drug-addicted HIV patient can be easily wiped away. Treatment for cases limited to the oral cavity generally consists of careful removal of the pseudomembrane, and in severe cases systemic antimycotics.

Right: Candida mycelia in culture.

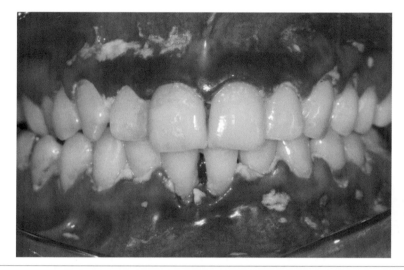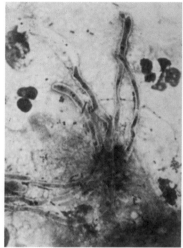

314 Atrophic, Erythematous Candidiasis
This 45-year-old, HIV-infected homosexual male exhibits reddish lesions in the middle of the palate. Similar alterations can also be observed on the edentulous alveolar ridge, attached gingiva and the dorsum of the tongue. The lesions may be painful.

Medicinal treatment involves *topical* rinsing with CHX, and *systemic* administration of the antimycotic Diflucan (Fluconazol).

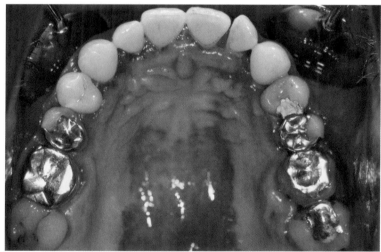

315 Angular Cheilitis (Perlèche)
Typical fissures at the corner of the mouth in a 32-year-old heterosexual, HIV-positive patient (promiscuity). These lesions are very painful and render dental treatment difficult. There is an association between *Candida albicans* and *Streptococcus aureus*. Perlèche is also observed in immunodeficient elderly individuals, as well as patients with severe overbite. The treatment consists of topical antimycotic agents (see above).

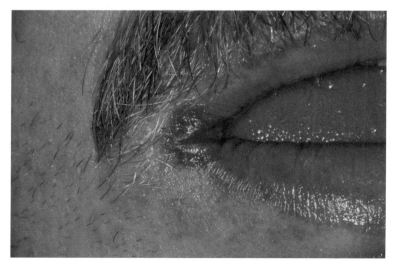

Viral Infections

Human Herpes Viruses (HHV)

- H. simplex virus   HHV-1
  Type 1 (HSV-1)
- H. simplex virus   HHV-2
  Type 2 (HSV-2)
- Varicella zoster   HHV-3
  virus (VZV)
- Epstein-Barr   HHV-4
  virus (EBV)

- Cytomegalovirus   HHV-5
  (CMV)
- Human herpes   HHV-6
  virus type 6
- Human herpes   HHV-7
  virus type 7
- Human herpes   HHV-8
  virus type 8

Viruses that are latent and which can also be found in "healthy" tissue usually are limited to ectodermal structures (skin, mucosa, retina etc). The primary infection usually occurs early in childhood through contact or droplet transfer. It can remain as a so-called latent infection throughout life.

The clinical manifestations of viruses in the oral mucosa are extraordinarily variable. Blisters, leukoplakic lesions on the tongue ("hairy leukoplakia"), localized and often expansive ulcerations and wart-like lesions have been described.

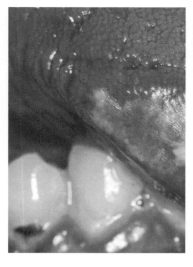
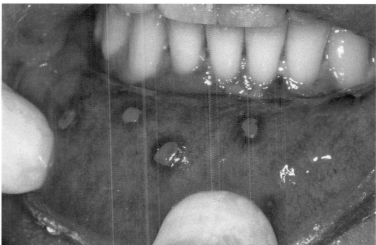
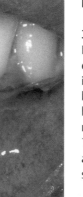

Human Herpes Viruses

316 Herpetic Stomatitis
Multiple blisters surrounded by erythema were caused by HSV-1 in this 40-year-old, HIV-positive homosexual patient. When the blisters burst, painful ulcerations remain.
Therapy: Topical analgesics and anti-inflammatory medicaments; systemic Aciclovir (e. g., Zovirax).

Left: Hairy leukoplakia on the lateral tongue border (Epstein-Barr virus, EBV).

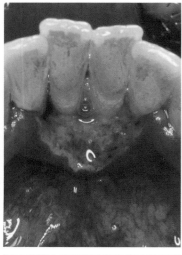
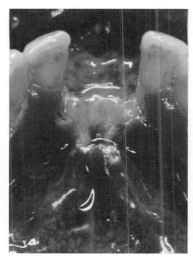
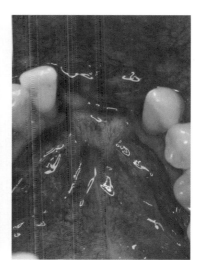

317 Expansive Ulceration
Left: 28-year-old, HIV-positive homosexual with expansive ulceration and advanced attachment loss in the mandible.

Middle: After gross debridement of the soft tissue and extraction of 41 and 31. Despite treatment, the ulcer became larger. Suspicion of cytomegalovirus infection (CMV, smear).

Right: CMV infection confirmed. Extraction of tooth 42 and systemic therapy. Ulcer healed.

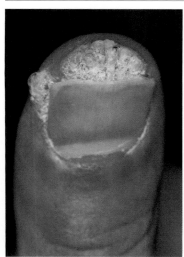
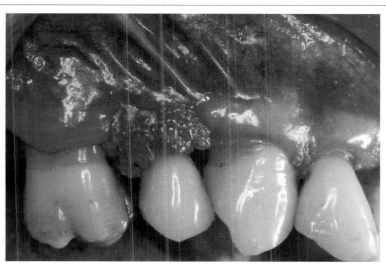

Human Papilloma Virus (HPV)

318 Verrucae (Wart)
Wart on the gingiva of a 42-year-old, HIV-positive homosexual, caused by HPV. This lesion was removed using the CO_2 laser.

Left: Similar wart, caused by the same virus on the fingertip and nail bed.

Neoplasms

- Kaposi sarcoma
  ○ Non-Hodgkin lymphoma
  ○ Spinal cell carcinoma

The most common neoplasm in HIV disease is the *Kaposi sarcoma*. It is an angiosarcoma of the endothelium of blood and lymph vessels, and can appear ubiquitously. The affected sites are dark red to bluish, with varying color intensity; they may be flat or exophytic in appearance; they are painless. Kaposi sarcoma of the oral cavity is observed frequent-

ly bilaterally on the hard palate corresponding to the course of the palatine arteries (Fig. 319), but is also observed on the soft palate, the gingiva (Fig. 320) and the buccal mucosa.
The etiology has been only partially elucidated. While the participation of the human herpes virus type 8 (HHV-8) is certain, the influence of angiogenic factors from mononuclear cells is only suspected. The Kaposi sarcoma is found in 10–20 % of all HIV disease. It is more common in homosexuals than in drug dependent patients (Grassi & Hämmerle 1991, Reichart & Philipsen 1998).

319 "Flat" Kaposi Sarcoma on the Palate
34-year-old homosexual with end-stage AIDS.
There is no proven therapy. Laser surgery has been recommended for lesions in the oral cavity, and radiotherapy for skin lesions. Systemically administered drugs such as cytostatics and Interferon may be considered.

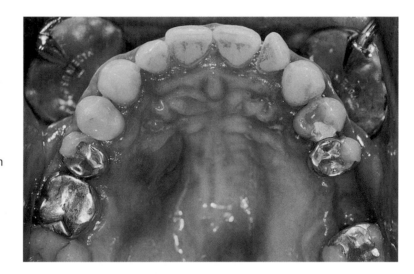

320 Aggressive, Exophytically Growing Kaposi Sarcoma on the Gingiva
40-year-old homosexual with end-stage AIDS. Several months after this photograph, the patient died.

Right: Less pigmented and pronounced Kaposi sarcoma on the gingiva between teeth 11 and 21. The exophytic tissue can be "lifted."

Courtesy *M. Grassi*

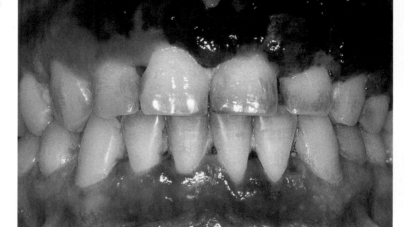
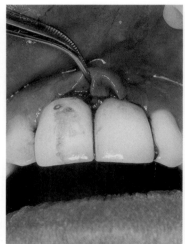

321 Histology of Kaposi Sarcoma
Left: Biopsy from the palate. Note keratinized epithelium. Blue-stained hemosiderin is observed within the connective tissue. The pigment derives from extravascular, dead erythrocytes (Berlin blue, x32).

Right: Large tumor cells exhibiting a vortex arrangement. Note also the proliferating capillaries (HE, x80).

Courtesy *S. Büchner*

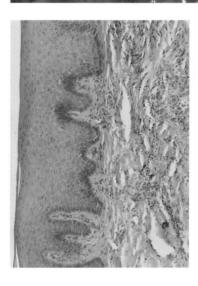
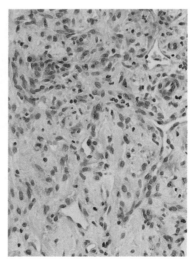

HIV-Associated Lesions of Unknown Etiology

- Ulcers
- Aphthae
- Saliva gland disorders (xerostomia)
- Tissue hemorrhage (thrombocytopenia)
- Oral pigmentations

Ulcers of unknown etiology may occur in the region of the marginal gingiva as localized, expansive and sharply demarcated lesions. They can persist for long periods of time and, like aphthae, be extremely painful. The etiology of some ulcerous alterations is known, e.g., the necrotizing, ulcerative periodontitis (NUP), and the cytomegalovirus infection. Large, recurrent *aphthae* are more frequently observed in patients with compromised immune function. The etiology is unknown.

Saliva gland disorders and the resultant xerostomia as well as rampant caries occur in up to 50% of HIV-infected children. The saliva glands in adults are less frequently affected. Especially the parotid gland is often enlarged. Such glands produce less saliva. This symptom is frequently coupled with lymphadenopathy.

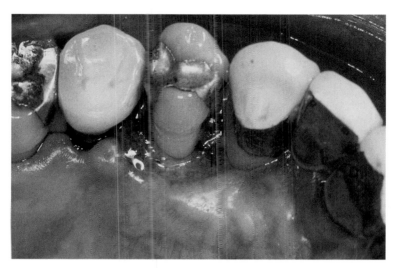

322 Ulceration
In this 40-year-old male one observes a broad healing ulceration on the palatal margin of tooth 14. Because of this lesion and the expansive aphthae in this patient (Fig. 323), the dentist requested an HIV test. The result was positive.

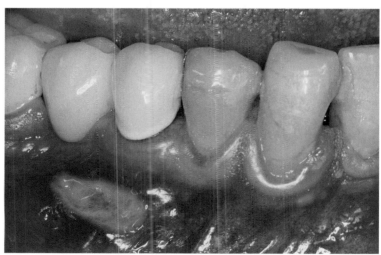

323 Expansive Aphthae
The ulcer on the mucosa is coated with fibrin and the margins are erythematous. Causal treatment is not possible. Therapy is polypragmatic and symptomatic, involving rinsing solutions. Positive effects may also be obtained using tinctures and ointments that disinfect, anesthetize, cauterize or reduce inflammation (corticosteroids).

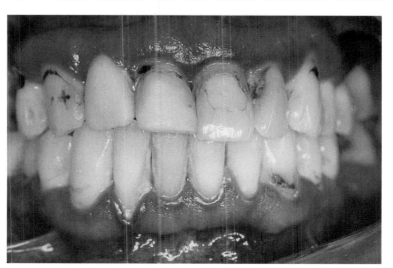

324 Caries with Xerostomia
This 42-year-old, HIV-positive homosexual exhibited bilateral enlargement of the parotid glands, which led to pronounced xerostomia. As a result, rampant caries developed throughout the dentition.
Restorative treatment and intensive preventive measures are highly indicated (oral hygiene, fluoridation, nutritional counseling, and possibly also saliva-stimulating sugar-free chewing gum).

Invasion and Replication of the HI Virus—Hurdles for Systemic Medical Treatment

HIV affects monocytes/macrophages (MΦ) and T4-lymphocytes via CD4-receptors and co-receptors (Fig. 325). The replication within the T4-lymphocytes is depicted in Fig. 326.

The best way to conquer the HIV disease worldwide, and in a financially feasible manner, would be immunization. This is not yet possible (p. 149, vaccines). The pharmaceutical treatments used today and in development are targeted to inhibit the "docking" of the virus on target cells, and breaking the replication cycle. In the foreground today is blocking the reverse transcriptase (RT), which transforms viral RNA into DNA. An additional therapeutic possibility is the inhibition of proteases. These are necessary at the end of the replication cycle, for modification of the synthesized virus proteins. Other theoretical possibilities for therapy are depicted in Fig. 328.

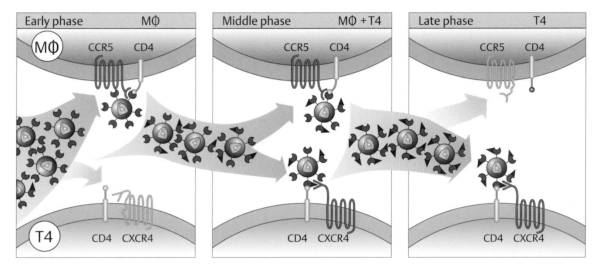

325 Tropism of HIV

HIV strains exhibit affinity for macrophages and T-cells, and following infection they bind specifically via the HIV surface glycoprotein gp/20 (Fig. 302) to CD4 receptors on T4 cells and monocytes/macrophages.

A consequence of this binding is that the "knob" is removed, and a harpoon-like binding area (gp41) on the viral membrane is exposed. Endocytosis then occurs if corresponding co-receptors are present (MΦ: **CCR-5**, T4 cell: **CXCR4**; Chemoreceptors!).

326 HIV Replication Cycle in the T4 Cell

- **A** HIV "docking" on specific receptors.
  Example: T-helper cell
  - CD4 receptor
  - Co-receptor CXCR4
  - "Viral harpoon" binds the virus to T4 cells
- **B** Endocytosis and release of the single-strand viral RNA
- **C** Transcription of the RNA into host-readable DNA by **Reverse Transcriptase (RT)**
- **D** Integration of the "pro-virus" DNA into the host DNA by **Integrase (IN)**
- **E** Induced copying of ...
  - virus RNA = transcription
  - viral structural elements = translation
- **F** Initial congregation of viral RNA and capsule proteins
- **G** Budding of the immature HIV, modification of the structural proteins via **Proteases (PR)**
- **H** Maturation into the infectious virus

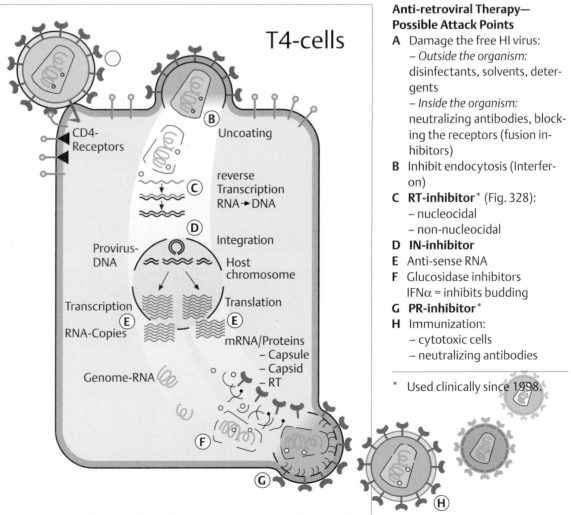

Anti-retroviral Therapy— Possible Attack Points

- **A** Damage the free HI virus:
  - *Outside the organism:* disinfectants, solvents, detergents
  - *Inside the organism:* neutralizing antibodies, blocking the receptors (fusion inhibitors)
- **B** Inhibit endocytosis (Interferon)
- **C** **RT-inhibitor*** (Fig. 328):
  - nucleocidal
  - non-nucleocidal
- **D** **IN-inhibitor**
- **E** Anti-sense RNA
- **F** Glucosidase inhibitors IFNα = inhibits budding
- **G** **PR-inhibitor***
- **H** Immunization:
  - cytotoxic cells
  - neutralizing antibodies

---

* Used clinically since 1998.

Treatment of the HIV Patient—Pharmacologic Aspects

Antiretroviral Medicines

Groups of drugs (Fig. 328) have existed for several years that have the capacity to reduce the viral load in blood plasma; especially the "triple therapy", a combination of three drugs (today even four and more). This drug regimen must be taken over the long term; it is extremely cost intensive, brings with it many serious side effects and is therefore compliance dependent. This treatment regimen is referred to as "HAART" (*highly active anti-retroviral therapy*). For compliant HIV-infected patients, this drug regimen can significantly increase post-infection lifespan.

Vaccines

Active or passive vaccines with the capability of immunizing healthy individuals or stopping further spread of HIV remain in the research stages and are not yet ready for use. But the clock is running quickly: Only an effective vaccine will be financially feasible worldwide and promise the capability to reduce the developing AIDS pandemic in Third World countries. To date the most promising are genetic vaccines, e.g., directly injected plasmid-bound DNA of certain HIV genes, which elicit a potent host immune response (Kennedy 1997, Weinert & Kennedy 1999).

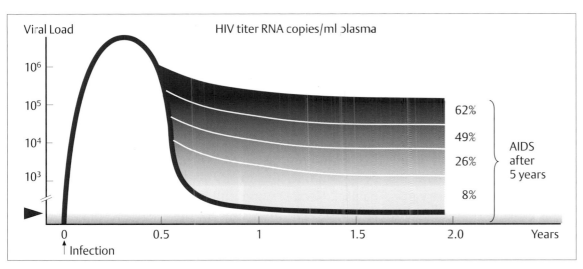

327 Viral Load and Average Five-year Survival Rate for HIV-positive Persons (Mellors 1996)
The goal of anti-retroviral therapy is the elimination of virus particles from the blood (i.e., below the level of detection, which is becoming lower and lower because of more precise test methods). Success is acknowledged today when the level of viral RNA copies is less than 5,000 per ml of plasma

RT I	Nucleoside analogs	
Videx	Didanosine	**ddl**
Epivir	Lamivudine	**3TC**
Zerit	Stavudine	**d4T**
Hivid	Zalcitabine	**ddC**
Retrovir	Zidovudine	**AZT**
Combivir	AZT + 3TC	
Ziagen	Abacavir	
Sustiva	Efavirenz	

RT I	Non-nucleoside analogs
Rescriptor	Delavirdine
Viramune	Nevirapine
Stocrin	Efavirenz

PR I	Protease inhibitors
Crixivan	Incinavir
Viracept	Ne finavir
Norvir	Ritonavir
Invirase	Saquinavir a (Hartgel)
Fortovase	Sacuinavir b (Softgel)
Agenerase	Amprenavir

328 Antiretroviral Medicaments
Most widely employed today are agents that inhibit the viral enzyme *reverse transcriptase (RT)* and *proteases (PR)*. RT inhibitors prevent the translation of the viral RNA into DNA that can be read by host cells. PR inhibitors prevent the proper structural configuration of viral proteins, which—immediately following budding of the immature virus particles—are absolutely necessary for the definitive structure of the infectious virus.

The high mutation rate of HIV leads quickly to mutants that are resistant to an individual medicament.

On the other hand, the so-called "varying therapy" has been effective because it better prevents the development of resistance; these therapies, however, are often almost unbearable for the patients, who must consume up to 20 different tablets per day in precise intervals. In addition, as of **1998**, most of these medications are associated with severe side effects.

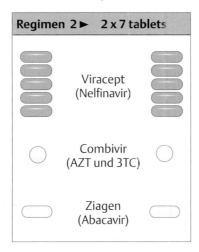

Regimen 1 ▶ 2 x 3 tablets
Zerit (Stavudine; d4T)
Viramune (Nevirapine)
Epivir (Lamivudine; 3TC)

Regimen 2 ▶ 2 x 7 tablets
Viracept (Nelfinavir)
Combivir (AZT und 3TC)
Ziagen (Abacavir)

Regimen 3 ▶ 2 x 13 tablets
Agenerase (Amprenavir)
Retrovir (Zidovudine)
Norvir (Ritonavir)
Epivir (Lamivudine; 3TC)

Lingual View of the Mandible

332 Initial Findings
This lingual view clearly reveals the extensive band of necrosis in the anterior, canine and premolar regions.

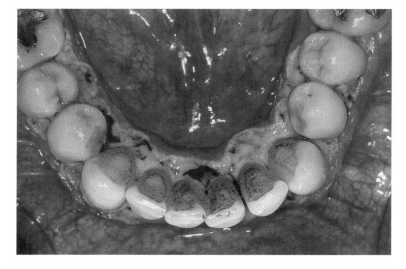

333 Following Removal of the Necrotic Tissue and Initial Calculus Removal
This photograph was taken immediately following removal of the necrotic tissue and supragingival calculus. The careful soft tissue treatment was performed with continuous irrigation using betadine solution (10 %). This agent not only has antimicrobial effects, it also reduces hemorrhage and provides mild surface anesthesia.

Right: Betadine solution (10 %) and syringe for irrigation.

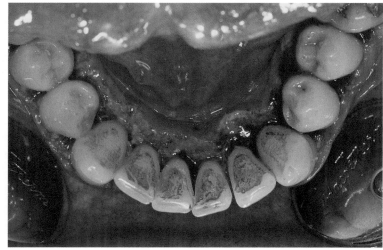

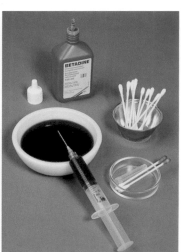

334 Four Days After Treatment
Tissue healing began immediately following the initial treatment. Four days later, the formerly ulcerated tissue has already begun to re-epithelialize. The patient was now free of pain.

Right: He continued daily rinses with CHX and took his metronidazol (Flagyl) for an additional 3 days (total of 7 days). Purely mechanical oral hygiene was re-instituted, checked and corrected.

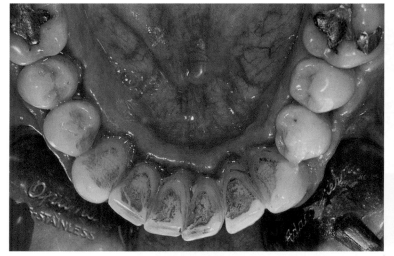

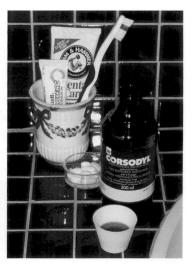

335 Four Years Later
Clinical photograph taken during a recall appointment.
In the interim, new restorations were placed.

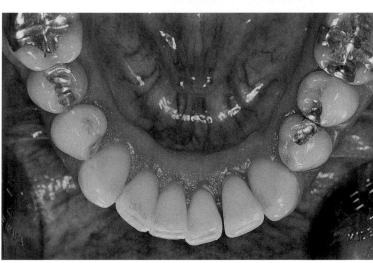

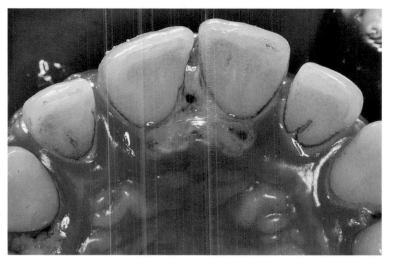

Palatal View of the Maxillary Anterior Region

336 Initial Situation; Same Patient
Pronounced ulceration in the region of teeth 11 and 21; both were highly mobile. Expansive ulceration such as this could be caused by the cytomegalovirus. These can only be successfully treated in combination with a systemic anti-viral (herpes-) approach. When this case was first seen (1990), that approach was not available.

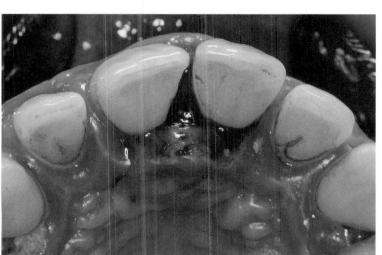

337 Following Soft Tissue Debridement
The clinical view clearly shows that the necrotic tissue has been mechanically removed. A deep crater remains between the incisors. Subepithelial connective tissue has been denuded over a large area.

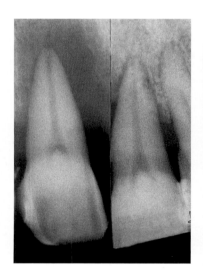
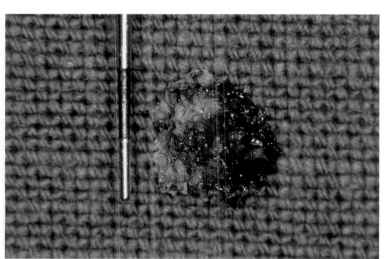

338 Bone Sequester
An osseous sequester with a diameter of ca. 6 mm was removed from between teeth 11 and 21.

Left: Periapical radiograph taken 5 months after initial therapy, immediately following removal of the bone sequester. The radiolucency in this film is considerably larger than the size of the sequester itself.

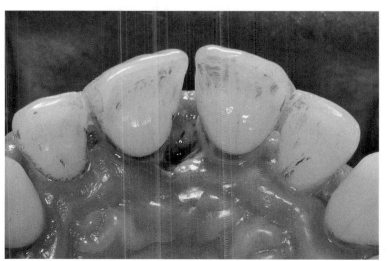

339 Maxillary Anterior Palatal View Immediately After Sequester Removal
Deep interdental crater with gingival retraction. Tooth 11 exhibited a mobility of grade 4, tooth 21, grade 3. The treatment plan included extraction of all four anterior teeth.

The expansive primary ulceration, the sequester formation and the remaining large defect could be attributed to infection with cytomegalovirus.

**Prosthetic Restoration
of the Maxilla**

**340 Cast Framework Partial
Denture**
Immediately after extraction of
the anterior teeth, a removable
acrylic resin temporary denture
was seated. It was replaced 8
months later by a cast framework
partial denture (chrome-cobalt).

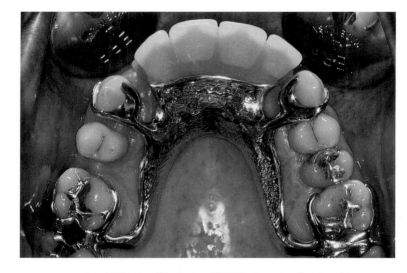

**341 Irritation of the Mucosa
by the Prosthesis**
Mucosal erythema beneath the
prosthesis became more severe
over time. Allergic and toxicologic
tests were *negative*. It is likely that
mechanical and microbial irritations were the causes of this severe, localized inflammation in a
patient with reduced immune response capacity.

Right: Fixed bridge (titanium-
acrylic). The bridge was constructed to make plaque control
as simple as possible.

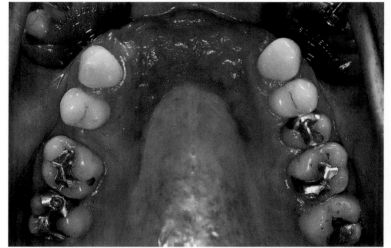
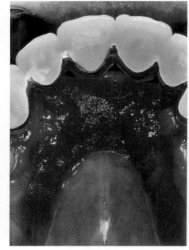

**Seven Years After Completion
of Treatment**

342 Maxillary Bridge
The mucosal erythema completely disappeared a months after
seating the fixed bridge. This type
of anterior bridge has been completely free of complications.

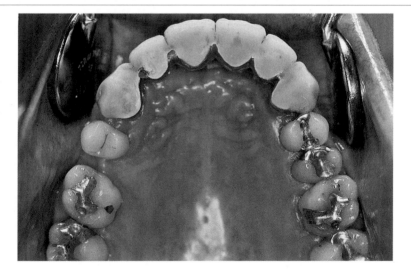

343 Mandible
With "more or less" regular recall
every 4–6 months, the patient's
home care is of varying quality.
Since the beginning of his dental
treatment, he also participated in
a methadone program; this drug
leads to reduced saliva flow and,
despite regular fluoride application, new caries developed.
When this photograph was taken,
the patient had been on a "triple
therapy" with anti-retroviral
medicaments for a 2-year period
(p. 149).

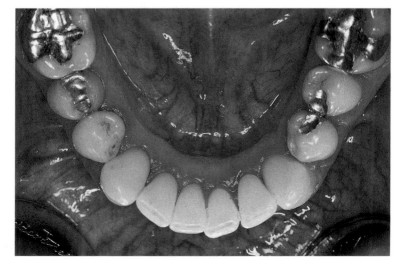

Gingival Recession

Type VIII B 1

Recession of the marginal gingiva (classified as Type VIII B 1) may result from various etiologies, and can occur in various clinical manifestations, including combined forms:

- *"Classical" recession* occurs in the absence of any infection, is inflammation-free, and is usually localized to the facial surfaces. It is the most common type of gingival recession, normally without loss of the interdental papillae (Figs. 349–350).
- Recession attendant to *untreated periodontitis* (most often the chronic forms): It progresses slowly, often over many years, and involves both marginal gingiva and papillae (Fig. 358).
- Loss of the marginal and interdental gingiva often occurs following *periodontitis therapy*, especially when resective treatment methods are employed (Fig. 359).
- Recession is a manifestation of the involution of aging, with retraction/recession of marginal and usually also the interdental gingiva (Fig. 360).

"Classical" Recession

Classical recession accounts for 5–10 % of all periodontal attachment loss. The term recession is defined as an *inflammation-free* clinical condition characterized by apical retreat of the facial and less often of the oral gingiva. Despite recession of the gingival margin, the interdental papillae usually fill the entire embrasure area in younger patients. Recession is usually localized to one or several teeth; generalized gingival recession is rare. Teeth exhibiting classical gingival recession are not excessively *mobile*. The periodontal supporting structures are generally of excellent quality. Teeth are never lost due to classical gingival recession alone! If the patient's oral hygiene is inadequate, secondary inflammation and eventually pocket formation (periodontitis) may ensue.

Etiology: A primary factor is purely the morphology and the anatomy of the situation. The facial plate of bone overlying the root is usually very thin. Not infrequently, the root surface is completely denuded of alveolar bone (*dehiscence*), or exhibits *fenestrations* in the thin osseous lamella. Anterior teeth and premolars are most frequently affected.
Recession is initiated as a consequence of the morphologic/anatomic situation, and the following etiologic factors:

- Improper, traumatic tooth brushing, e.g., horizontal scrubbing, excessive force (Mierau & Fiebig 1986, 1987)
- Mild, chronic inflammation that may be only slightly visible clinically (Wennström et al. 1987a)
- Frenum pulls, especially when fibers of the frenum attach near the gingival margin
- Orthodontic treatment (tooth movement labially; arch expansion; Foushee et al. 1985; Wennström et al. 1987a)
- Excessive periodontal scaling (Caution at recall!)
- Functional disturbances (e.g., bruxism) as the cause for gingival recession continue to cause heated discussion.

"Classical" recession is illustrated in the following pages graphically, on skull preparations and clinically.

Radiographically, pure gingival recession localized to the facial surfaces of teeth cannot be diagnosed.

Therapy: With scrupulous and *proper* oral hygiene, recession can be halted. An atraumatic tooth brushing technique with a soft manual brush or a sonic device should be recommended.
Severe types of recession may require mucogingival surgery.

Fenestration and Dehiscence of the Alveolar Bone

In a healthy periodontium the facial margin of the alveolar crest lies approximately 2 mm apical to the gingival margin, which courses near to the cementoenamel junction. The facial aspect of the alveolar bone covering the root is usually very thin. As revealed by a flap operation or on a skull preparation the coronal portion of the root often is not covered by bone (*dehiscence*) or there is a *fenestration* of the facial bony plate. Towards the apex, the facial plate of bone becomes thicker and trabecular bone fills the interval between the facial cortical plate and cribriform plate. In these thicker areas, recession generally stops spontaneously.

In *elderly* individuals, especially in those who have practiced excessive interdental hygiene for many years, recession of facial periodontal tissues may appear in combination with horizontal bone loss in the interdental area. In such cases, the interdental papillae usually also recede. Nevertheless, no *true* periodontal pockets are in evidence.

344 Normal Periodontium and Various Manifestations of Recession as Viewed in Orofacial Section
Recession (blue), junctional epithelium (**JE**), minimal PD (red). The mucogingival line (arrowheads) and the CEJ are indicated.
A   Gingiva and normal bone
B   Simultaneous recession of bone and gingiva, fenestration
C   Bony dehiscence more pronounced than gingival recession
D   Recession with formation of McCall's festoon (Fig. 350).

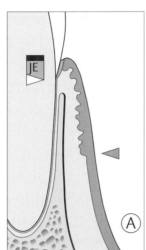
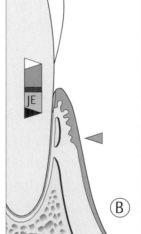
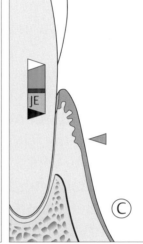
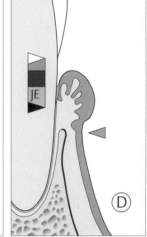

Skull Observations

345 Fenestration (left)
Adjacent to the fenestration on tooth 13 (circle), dehiscences and horizontal bone loss in the interdental areas.

346 Dehiscence (right)
A pronounced dehiscence that extends almost to the apex is observed on the facial of 13. The other teeth exhibit dehiscences of lesser severity. Generalized interdental bone loss is also in evidence (right).

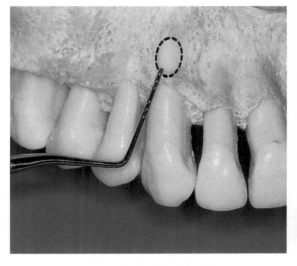
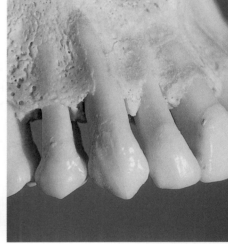

Findings During Surgery

347 Multiple Fenestrations
During the course of an Edlan operation, large fenestrations on teeth 16, 15 13 and 12 became visible after flap reflection (left).

348 Dehiscence on Tooth 13
During an extension operation using FGG, an unexpected osseous dehiscence was encountered, which had not been detected by probing. The dehiscence was more severe than the orginal gingival recession (right).

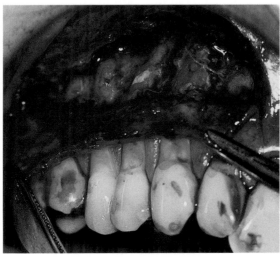
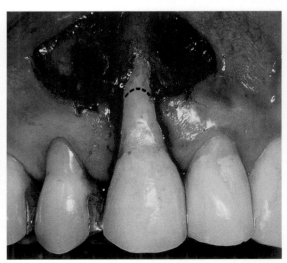

Clinical Symptoms

- Gingival recession (of the entire gingival margin)
- Stillman cleft
- McCall's festoon

The clinical manifestations of recession are numerous. Gingival recession usually begins with a gradual apical migration of the entire *facial aspect* of the gingiva, revealing the CEJ. Less frequently, the first sign of recession is the relatively rapid formation of a small groove in the gingiva, a so-called *Stillman cleft*. This can expand into pronounced recession. As a consequence of recession, the remaining attached gingiva may become somewhat thickened and rolled, a non-inflammatory fibrotic response known as *McCall's festoon* (Fig. 350).

If the recession progresses to the mucogingival line, secondary inflammation of the gingival margin often occurs (Fig. 351).

Gingival recession can lead to esthetic considerations in the maxillary anterior segment. As root surfaces are exposed, cervical sensitivity may also become a problem. Gingival recession is often observed on teeth that exhibit wedge-shape defects at the cervical area (p. 164).

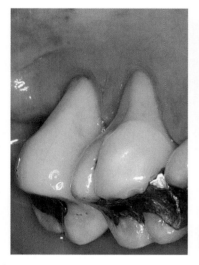
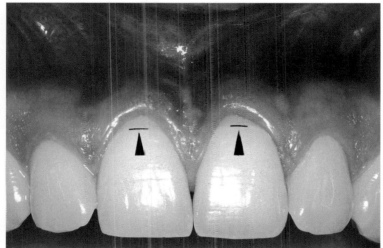

349 Initial Recession
Early exposure of the cementoenamel junction (arrows) due to recession of the gingival margin. The mobile oral mucosa has been stained with Schiller iodine solution (see Fig. 363).

Palatal Recession (left)
Gingival recession on the palatal or lingual surfaces is considerably less common than on facial surfaces (morphology).

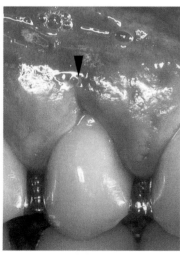
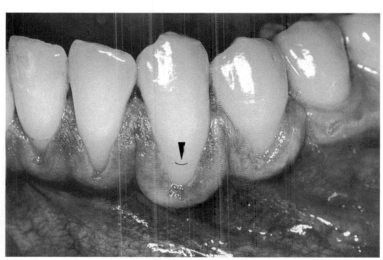

350 McCall's Festoons
The attached gingiva consists of nothing more than a collar-like, fibrous thickening (arrow). This *may* be a tissue response to further recession beyond the mucogingival line.

Stillman Cleft (left)
Cleft-like defect of traumatic etiology. Such clefts may spread laterally, creating an area of gingival recession. The exposed root surface may be extremely sensitive. Such clefts are often covered with plaque.

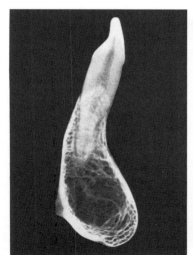
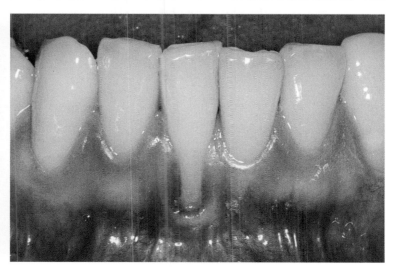

351 Severe Localized Recession
The root of this tooth has been denuded all the way down to the mucogingival line. The gingival margin is secondarily inflamed. Following initial therapy, mucogingival surgery for covering the exposed root was indicated (Miller class II; p. 163).
Dehiscence of the Alveolar Process (left)
Orofacial section through an anterior tooth, as viewed in the radiograph. Remarkably little bone surrounds the tooth, facially and lingually.

Recession—Localized

A 26-year-old male presented to the clinic with a chief complaint of recession on his maxillary canines. His oral hygiene was impeccable; he claimed to brush his teeth four times a day. Neither a dentist nor a dental hygienist had ever observed or corrected his tooth brushing technique.

Findings:

API: 10 %   PBI: 0.8

Figure 353 depicts probing depths, tooth mobility and areas of recession.

Diagnosis: Pronounced facial gingival recession on canines. Initial generalized gingival recession.

Therapy: Oral hygiene instruction, emphasizing a gentle technique. Study models provide a way to measure any progression of the gingival recession. If the esthetic situation is of great concern, one may consider surgical intervention to cover the recession, e. g., with a connective tissue graft (CTG) on tooth 23.

Recall: 6 months or longer.

Prognosis: Good.

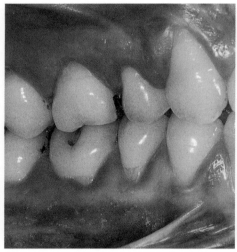
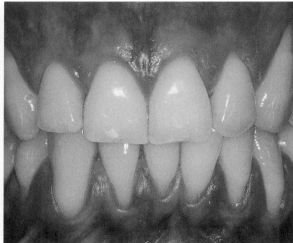
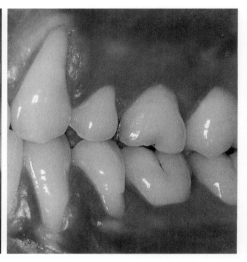

352 Clinical Overview (above)
The gingival recessions are of varying severity, with pronounced areas over the canines. The papillae still fill the interdental spaces. In the molar segments, mild marginal inflammation is noted. Tooth 35 exhibits a wedge-shaped defect.

353 Probing Depths, Recession (Re), Tooth Mobility (TM; right)
The classical recession is associated with neither pathologically deepened pockets nor elevated tooth mobility.

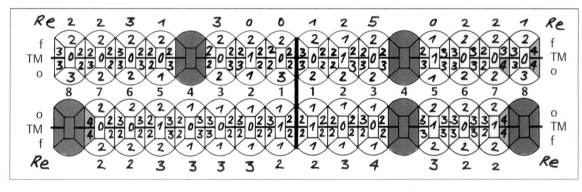

354 Radiographic Survey
Facial osseous dehiscences are not visible on the radiograph (see clinical picture of the canines). Recession cannot be diagnosed using radiographs alone. In young patients, no loss of interdental septal height is noted.

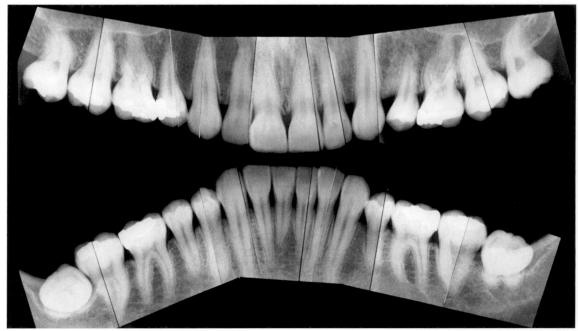

Recession—Generalized

This 43-year-old female was worried that her teeth appeared to be getting longer. Wedge-shaped defects were in evidence on all canines and premolars; the patient experienced cervical sensitivity in these areas from time to time. She expressed the desire to have her "gum condition" treated, if possible.

Findings:

API: 20 %   PBI: 1.0

Probing depths, recession, tooth mobility: see Fig. 356.

Diagnosis: Generalized, advanced facial recession. Slight loss of periodontal supporting structures in the interdental areas, but without significant pocket formation.

Therapy: Change home care technique; fabricate study models; monitor at regular intervals of 3–6 months. If the recession progresses, mucogingival surgery to halt or cover the recessions.

Recall: 6 months or longer, comparing measurements on sequential study models.

Prognosis: Good, if secondary inflammation is avoided and proper oral hygiene is practiced.

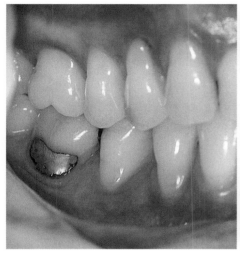
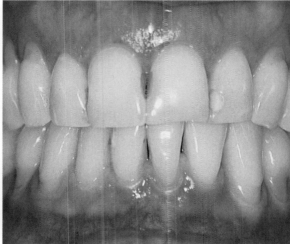
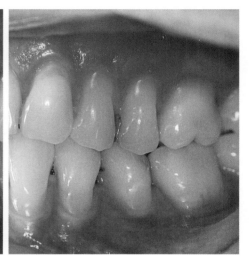

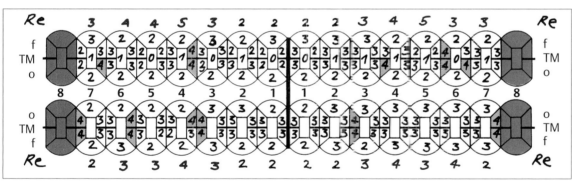

355 Clinical Overview (above)
Generalized gingival recession is apparent in this middle-aged female. The interdental papillae have also receded slightly. The interdental spaces have begun to "open."

356 Probing Depths, Facial recession (Re), Tooth Mobility (TM; schematic, left)
In the mandibular premolar area, the facial attached gingival is almost completely absent due to the gingival recession. In this area, attachment loss continued slowly despite changing the patient's brushing technique.

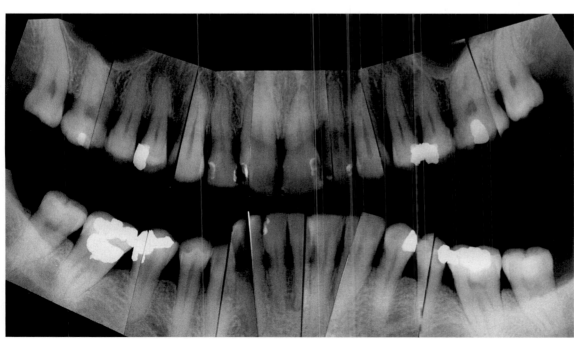

357 Radiographic Survey
Mild generalized, horizontal reduction of the interdental septal height is noted. The more advanced bone loss on the facial surfaces is not visible radiographically.

Clinical Situations Resembling Recession

In addition to classical gingival recession, there are other forms of *clinically observable* attachment loss:

- *Shrinkage (recession) of the gingiva as a consequence of untreated periodontitis*
- Symptom of periodontitis (p. 105)
- *Condition following periodontal therapy:* "Long teeth," open interdental spaces and cervical sensitivity are often the uncomfortable consequences of treatment for advanced periodontal disease.

- *Recession of the entire periodontium in the elderly:* This condition is *not* the rule. It may be caused by mild chronic inflammation and shrinkage; it can be enhanced by improper (overzealous) tooth brushing technique or other iatrogenic irritation.
- *Classical recession with a superimposed secondary periodontitis:* This combination seldom occurs, because patients who practice proper oral hygiene usually exhibit neither plaque accumulation nor inflammation.

358 "Recession" (Shrinkage) in a Case of Untreated Periodontitis
This 32-year-old female with periodontitis presented with 5–6 mm pockets in the interdental areas. In addition, she exhibited 4–5 mm of gingival recession; thus, the true measure of attachment loss was 9–11 mm. This uncommon degree of gingival recession appeared to have been enhanced by improper tooth brushing technique (note wedge-shaped defects).

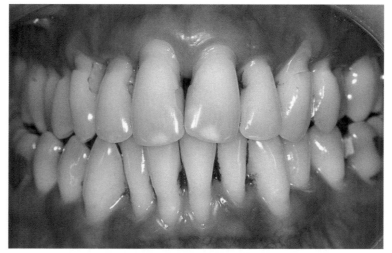

Similar Clinical Manifestations
– at Various Ages
– with Varying Etiologies

32-year-old
_____
Periodontitis

359 Clinical Picture Following Periodontal Therapy
In this 36-year-old female with advanced periodontitis (9 mm pockets) the esthetic consequences of radical surgical intervention (primarily resective, radical surgical operations) were severe. Although the "pocket reduction" was successful, the esthetic result was considerably less than favorable.

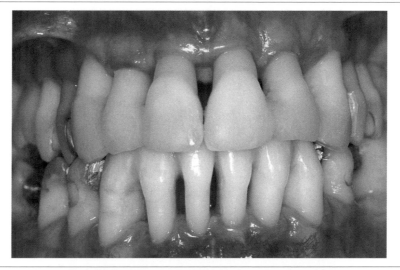

36-year-old
_____
Therapy

360 Gingival "Shrinkage" in an Elderly Male
This 81-year-old man exhibited no periodontal pockets. Throughout the patient's life, the dentist had performed only restorative treatment. The patient had taken care of the periodontal "treatment" by himself, through vigorous brushing and a coarse diet (note wedge-shaped defects and abrasion).

Courtesy G. Cimasoni

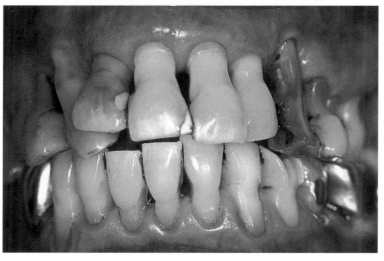

81-year-old
_____
Age

Recession—Diagnosis

For many patients, gingival recession is the primary reason for seeking dental care. These patients are disturbed by the poor esthetics of gingival recession, they confuse recession with periodontitis, and they fear tooth loss.

Both dentist and patient can readily recognize gingival recession. Nevertheless, especially for treatment planning, precise data collection must be made, for example, using exact measurement methods. The dentist must clarify whether the recession is "classical" and without inflammation or pocket formation, or whether the clinical symptom is of untreated periodontitis (shrinkage), or the result of periodontal therapy (radical surgical procedures). The width of the remaining attached gingiva is of less importance, but if it is completely absent and if the mobile mucosa (labial or buccal frena) extends directly over the area of recession, the result can be an uncontrollable progression of the gingival recession.

Probing of the sulcus, use of the "roll test" with probe or finger, and staining the mobile mucosa are examinations that can be performed to predict whether or not complications will ultimately result from the recession.

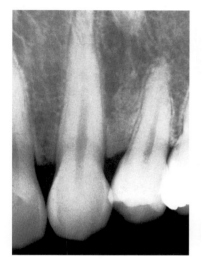

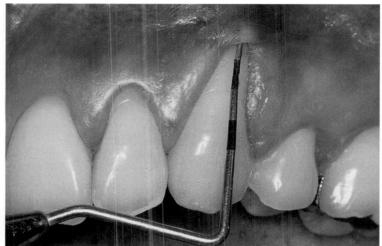

361 Attachment Loss Due to Recession—Toothbrush Injury
In this case, the facial gingival recession from the cementoenamel junction to the gingival margin was 5 mm. It appeared as though absolutely no attached gingiva was present. In addition, the typical McCall's festoon was not in evidence, which would usually be viewed as a reparative response to the minimal gingival width.

Left: The radiograph does not permit diagnosis of facial bone loss.

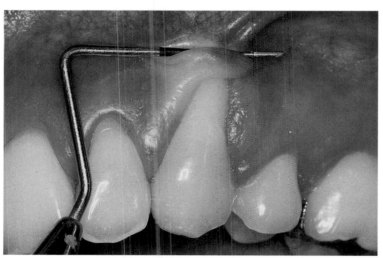

362 "Roll Test"
Using the finger or a periodontal probe, the mobile mucosa is displaced toward the area of recession. This permits verification of whether or not attached gingiva provides any resistance against the roll test.
In the case depicted here, the mobile oral mucosa extends all the way to the gingival margin.

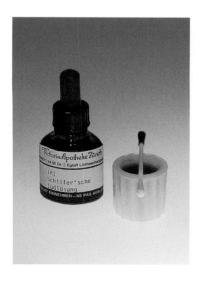

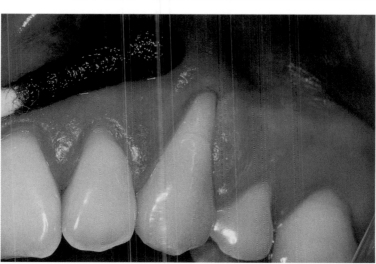

363 Iodine Test
Both gingiva and oral mucosa are painted with Schiller iodine solution (diluted aqueous iodine-calcium iodide) or diluted Lugol solution. The glycogen-containing mobile mucosa takes on a brown coloration, while the attached, glycogen-free gingiva remains unstained.
In this case, the iodine test clearly shows that there is *no* attached gingiva over tooth 23.

Left: Schiller iodine solution.

Measurement of Recession (Jahnke)

Occasionally more precise methods are needed to more exactly define areas of recession, e.g., for scientific clinical studies. In an effort to quantitate gingival recession, Jahnke et al. (1993) measured not only the *vertical* extent of recession in millimeters from the cementoenamel junction to the gingival margin (measurement 1), but also the probing depth (4), which together with the recession provides a measure of attachment loss or the attachment level (2). In addition to the width of the keratinized gingiva (3), the *horizontal* expanse of the recession (5) and the adjacent papillae (6) are of significance for surgical treatment of the recession.

Classification of Recession (Miller)

Also with an eye toward treatment, P. D. Miller (1985) devised a "classification of gingival recession." Without precisely measuring the extent and the various localizations of gingival recession, Miller described recession on the one hand with regard to its breadth and depth in relation to the gingival margin and the remaining attached gingiva; on the other hand, he described the loss of papillae, i.e., the interdental tissues.

The Miller classes I–IV are significant in defining the possibilities and boundaries of surgical therapeutic modalities (e.g., covering recession).

364 Measurement of the Recession and the Surrounding Gingiva Tissue

This figure considers only the "classical" recession (length and width) and its relationship to the attached gingiva, the sulcus depth and the width of the adjacent papillae. These parameters are of significance for any anticipated surgical procedures.

Recession of the papillae themselves, which is important both for treatment and especially for the prognosis following treatment, is not considered. The "Jahnke measurements" are primarily used in scientific (computerized) investigations of gingival recession.

Modified from *P. Jahnke et al. 1993*

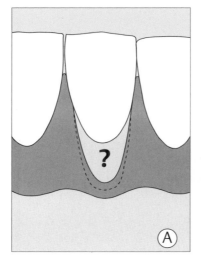 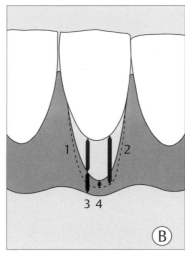 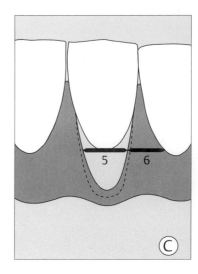

Recession: Millimeter Measurements (Jahnke et al. 1993)

- **Vertical Measurements**

    1 vertical recession
    2 probing attachment level
    3 width of keratinized tissue
    4 probing (pocket) depth

- **Horizontal Measurements**

    5 defect width at the level of cementoenamel junction (CEJ)
    6 width of interdental papilla at the CEJ

365 Clinical Measurement of the Three Most Important Parameters

1 & 2 Vertical recession and attachment level (left)
5   Horizontal recession/width (middle)
6   Width of papilla (right)

For a surgical procedure to cover areas of recession, it is the mass of surrounding tissue and not the expanse of the recession itself that is most important (nutrition for the graft).

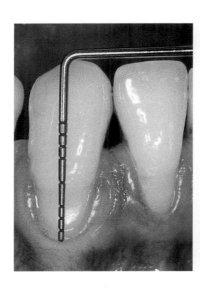 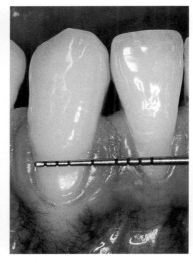 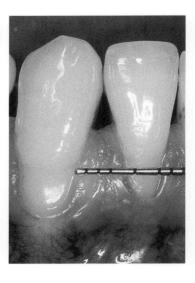

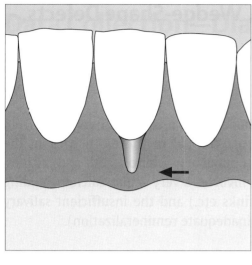

I

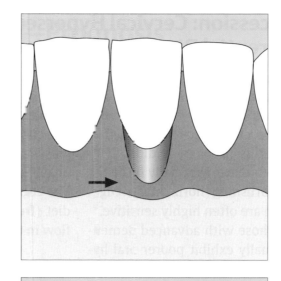

Classification of Recession (Miller, 1985)

366 Class I
Narrow *(left)* or wide *(right)*, localized "classical" recession isolated to the facial surface, with papillae filling the interdental areas. The defects do not extend to the mucogingival line.

Therapy: Complete, 100 % coverage of this type of recession can be achieved, e. g., by use of a free connective tissue graft.

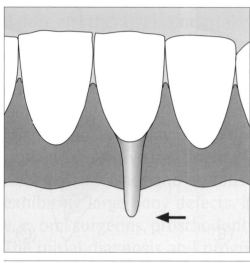

II

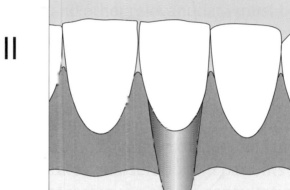

367 Class II
Narrow and wide, facially localized "classical" recessions, which extend beyond the mucogingival line into the mobile mucosa. The papillae remain essentially intact.

Therapy: Complete coverage of the root surface can still be achieved. With such deep recessions, guided tissue regeneration (GTR) with membranes can be employed instead of a connective tissue graft.

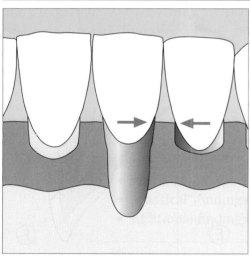

III

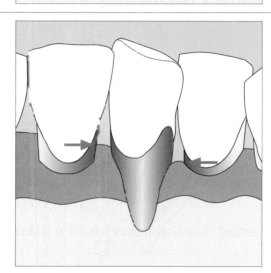

368 Class III
Broad recessions that extend beyond the mucogingival line into the mobile mucosa. The interdental papillae may be lost due to "shrinkage" and malpositioned teeth.

Therapy: Complete regeneration of such tissue defects is not possible; the facial root surface can, at best, be partially covered, and rebuilding the papillae is hopeless.

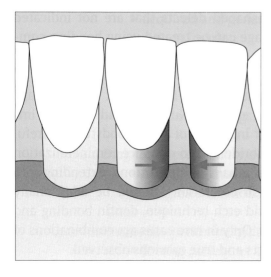

IV

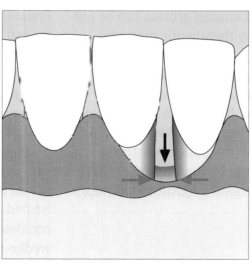

369 Class IV
Left: Loss of periodontal hard (bone) and soft tissues around the entire tooth. The loss of tissue may be due to periodontitis, or to radical, resective periodontitis therapy.

Right: This type of tissue loss is frequently observed after repeated acute exacerbations of ulcerative gingivoperiodontitis.

Therapy: Regeneration of the lost tissues by surgical procedures is only rarely possible.

Data Collection—Examinations

Before performing extensive periodontal examinations, every patient should be subjected to a screening exam (e.g., PSR index, p. 73); this takes only a few minutes, and reveals whether periodontal lesions are present or whether other oral problems predominate.

If periodontal tissue destruction is detected, more extensive examinations are indicated. First among these are the "classic" examinations such as periodontal probing or measurement of attachment level (Fig. 383).

If there is evidence of special forms of disease, their etiologies and clinical course, additional facultative examinations should be performed. Such exams are especially indicated when one encounters:

- copious hemorrhage with slight plaque accumulation
- symptoms of disease activity (pus)
- advanced attachment loss in young patients
- elevated tooth mobility with mild bone loss
- suspicion of a systemic disease.

Only after collection and evaluation of these exams will it be possible to establish a more precise differential diagnosis (e.g., aggressive periodontitis).

372 Checklist of Obligatory and Supplemental Clinical Findings

Obligatory

The obligatory, "classical" clinical findings must be recorded for every periodontitis patient before initiating therapy. This requires a special periodontal chart, which may be enhanced by additional forms for the history, hygiene index, gingival indices and functional analyses. Such data collection can be performed using traditional data collection forms or, today, using computer-enhanced and -printed data collection forms. In either case, most important is that the obligatory examinations be performed systematically, and that data be collected for each individual tooth.

Supplemental

In severe cases, e.g., in aggressive, progressive forms of periodontitis, and/or with the existence of severe functional disturbances and anticipated major reconstructions, *supplemental* examinations will be necessary. Such examinations, and their necessity, will be determined and selected for each individual patient.

Beyond data collection, contemporary tests for specific bacteria and for host response in aggressive periodontitis cases provide an improved estimation of the risk potential and more targeted treatment planning (additional systemic medication?) and a more precise prognosis.

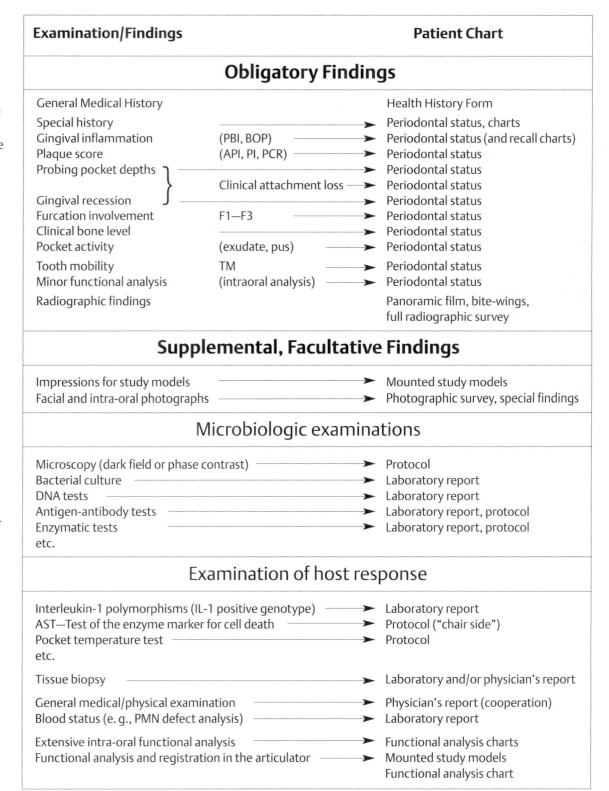

Examination/Findings		Patient Chart
Obligatory Findings		
General Medical History		Health History Form
Special history		Periodontal status, charts
Gingival inflammation	(PBI, BOP)	Periodontal status (and recall charts)
Plaque score	(API, PI, PCR)	Periodontal status
Probing pocket depths		Periodontal status
	Clinical attachment loss	Periodontal status
Gingival recession		Periodontal status
Furcation involvement	F1—F3	Periodontal status
Clinical bone level		Periodontal status
Pocket activity	(exudate, pus)	Periodontal status
Tooth mobility	TM	Periodontal status
Minor functional analysis	(intraoral analysis)	Periodontal status
Radiographic findings		Panoramic film, bite-wings, full radiographic survey
Supplemental, Facultative Findings		
Impressions for study models		Mounted study models
Facial and intra-oral photographs		Photographic survey, special findings
Microbiologic examinations		
Microscopy (dark field or phase contrast)		Protocol
Bacterial culture		Laboratory report
DNA tests		Laboratory report
Antigen-antibody tests		Laboratory report, protocol
Enzymatic tests		Laboratory report, protocol
etc.		
Examination of host response		
Interleukin-1 polymorphisms (IL-1 positive genotype)		Laboratory report
AST—Test of the enzyme marker for cell death		Protocol ("chair side")
Pocket temperature test		Protocol
etc.		
Tissue biopsy		Laboratory and/or physician's report
General medical/physical examination		Physician's report (cooperation)
Blood status (e. g., PMN defect analysis)		Laboratory report
Extensive intra-oral functional analysis		Functional analysis charts
Functional analysis and registration in the articulator		Mounted study models Functional analysis chart

General Patient Health History

Each and every patient examination begins with the collection of the systemic, medical history. This is simplified by use of a health questionnaire, but such questionnaires do not replace a face-to-face discussion of the patient's history. The health questionnaire must be rendered complete through targeted questioning. It is very important, today, to ascertain acquired and genetic risk factors.

The general medical history serves to protect patients with systemic diseases, and also protects the dentist and dental team from potentially dangerous infections (p. 211).

Special Patient Health History

In addition to questions concerning the general health of the patient, special areas of the patient's background must be investigated: What was the patient's motivation to seek out the dentist? What oral complaints does the patient have, and what does she/he expect from the dentist? Are caries, periodontal, or prosthetic problems of prime importance? Is the oral mucosa diseased? Is the patient experiencing pain? And last but not least: Does the patient complain of esthetic problems with teeth which are too dark, or large interdental spaces, tooth positional anomalies, "long teeth," or excessively visible gingivae?

Medical History Questionnaire

Please fill out this form correctly and completely—thank you! Your responses are important and will be kept in complete confidence.—You are aware of the physician's code of confidence –

Family name .... Given name ....

Street address .... City and zip code ....

Profession .... Date of birth ....

Home telephone .... Business phone ....

Physician ....

Reason for this consultation ....

Do you now have, or have you experienced ...	**Yes**	**No**
– Chest pain on exertion (Angina pectoris)	❏	❏
– A heart attack ... (when?)	❏	❏
– Heart valve failure/artificial heart valve	❏	❏
– High blood pressure	❏	❏
– Elevated bleeding tendency ... (Quick?/INR?)	❏	❏
– Stroke	❏	❏
– Epilepsy	❏	❏
– Bronchial asthma	❏	❏
– Lung problems, chronic coughing	❏	❏
– Allergic reactions ... (medicines?, other allergies?)	❏	❏
– Diabetes mellitus	❏	❏
Do you require insulin?	❏	❏
– Thyroid disease	❏	❏
– Liver disease	❏	❏
– Kidney disease	❏	❏
– Malignant diseases (leukemia, carcinoma, other)	❏	❏
– Infectious diseases	❏	❏
Hepatitis/jaundice	❏	❏
HIV—positive (AIDS)	❏	❏
Others, specify	❏	❏

Additional information ...

– Do you require antibiotic coverage before dental treatment? | ❏ | ❏
– Are you currently taking any medications prescribed by a physician? | ❏ | ❏
   Other medications? .... | ❏ | ❏
– Are you a smoker? How many cigarettes per day? | ❏ | ❏
– For women only: Are you currently pregnant? (week, month?) | ❏ | ❏

Date: .... Signature: ....

373 Medical History Form
For new patients, the top section of the questionnaire contains the important personal data, which can subsequently be entered into the comprehensive, computerized office database.

The medical history form should be completed by the patient in the waiting room, to save time.

The medical history form comprises ca. 20 questions about the patient's medical history, which can be answered *yes* or *no*. By signing the form, the patient acknowledges the validity of her/his answers.

As mentioned previously, the dentist or dental hygienist should discuss the medical history form with the patient in order to enhance information.

In the case of severe systemic diseases, the prudent dentist will consult the patient's physician.

All information provided by the patient must be held in strict confidence.

Classic Clinical Findings

Following collection of the systemic and special medical histories, the clinical examinations are performed. Recording of the "classic" findings (gold standard) remains of primary importance. It begins with a visual diagnosis. The entire oral cavity is inspected using a mirror. Even such a cursory inspection can reveal numerous manifestations of potential disease, e.g., plaque accumulation, gingivitis, gingival recession (Fig. 374). Brief inspection, however, can also lead to incorrect conclusions. For example, severe gingivitis may be incorrectly interpreted as periodontitis, or healthy appearing gingiva may mask true attachment loss. The important early diagnosis of periodontitis, including the existence of true periodontal pockets (clinical attachment loss, alveolar bone defects) can only be determined using the periodontal probe.

The clinical examination must be enhanced by radiographic diagnosis as well as vitality testing of all teeth. Elevated tooth mobility should be compared to the clinical findings (functional analysis, p. 174).

374 Cursory Inspection – Useless?
A brief inspection of the oral cavity reveals what appear to be healthy gingival conditions. However, such inspection can reveal only superficial alterations of the oral mucosa and teeth (see right), but reveal nothing in the *periodontal area*. On the other hand, visual inspection can be life saving: a *carcinoma screening*, e. g., floor of the mouth, palate, lateral lingual borders should be routinely performed, especially in heavy smokers (stomatitis, leukoplakia).

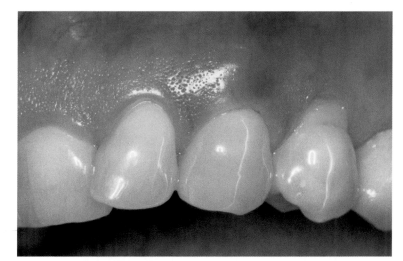

Teeth
- Condition of the hard structures
- Plaque accumulation
- Restorations (oral hygiene)

Gingiva
- Erythema
- Swelling
- Ulceration
- Recession

Oral Mucosa
- Effluorescences
- Discolorations
- Precancerous areas
- Tumors

375 Pocket Probing
In the same case (above), periodontal probing reveals that advanced periodontitis (labial attachment loss) is present in this area of healthy appearing gingiva.

Right: The surgical site reveals:
- Loss of 3 mm of bone
- Burnished calculus in . . .
- . . . a shallow buccal groove on the root surface

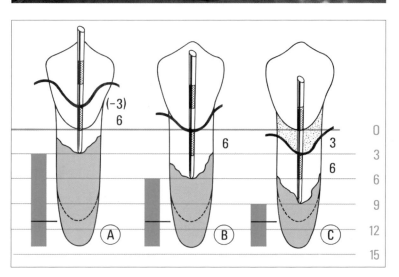

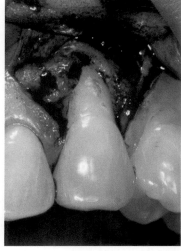

376 "Probing Depth 6 mm ..."
This statement provides no information concerning attachment loss or how much attachment remains on a tooth (blue columns):

A   6 mm probing depth
  − 3 mm pseudopocket
  = 3 mm true attachment loss
B   6 mm probing depth
  = 6 mm true attachment loss
C   3 mm gingival recession
  + 6 mm probing depth
  = 9 mm true attachment loss

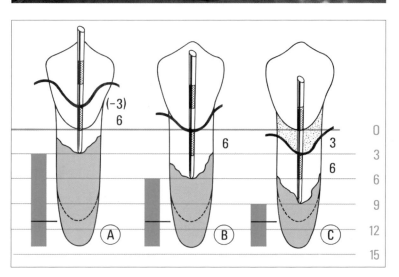

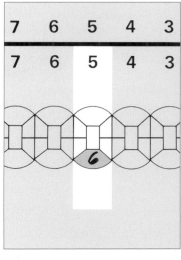

Pocket Probing—Probing Depth, Clinical Attachment Loss

The primary symptoms of periodontitis are loss of tooth-supporting tissues ("attachment loss") and the formation of true gingival and/or bony pockets. It is for this reason that any clinical examination of a periodontitis patient must include the measurement of pocket probing depths and attachment loss. Unfortunately, the significance of these *clinical* measurements is only relative, and not always congruent with the anatomic-histologic realities (Armitage et al. 1977, van der Velden and Vries 1980, van der Velden et al. 1986); the clinical measurements are much more dependent upon the state of health of the periodontium (tissue resistance).

The tip of the periodontal probe always penetrates into tissue that is below the sulcus or pocket fundus, even when the recommended probing force of 0.20–0.25 N is applied. With healthy gingiva and a normal junctional epithelium, the sulcus is histologically a maximum of 0.5 mm deep, but periodontal probing routinely yields a 2.5 mm measurement. The probe penetrates intraepithelially *into* the junctional epithelium. If gingivitis or periodontitis are present, the probe tip perforates the pocket epithelium and the infiltrated, vascular connective tissue (hemorrhage!) to the first intact collagen fibers that insert into cementum.

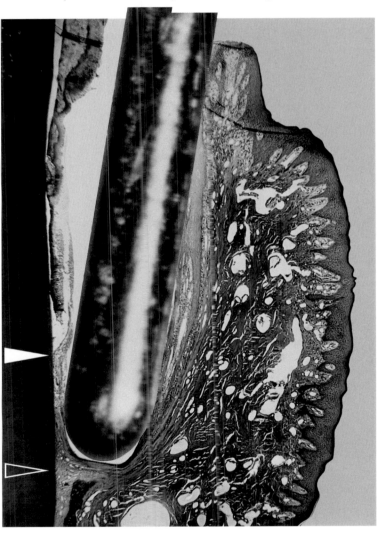

377 Probing Depth versus Pocket Depth
This photomontage depicts a periodontal probe within a shallow, supracrestal pocket, with anatomically accurate spatial relationships.

The pocket epithelium is perforated, and the gingiva is severely deflected laterally. It is only the healthy collagenous fiber bundles and/or alveolar crest of bone that stop the probe tip from further penetration.

White Arrow   pocket fundus
Empty Arrow   probing depth

The *measurement error* between the true, histologic pocket depth and the clinical measurement (probing depth) can be up to 2 mm in severe periodontitis. For initial data collection, such error is usually of no consequence, but must be considered for the "before and after" comparisons following periodontal therapy. In most cases, the therapeutic result will be overstated, revealing an exaggerated reduction of probing depth.

Courtesy of G. Armitage

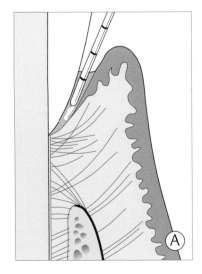

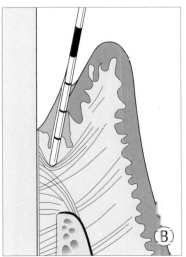

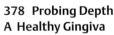

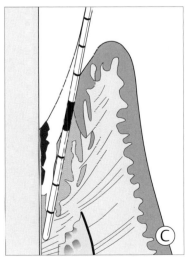

378 Probing Depth
A Healthy Gingiva
The probe tip remains in the junctional epithelium (pink) and no hemorrhage is elicited. PD ca. 2.5 mm.
B Gingivitis
The probe tip perforates the junctional epithelium (bleeding) and stops only when it encounters collagen fibers.
C Periodontitis
The probe tip perforates the junctional epithelium (bleeding) and is stopped only by contact with bone. PD 7.5 mm.

Pocket Probing—Periodontal Probes

For the measurement of pocket probing depths, an enormous variety of instruments is available. When used properly, most of these instruments fulfill their purpose; however, probes for use in routine daily practice and for scientific investigations can be differentiated.

Special plastic probes are used when "pockets" around a dental implant must be measured (mucositis, peri-implantitis).

The trend today is toward periodontal probes with simple millimeter markings, e.g., at 1 mm intervals. It is important that the readability of the probe is maintained.

Also today, periodontal probes with a tip diameter of 0.5–0.6 mm and a *rounded* tip are preferred.

The recommended probing force is ca. 0.20–0.25 Newtons (ca. 25 gm). Each dentist and dental hygienist should test her/his probing force using a laboratory scale, or if this is not available then using the nail bed (pain!): Research has shown that the probing force is generally too great, leading to incorrect measurements. A further important clinical observation is that the periodontal probe tip may be impeded by subgingival calculus and therefore not reveal the true and maximum pocket probing depth.

379 Periodontal Probes with Various Millimeter Indications
Metal probes with precise measurement indicators in mm.
From left to right:

- **CPITN/WHO Probe** (Deppeler): 0.5 (ball): 3.5, 5.5, (8.5, 11.5)
- **CP 12** (Hu-Friedy): 3, 6, 9, 12
- **GC-American:** 3, 6, 9, 12
- **UNC 15** (Hu-Friedy): millimeter markings, and a wide, black marking at 5, 10 and 15 mm

Right: UNC 15, enlarged.

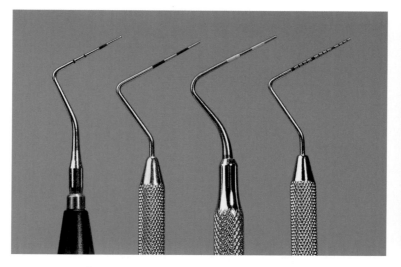
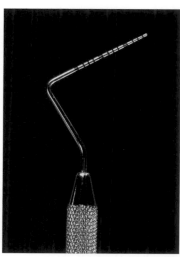

380 Plastic Probes
Sterilizable probes for pocket depth measurement around dental implants.
From left to right:

- **Deppeler:** 3, 6, 9, 12
- **Hu-Friedy:** 3, 6, 9, 12
- **Hawe:** 3, 5, 7, 10
- **Hawe "Click Probe":** 3, 5, 7, 10

Right: **Esro "Peep Probe":** 3, 6, 9, 12. When a force of ca. 0.20 N is applied, this probe provides an acoustic signal.

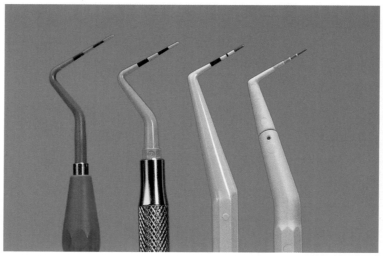
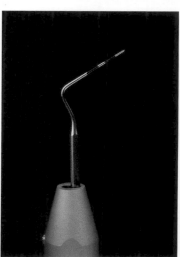

381 Florida Probe System
The *titanium tip* (diameter 0.45 mm) of this electronic probe measures pockets around teeth and implants with a normalized force of 0.25 N and with a precision of 0.2 mm.
Comparison: UNC 15 probe.

Right: The three probes of the Florida System measure from different reference points:

- **Disc Probe**
- **Stent Probe**
- **PD Probe ("Pocket Depth")**

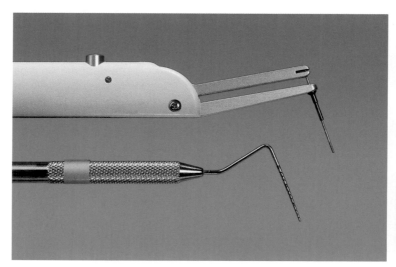
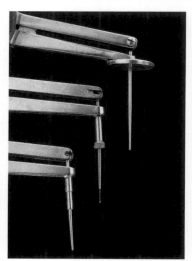

Pocket Probing Depths—Interpretation of the Measured Values

During the clinical examination of a periodontitis patient, the consideration of *pocket depth* receives high consideration, but the actual histologic depth of pockets *cannot* be determined clinically, because the probe tip always penetrates into the tissues. In the final analysis, the clinical probing results depend greatly upon the severity of the inflammation, i. e., the resistance offered by the periodontal tissues. On the other hand, the probe tip may also be inhibited by calculus, root irregularities etc.

In general, the following parameters can be ascertained with a periodontal probe, either mechanical or electronic:

- *Probing pocket depth*: Measurement from the gingival margin to the point at which the probe tip stops; inaccurate
- *Clinical attachment level* (CAL): Measurement from the cementoenamel junction (CEJ) to the point at which the probe tip stops (PDL fibers); more accurate
- *"Bone sounding," under anesthesia*: Measurement from the gingival margin to the alveolar crest
- *Recession*: Measurement from the cementoenamel junction (CEJ) to the gingival margin
- *Gingival swelling*: Measurement from the CEJ (often difficult to ascertain) to the coronal gingival margin.

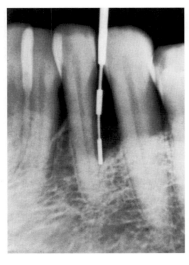

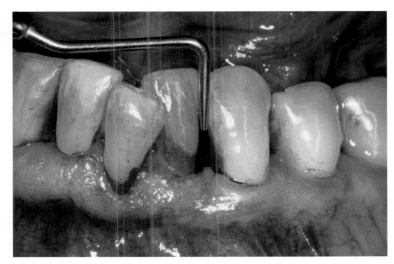

382 9 mm Deep Bony Pocket—Distal of Mandibular Left Lateral Incisor
The probe tip penetrates the remaining junctional epithelium and fundus of the pocket, and reaches the alveolar bone with only minimal pressure (ca. 0.25 N) in this case of inflamed periodontal tissues.
Advanced horizontal bone loss, with initial vertical, cup-shaped bone resorption.

Left: The probe tip appears to approach the osseous niveau.

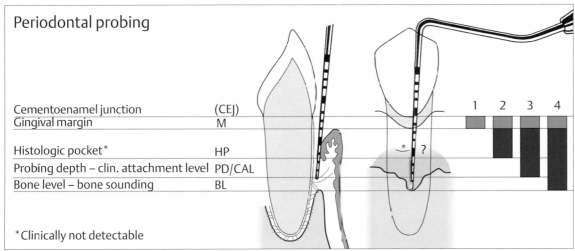

Periodontal probing

Cementoenamel junction	(CEJ)
Gingival margin	M
Histologic pocket*	HP
Probing depth – clin. attachment level	PD/CAL
Bone level – bone sounding	BL

*Clinically not detectable

383 Schematic Representation of Measurable Parameters
With the exception of gingival swelling, the above-mentioned measurement possibilities with a periodontal probe are depicted. The measurements shown here on the buccal aspect can be performed on at least six sites around each tooth (p. 194)!

The bar graph depicts:
1 Gingival recession (blue)
2 Histologic pocket fundus
3 Clinical probing depth
4 "Bone sounding"

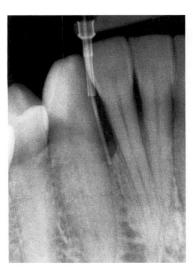

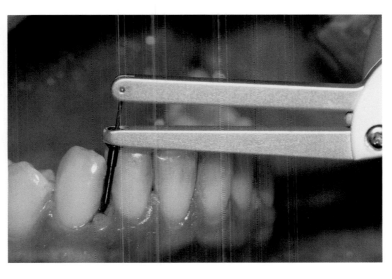

384 Florida Probe in situ
The probe exhibits a probing depth of 7 mm. It is clear that the guiding tube must approximate the gingival margin during this measurement.

Left: The thin (0.5 mm diameter) Florida Probe is depicted in a radiograph; the radiographic image is relatively small because the probe consists of titanium.

Furcation Involvement—Horizontal and Vertical Furcation Invasion

Root Surface Irregularities, Root Fusion, Enamel Projections

Treatment would be greatly facilitated if all tooth roots exhibited a round-oval profile! Very often, however, even single-rooted teeth exhibit concavities and the roots exhibit an hourglass shape. In the case of multirooted teeth, the practitioner must ascertain the exact location of the furcation (root trunk length, furcation entrance angle) and to what degree the furcation is already involved by attachment loss. On the other hand, one must also determine to what degree the individual roots are fused, a situation that often is accompanied by deep, narrow grooves along the root surface in the furcation area. Enamel projections and "pearls" in or near the furcation also deserve attention. Even the healthy root (cementum) surface is never smooth, rather it exhibits rough areas, and lacunae often occur in the apical region as well as in the furcations, where they are often pronounced (Schroeder & Rateitschak-Plüss 1983, Schroeder 1986).

The detection of such morphologic and pathologic peculiarities becomes more difficult as pocket depth increases, becomes narrower and more tortuous in the furcation region.

385 Special Probes for the Diagnosis of Furcations, Depressions and Grooves:

- **EX 3 CH** (HuFriedy): Fine and pointed, paired left-right, bent/curved, for checking surfaces, narrow grooves
- **PC-NT** 15 (HuFriedy): Right-angle probe; millimeter markings, with color-coding each 5 mm (5, 10, 15)
- **PQ 2N** (Nabers; HuFriedy): Color-coded furcation probe (markings at 3, 6, 9 and 12 mm)

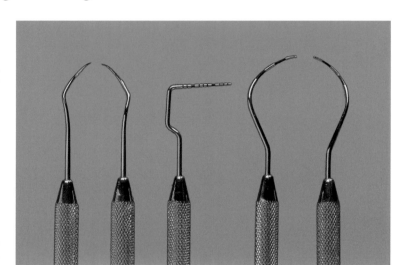

Severity of Furcation Involvement (cf. p. 306)

Horizontal (Grade 0–3)
F0 –
F1 up to 3 mm
F2 > 3 mm
F3 through-and-through between two roots

Vertical (Subclasses A–C)
A up to 3 mm
B 4–6 mm
C ≥ 7 mm
The length of the root trunk from the CEJ to the furcation roof must also be considered.

386 Section Through Maxilla
This view, with the cut root surfaces colored red, clearly depicts the enormous variations in root morphology. The narrow furcations, root fusions and hourglass shapes of some roots can also be observed. The interdental and interradicular osseous septa are also of varying dimensions.

387 Many Forms of Maxillary and Mandibular Molars (right)
The roots were sectioned horizontally about 4 mm apical to the cementoenamel junction. This view depicts clearly the variability of furcation areas as well as root fusions. It is easy to imagine the difficulties associated with root planing in such areas!

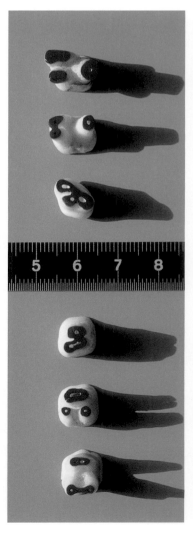

388 Section Through Mandible
Root morphology in the mandible is more uniform and less complicated than in the maxilla, but almost all of the roots exhibit some depressions labiolingually. Many molars also exhibit enamel projections ("pearls"). Particularly the mandibular molars exhibit variability in the length of the root trunk.

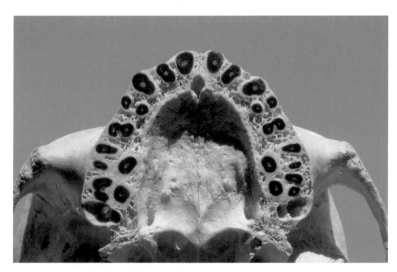

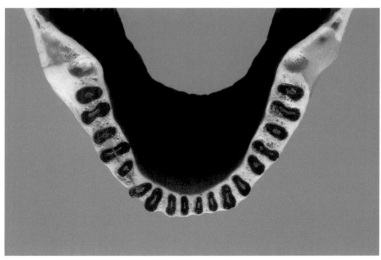

For diagnostic purposes, the blunt, straight periodontal probe alone is inadequate. Adjunct probes that are specially curved, blunt or pointed, are required (Fig. 385).

The clinical recognition and ascertainment of such root peculiarities is of importance, because furcations are some of the most difficult to treat plaque-retentive areas and retention areas for microorganisms.

Furthermore, when a flap procedure permits direct vision of the exposed root surfaces, the practitioner quickly realizes that nature has even more morphologic fantasy than was perhaps apparent at the initial examination. Morphologic peculiarities and the attachment loss picture are usually more pronounced than anticipated during the original data collection.

The radiograph can provide additional evidence of root peculiarities, but cannot precisely portray the variations in root morphologies that occur from tooth to tooth. The radiograph cannot replace the comprehensive examination of the root surface with a fine probe. Only high resolution computer tomography (CT) could display and reveal the three-dimensional characterization of this region.

Probing the Trifurcation of Tooth 17

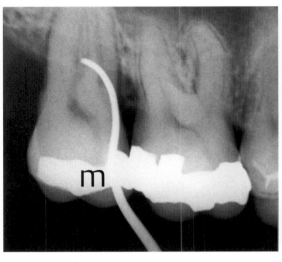

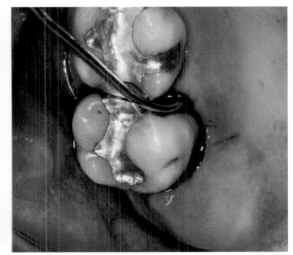

389 "Mesial" Furcation—m
In the radiographic, no furcation involvement is visible. However, using a Nabers-2 probe it is possible to probe the interradicular area of tooth 17 via the mesial furcation.

The mesial furcation can only be probed with certainty from a mesiopalatal approach.

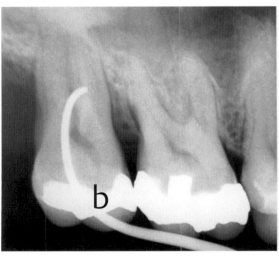

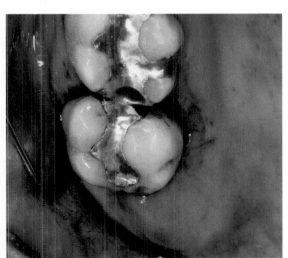

390 "Buccal" Furcation—b
Through the narrow buccal furcation, between the mesiobuccal and distobuccal roots, the probe tip reaches the roof of the furcation, and can also be guided into the interradicular area of the same tooth.

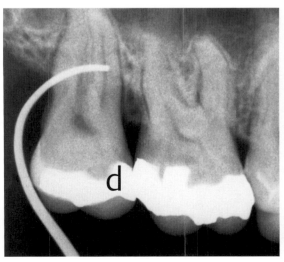

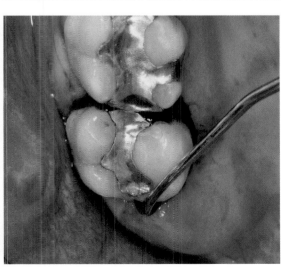

391 "Distal" Furcation—d
When the second molar is the most posterior tooth in an arch, the distal furcation can be probed from either distobuccal or distopalatal approaches. As shown, the Nabers-2 probe achieves the interradicular area from the distal approach.
→ Thus, tooth 17 is shown to exhibit three different class F3 furcation involvements: from the mesial, distal and buccal aspects.
These F3 lesions were treated periodontally and have remained stable for twenty years.

Tooth Mobility—Functional Analysis

Parafunctions (clenching and/or bruxing) do not cause gingivitis or periodontitis. Parafunctions can, however, lead to occlusal trauma and pathologic alterations within the periodontium, and therefore can accelerate the course of an *existing periodontitis* (Svanberg & Lindhe 1974, Polson et al. 1976a, b). Unphysiologic loading of the dentition can lead to elevated tooth mobility, without attachment loss. Parafunctions may be elicited by local *premature contacts*; parafunctions are frequently related to phases of stress.

According to Ramfjord (1979), "Occlusion-related periodontal trauma may elicit a deviation from periodontal health; therefore, periodontal comprehensive therapy should include treatment of traumatic lesions in the periodontium." Beyond their periodontal implications, functional disturbances may play a significant role in the etiology of myoarthropathology, and must therefore be eliminated before any prosthetic rehabilitation is initiated (Bumann & Lotzmann 2000).

392 Fremitus—Localization of Tooth Mobility
Any tooth mobility that is caused by premature contacts or traumatization of individual teeth can be clinically ascertained if the patient is asked to close in centric intercuspation and "tap" the teeth together while the clinician palpates the individual teeth with her/his fingertip. The etiology of locally elevated tooth mobility must be evaluated using additional tests. Here, the patient uses her own finger to "feel" her tooth mobility.

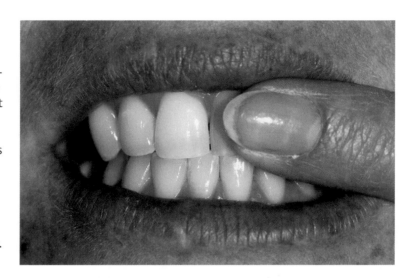

393 Manual Tooth Mobility Tests—TM Severity
With the patient's mouth open, each individual tooth is examined for its mobility, whereby the tooth is manipulated between an instrument and the clinician's fingernail using a force of ca. 5 N (ca. 500 g) in the oro-facial direction.

Right: In this *Atlas*, tooth mobility will be classified in four distinctly categorized degrees of severity, on the basis of previously performed electronic measurements.

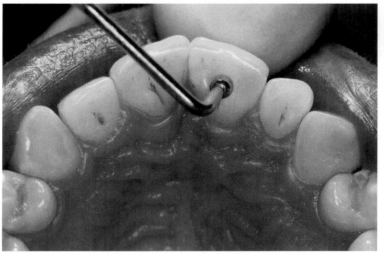

Tooth Mobility (TM)— Degrees of Tooth Mobility (H.R. Mühlemann 1975)
0   normal physiologic mobility
1   detectable mobility elevated mobility
2   visible mobility up to 0.5 mm
3   severe mobility up to 1 mm
4   extreme mobility vertical tooth mobility; tooth no longer functional

394 Hyperfunction and Inappropriate Function
Long-term and persisting parafunctions can exert negative influences upon the periodontium, tooth structure or the TMJ and masticatory musculature.

Left: Elevated tooth mobility and tooth migration, resulting from damage to the periodontal supporting structures.

Right: Excessive abrasion from severe parafunctions.

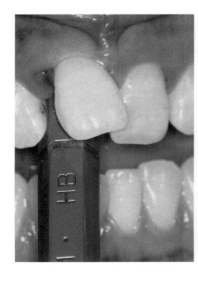
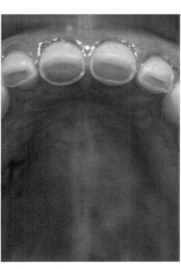

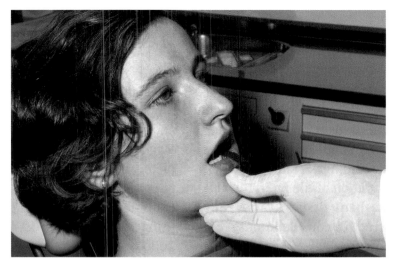

395 Manual Test for Premature Contacts in the Retruded Contact Position
With the patient seated upright, the clinician guides the mandible into its retruded position vis-à-vis the maxilla.

Excessive force in the retral direction can force the condyle backwards and downwards into an unphysiologic position. During this test, the mandibular condyle should achieve its zenith in the fossa.

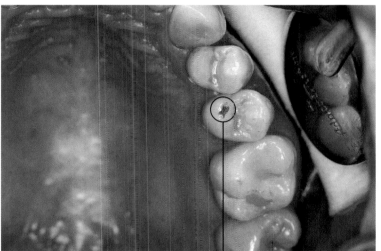

Marking a Premature Contact in Centric Relation (Retruded Contact Position) between Teeth 25 and 35.

396 Marking in the Maxilla on the Mesial Cusp of the Palatal Aspect of Tooth 25
This is a location in which premature contacts are relatively frequently observed.

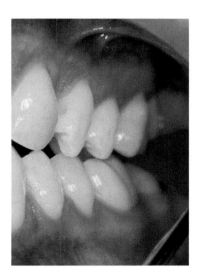

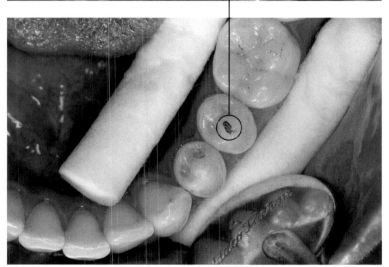

397 Marking in the Mandible on the Buccal Cusp of Tooth 35
Following the "tapping test" in retruded centric position, one notes contact solely between the left second maxillary premolar and its antagonist in the mandible.
When the patient bites together, the result is a *deviating movement* of the mandible anteriorly into *habitual occlusion* (intercuspation; centric occlusion).

Left: Lateral excursion to the left; no contact on tooth 25.

Centric Relation (CR)
– Initial "premature" contact $\dfrac{5}{5}$

– Deviation in   *1.5* mm *forward and right*

Articulation
– Contacts during lateral excursions $\dfrac{321}{321}$ $\dfrac{67}{67}$ B $\dfrac{7}{7}$ $\dfrac{1234}{1234}$

    toward......   right   left

      anteriorly **(B)** $\dfrac{21\;|\;12}{21\;|\;12}$ **(B)**

Parafunctions   Morphologic and functional
– Dental history   peculiarities
– Clinical examination   *None*

TMJ   *mild crepitus, left*

398 Most Important Entries into the "Minor Functional Analysis"
The chart entries shown here represent the case of a periodontally healthy female.

A minor "prophylactic" selective odontoplasty could, in this case, achieve an improvement of centric relation, by removing the premature contacts, as well as a reduction/elimination of the *balancing contacts* (**B**) between teeth 26, 27 and 36, 37 as well as 17, 47.

Bacterial Probe Test—Practical IAI PadoTest

The available DNA or RNA tests permit demonstration of three to eight of the most strongly associated marker bacteria for periodontitis.

Using the IAI PadoTest 4.5 — an RNA test, cf. p. 183 — the following four periodontopathogens can be demonstrated either site-specific or as pooled probes:

- *Aa/Actinobacillus actinomycetemcomitans*
- *Tf/Tannerella forsythia* (formerly *Bacteroides forsythus*)
- *Pg/Porphyromonas gingivalis*
- *Td/Treponema denticola*

In addition, this test provides supportive data regarding diagnosis and therapy (Fig. 420 and 421):
Quantitative:
- ML: Number and percentage composition of marker bacteria
- TBL/TML: Total load of all bacteria, i. e., the marker bacteria
- Statistical comparison of the results*
Qualitative:
- Typing of the pocket (Types 1–5)*

* Typing according to large field studies (Baehni et al. 1993).

417 Harvesting Pocket Flora Using a Paper Point
In most cases, the probes for bacterial tests are harvested from the deepest pockets in each quadrant (usually on molars). In the present "true" case, the sample is taken from the distal surface of tooth 12. The paper point is inserted to the fundus of the pocket and left *in situ* for 10 seconds.

Right: Thereafter, the paper point is placed into the color-coded transport vial, and the vial is tightly sealed.

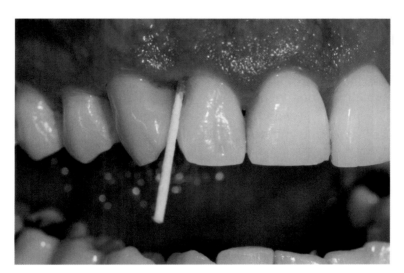
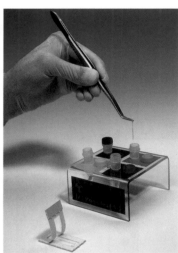

418 The IAI PadoTest 4.5 Kit for Harvesting Bacterial Samples
Paper points, transport vials and a convenient holder are included gratis in the commercially-available kit. The helpful *color-coding* is perpetuated throughout the four transport vials and the test stand, as well as the information forms and the final report (see p. 185) (red = quadrant 1 etc.).

Right: DNA probes are stable even in the dry condition, but the chemically more fragile RNA requires a stabilizing transport fluid.

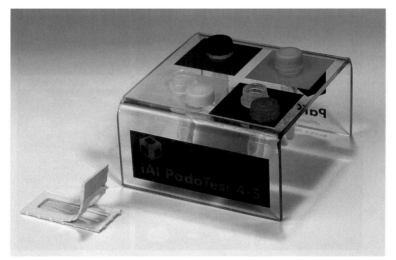
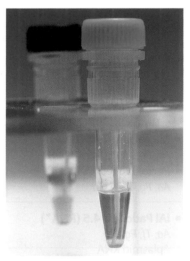

419 Transport to the Specialized Laboratory
The transport vials along with the pre-printed protocol form and often a coded patient name, as well as the noted site of sample harvest are sent using regular mail to the laboratory. The test results will be provided within a few days. The microflora of the individual pockets (sites) will be typified according to the reported field studies and the bacterial distribution reported therein (cf. Cluster/Socransky 1998; IAI/pocket types 1–5).

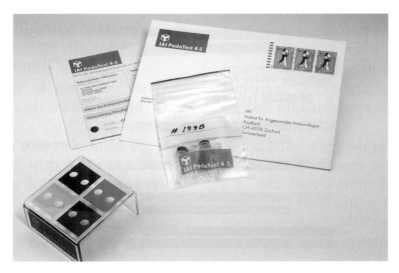
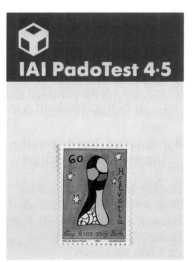

DNA/RNA Probe Tests—IAI PadoTest 4·5

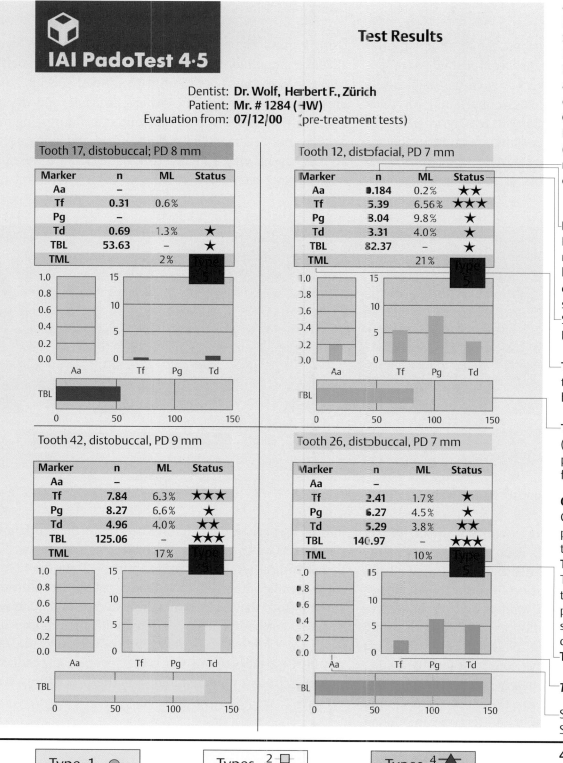

IAI PadoTest 4·5

Test Results

Dentist: **Dr. Wolf, Herbert F., Zürich**
Patient: **Mr. # 1284 (HW)**
Evaluation from: **07/12/00** (pre-treatment tests)

Tooth 17, distobuccal; PD 8 mm

Marker	n	ML	Status
Aa	–		
Tf	0.31	0.6%	
Pg	–		
Td	0.69	1.3%	★
TBL	53.63	–	★
TML		2%	Type 5

Tooth 12, distofacial, PD 7 mm

Marker	n	ML	Status
Aa	0.184	0.2%	★★
Tf	5.39	6.56%	★★★
Pg	3.04	9.8%	★
Td	3.31	4.0%	★
TBL	82.37	–	★
TML		21%	Type 5

Tooth 42, distobuccal, PD 9 mm

Marker	n	ML	Status
Aa	–		
Tf	7.84	6.3%	★★★
Pg	8.27	6.6%	★
Td	4.96	4.0%	★★
TBL	125.06	–	★★★
TML		17%	Type 5

Tooth 26, distobuccal, PD 7 mm

Marker	n	ML	Status
Aa	–		
Tf	2.41	1.7%	★
Pg	6.27	4.5%	★
Td	5.29	3.8%	★★
TBL	140.97	–	★★★
TML		10%	Type 5

420 Test Results and their Prognostic and Therapeutic Significance
In this case, the three deepest sites in the maxilla (teeth 17, 12, 26) and a very deep pocket in the mandible (tooth 42) were evaluated.

Quantitative Parameters,
Pocket on tooth 12 distobuccal (green table)
n = number of bacteria in millions, e. g., *Aa* about 180,000 entities; *Tf* about 5.4 million

ML = "marker load" in %. Percentage composition of the marker bacteria vis-à-vis the total bacterial load (**TBL**), e. g., in this case ca. 82,000,000; in comparison: percentage of *Aa* = 0.2 %
Statistical comparison ("Stars"). For details, see Fig. 421.

TML = "total marker load" in % of the entire count of *all* bacteria, here 21 %

TBL = "total bacterial load" (Total "pathogens + nonpathogens") The scale ranges from 0 to 150 million

Qualitative Parameters
Characterizing the periodontal pocket according to its colonization and microbial assortment in **Types 1–5.**
This characterization permits a true understanding of the complexity of the microbiological results, and provides a clue to the clinical significance.
Type 5 = pocket type

Tf, Pg, Td—"red complex," p. 37

Scale for ***Aa***: 0–1 million
Scale for *Tf, Pg, Td*: $0–15 \times 10^6$

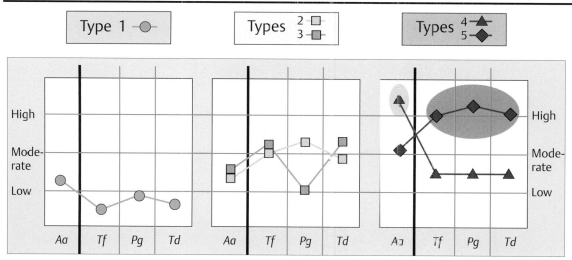

Type 1 ●
Types 2 ☐ 3 ☐
Types 4 ▲ 5 ◆

421 Pocket Type—Microbiologic Complexes
According to the distribution of the marker bacteria, five types can be distinguished:

	Therapy
Type 1	Simple therapy
Types 2 and 3	Moderately difficult
Types 4 and 5	complex

Types 1–3 can be treated purely mechanically. Types 4 (*Aa*!) and 5 ("red complex") demand adjunctive antibiotic therapy.

Immunological Tests—Antigen-Antibody Reactions

Antigen-Antibody Reaction

In contrast to the tests just described, the immunologic determination of bacteria can also be accomplished using specific *antigens* (Ag), *surface markers* (structures such as pili, fimbria; usually carbohydrates or glycoproteins), to which specific monoclonal antibodies (Ab) attach. In order to render the Ag-Ab binding visible, specially prepared antibodies with so-called reporter molecules (RM) are tagged. This can be done using enzyme-like colors or substances that fluoresce.

Direct and Indirect Immunofluorescence

Using immunofluorescence, the Ag-Ab reaction can be visualized using a *fluorescence microscope*. The bacteria affixed to the microscope slide bind to the added specific antibodies via their type-specific *surface antigens*, and the antibodies are rendered visible in UV light as fluorescing molecules (Gmür & Guggenheim 1994). Dead *and* living bacteria are seen in this way, and new techniques make it possible to differentiate even on the basis of color (Netuschil et al. 1996).

422 Immunofluorescence
D—direct (left):
The specific antibody (yellow), tagged with a fluorescent enzyme, docks with the red, triangular antigens (Ag).

I—indirect (right)
In a second step, several tagged (green) antibodies bind to the non-tagged yellow; this permits the fluorescence to be clearly visualized in UV-light (Ag-Ab reaction).

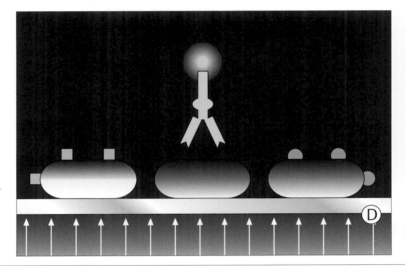
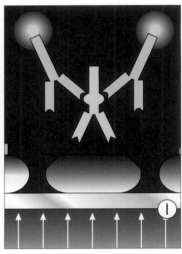

EIA/ELISA—Enzyme-Linked Immunosorbent Assay

An immediate chairside test for identification of marker bacteria in periodontitis patients is no longer commercially available. In fact, immunologic tests that would elicit a color reaction would be an ideal solution to avoid the expensive and time-consuming laboratory studies and the expensive apparatus needed for immunofluorescence investigations. In recent years, the quite good Evalusite Test was made available (Kodak/semiquantitative color test for the marker bacteria *Aa*, *Pg*, *Pi*), but unfortunately it has been removed from the market. Practitioners are therefore reconciled to waiting for a similar reliable chairside test system. Today,

immunological test procedures are performed in laboratories according to the two procedures shown below: "antibody capture" (A) or "antigen capture" (B). In the first case (A) a specific monoclonal antibody (yellow) "captures" the antigen (red) that is fixed in a minicuvette, and upon which a second antibody becomes affixed with the reporter molecule (RM). Following a rinsing procedure, only the Ag-Ab complex participates in the color reaction. Procedure (B) proceeds in a similar manner, but the procedures are reversed.

423 Immunological Tests, Color Reactions—EIA and ELISA

A "Antibody Capture"

B "Antigen Capture"

1 Specific antigen (red)
2 Primary antibody (yellow):
   Ag-Ab reaction
3 Secondary antibody (green or orange) carry reporter molecules
4 Reporter molecules (RM) elicit the *color reaction*

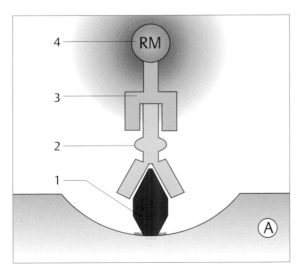
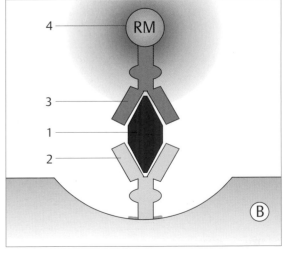

Enzymatic Bacterial Tests—BANA Test

Certain periodontopathic bacteria (including the "red complex": *Tf, Pg, Td*; pp. 37, 191; but not *Aa*) produce in their metabolism a trypsin-like enzyme, a peptidase, which has the ability to degrade BANA (Loesche et al. 1992). BANA stands for *N-α-benzoyl-DL-arginine-2-naphthylamide,* a synthetic substrate that is hydrolyzed by the above-mentioned bacterial peptidase. One of the breakdown products is β-naphthylamide, which becomes visible due to a color reaction and therefore provides evidence of the pathogenic bacteria.

The BANA test (e. g., Dentocheck; Butler) is relatively inexpensive and can also be performed by auxiliary personnel in the practice. A *strong positive* test is an indication that antibiotics against obligate anaerobes should be used in addition to mechanical *pocket treatment* (pocket Type 5; p. 185). Unfortunately, the robust and difficult to eliminate *Aa* is not identified by the BANA test. An additional disadvantage is that other, less-pathogenic pocket flora may also be BANA positive. These facts demonstrate the limitations of this bacterial test.

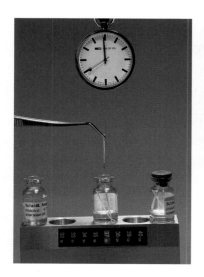

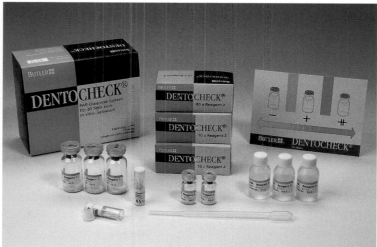

424 DentoCheck
(Butler/Heico Dent)
The kit contains materials for 30 tests/test sites:

- Reagents 1, 2 and 3
- 100 paper points
- 1 pipette
- Color scale
- Detailed instructions

Left: Using 3 paper points, plaque samples from the deepest pockets are harvested and then processed according to the laboratory protocol.

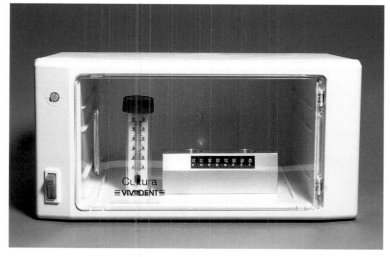

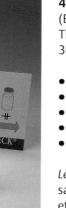

425 Incubation Chamber, Aluminum Block, Thermometer, Stopwatch. . .
. . . must be available. The incubation chamber and the aluminum block must be brought to 37° C before the test is initiated.

Left: BANA-positive are the "companions of the red complex" (cf. p. 37; Socransky et al. 1998). Depending on the concentrations of these microorganisms, the test will reveal negative, weakly positive or strongly positive.

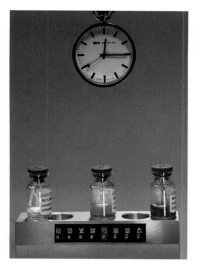

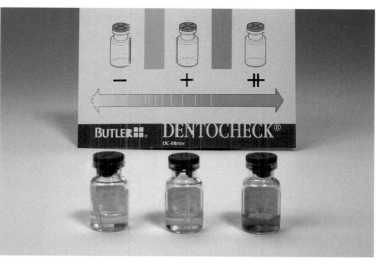

426 Evaluation of the BANA-Test
In comparison to the color scale, the presence and quantity of BANA-positive bacterial flora can be estimated.

Left: The reaction time (15 min at 37° C) must be carefully adhered to.
The following tests are commercially available:

- **Dentocheck**
- **Perioscan**
- **Periocheck**

Tests of the Host Response—Risks

- **Risk Factors**
- **Severity Factors**
- **Progression Factors**

All of the tests described thus far are based on clinical parameters and directly or indirectly on the identification of periodontopathic bacteria. The tests described below provide indications of the host response to the microbial infection.

Many indicators can signal on-going periodontal destruction, including PMN defects, high titers of antibodies against periodontopathogens, enzymes such as aspartate aminotransferase (AST; Persson et al. 1995), elevated inflammatory mediators (PGE2) and others. Also, the measurement of subgingival temperature (e. g., PerioTemp System) can indicate the existence of inflammation, but not necessarily provide information about the progression of the disease (Kohlhurst et al. 1991, Fedi & Killoy 1992, Trejo et al. 1994).

None of the current methods for testing host response have yet achieved routine utilization in practice.

**427 Enzyme Test—
Hawe Periomonitor**
This practical test measures the amount of aspartate aminotransferase (AST) in the *sulcus fluid*. AST is an intracellular enzyme, which is released upon cell death and can therefore be correlated with the amount of tissue destruction. The test is based on a color reaction.

Right: Sulcus fluid strips remain *in situ* for 30 seconds.

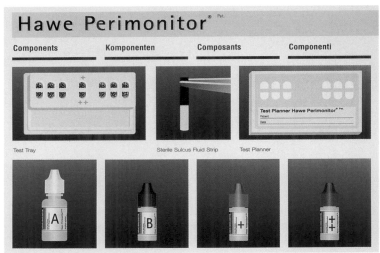
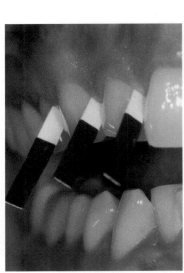

**428 Subgingival Temperature
– PerioTemp System**
(Abiodent, Inc.)
Heat is one of the cardinal symptoms of inflammation ("calor"). The temperature at the base of a periodontal pocket can be measured using a fine, graduated, sterile temperature probe. The instrument provides a color scale depicting all 32 teeth, displaying green-red when the average subgingival temperature exceeds 35.5° C. The measured values can also be printed out (left).

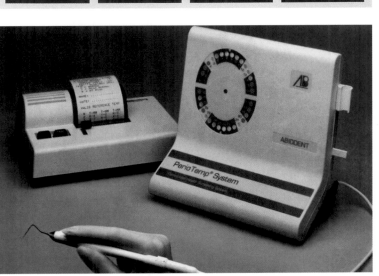

Genetic Risk—Test for IL-1 Gene Polymorphism

In the chapter on etiology and pathogenesis (pp. 41–66) the *enormous* significance of the various host defense mechanisms against microbial infection was extensively portrayed. It was demonstrated that inflammatory reactions are regulated by numerous messenger substances and enzymes such as prostaglandins, metalloproteinases and certain cytokines. One of these cytokines is one of the most powerful general activators: Interleukin 1 (IL-1). It exists as IL-1α and IL-1β, whose production is coded for by the two genes *IL-1A* and *IL-1B* (both on chromosome 2).

IL-1 Gene Polymorphism

Mutations of an individual base pair ("single nucleotide polymorphism"; SNP) are quite common; the normal base sequence in the gene is termed *Allele 1*, and the less common or altered as *Allele 2*. Both IL-1 genes can exhibit the SNP: The base cytosine (pairing with guanine, Fig. 430) is then replaced by thymine (pairing with adenine). Polymorphisms are not representative of major genetic alterations (gene defects, cf. p. 54), and their effects are therefore usually mild.

Note: This local overproduction by hyperactive MΦ can be additionally elevated as a result of the *autocrine* (self-stimulating) effect of IL-1 (Deschner 2002).

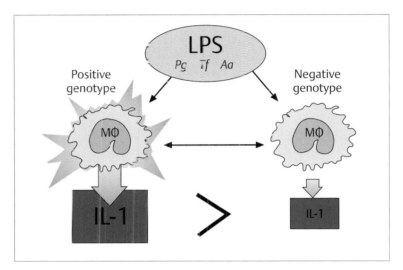

429 Differences in Monocyte Stimulation with IL-1-positive and IL-1-negative Genotype
Monocytes/Macrophages determine for the most part the severity of the local inflammatory reaction to the corresponding irritant.

With an IL-1-positive genotype, the monocytes are provoked to up to 4 times higher production of IL-1 by lipopolysaccharide (LPS) from gram-negative anaerobes (*Pg, Tf, Td*).

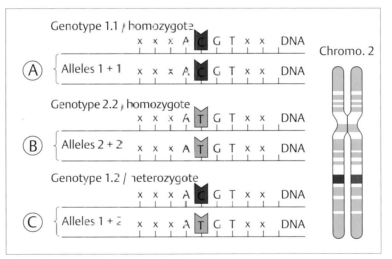

430 Polymorphism—Genotype
The chromosomes of tissue cells are present in two categories (diploid, one each from the mother and the father). Therefore in a SNP, three variants per gene are possible (**A, B** and **C**):

A 2 times **C** (Cytosine: "normal")
= Allele 1 & 1, homozygote

B 2 times **T** (Thymine; *SNP*)
= Allele 2 & 2, homozygote

C 1 time **C** and 1 time **T**
= Alleles 1 & 2, heterozygote

Effect upon the Periodontium

The general effect of a positive IL-1 genotype is depicted in Figure 429.

Definition: The "IL-1-positive genotype" ("positive" with regard to SNP) is allocated to those individuals who possess the Allele 2 homozygote in one gene or at least heterozygosity in both IL genes (genes *IL-1A* and *IL-1B*; see above).

The elevated susceptibility to periodontal inflammation that is associated with the IL-positive genotype does not manifest itself immediately in the young persons, as long as no additional risk factors such as smoking, poor oral hygiene, systemic diseases such as diabetes mellitus (DM) etc. are present (Kornman et al. 1997). But if risks exist over a longer period of time, the IL-1 polymorphism accelerates and accentuates periodontitis to a great degree ("severity factor"; odds ratio ca. 1.5–2).

In difficult cases or in patients with high or multiple risk factors, the test for the existence of the IL-1 gene polymorphism is indicated.

Prevention—Prophylaxis

Dentistry: Caries, Gingivitis, Periodontitis

Maintenance of Health and Prevention of Disease ...

... are the noblest goals of modern medicine! For the patient, prevention is more comfortable, simpler to perform and, last but not least, less costly than treatment. The cost "explosion" in all disciplines of diagnostic and therapeutic medicine is enormous. It is scarcely possible to finance such costs regardless of whether socialized medicine or private insurance or direct payment by patients are invoked. Ethical, social and scientific facts demand that we move toward prevention.

Dentistry

Prevention of the ubiquitous inflammatory periodontal diseases should benefit every socioeconomic segment of society and every age group. Children, young persons and young adults in particular should be exposed to preventive measures. At the same time, they must be educated concerning the importance of their own responsibility in personal health care. Long-term preventive awareness and behavior demand insight, will and persistence from the patient (compliance). This can only be expected if the dental team, dental educators etc. continually make known the possibilities and the enormous importance of prevention, and thereby motivate the patient toward maintenance of health. This demands especially that the dentist not only possess current knowledge of new developments in periodontal diagnosis and treatment possibilities, the dentist must also recognize and keep abreast of systemic medical relationships, and communicate these to all patients.

Definition: Prevention—Prophylaxis

Prevention: Medical and dental measures to inhibit disease initiation
- *Primary prevention*: "Strengthening" health—inhibition of a disease, e.g., through vaccination; in dentistry, e.g., patient information, oral hygiene instruction, prophylactic measures
- *Secondary prevention*: Early detection and treatment of diseases, e.g., comprehensive diagnosis of the disease, and anti-infectious therapy
- *Tertiary prevention*: Stopping and preventing the recurrence of an already treated/healed disease, e.g., through regular recall
(SPC—"supportive periodontal care")

Prophylaxis: Prevention of diseases (individual and collective)
- *Oral prophylaxis*: Mechanical removal of deposits, plaque and calculus
- *Antibiotic prophylaxis*

Prevention of Gingivitis and Periodontitis

In recent years it has been demonstrated in well-documented studies that prevention of periodontitis can be successful if performed consistently and appropriately (Axelsson & Lindhe 1977, 1981a, b; Axelsson 1982, 1998, 2002).

The primary etiologic agent for gingivitis and periodontitis is the *microbial biofilm.* In the absence of biofilm, marginal inflammation will not develop. Therefore, prevention and prophylaxis involves, as always, the elimination of plaque and calculus, and motivation of the patient toward adequate oral hygiene.

From a somewhat broader prospective, prevention of periodontal disease encompasses several additional measures that are also targeted toward elimination of plaque, but indirectly. This is termed *anti-infectious therapy,* and includes the elimination of natural plaque-retentive areas (crowding, etc.) and above all the elimination of iatrogenic irritants. An overhanging restoration or a poorly adapted crown margin make oral hygiene in the interdental area impossible. Dental floss is ineffective in such cases; it tears and becomes lodged in the defective restoration. The possibility for satisfactory hygiene in each individual patient must be created by the dentist and the auxiliary dental personnel. Finally, the margins of restorations and reconstructions must be placed supragingivally whenever this is esthetically feasible in order to enhance prevention of gingival inflammation.

Total freedom from plaque is only a utopic goal. The reality is that, for each patient, an individual optimum hygiene level (plaque index) must be achieved, one which can be maintained consistently over the years, dependent upon the patient's own degree of motivation and above all the recall interval. It has been demonstrated again and again that the gingival and periodontal conditions, even in large groups of patients, do not deteriorate if an appropriate recall interval is established and maintained for the individual patient (Ramfjord et al. 1975, 1982; Rosling et al. 1976a; Axelsson & Lindhe 1981a, b; Axelsson 1982, 1998, 2002; Manser & Rateitschak 1997).

In the absence of microorganisms, there will be no gingivitis or periodontitis; on the other hand, the existence of plaque bacteria alone does not in every case lead to periodontitis. The susceptibility of the patient, her/his immune status, the existence of non-alterable (usually genetically-determined) and alterable risk factors, and the host's response to the infection are what determine the initiation and progression of periodontitis.

"Prevention," then, extends beyond elimination of the infection—as far as this is possible—and to *influencing the host* itself. Any strengthening of the immune system has, heretofore, been possible only in minute measure, and true gene manipulation stands far in the future. Most likely, the future will hold the possibility to suppress pro-inflammatory mediators or, on the other hand, to stimulate anti-inflammatory mediators. Possible already today is the effort to influence and therefore reduce *alterable risk factors.* Systemic diseases that enhance or even elicit periodontitis must be appropriately treated; e. g., diabetes must be optimally controlled. Most especially, smokers must eliminate the high risk of tobacco use. The goal is a generally healthy lifestyle, with a minimum of stress.

Dental/oral prevention cannot simply be a casual endeavor. It demands time—considerable time—from both the patient and the practitioner. This is usually underestimated, and the consequences may render treatment success problematic.

The practical performance of prevention for gingivitis and periodontitis is for the most part identical to the measures described in the chapter "Initial and Phase-1 Therapy" (pp. 211–252), and will not be further discussed in this brief treatise on "Prevention."

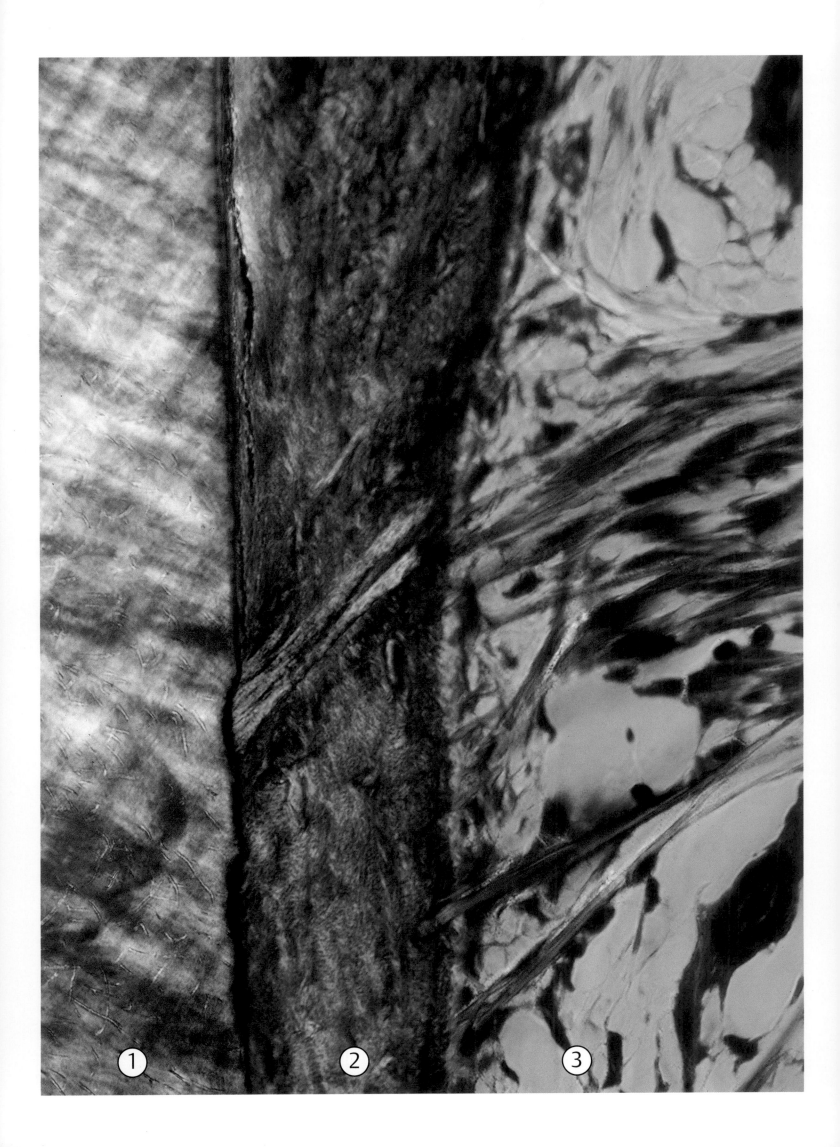

Treatment of Inflammatory Periodontal Diseases - Introduction

- **Gingivitis**
- **Periodontitis**

Gingivitis and periodontitis are elicited primarily by bacteria. As a consequence, the treatment must have a primarily anti-infectious nature. Reduction or elimination of the infection results for the most part from mechanical treatment of affected teeth and root surfaces as well as the gingival soft tissue. In special cases, support via topical or systemic medications may be indicated. Alterable risk factors must be eliminated as much as possible.

This section deals with the following constituents of periodontal therapy:

- Concepts of periodontal therapy: methods, goals, outcomes
- Periodontal healing, treatment planning, course of treatment

"Phase 0" Therapy **Systemic Pre-treatment**

- Periodontal emergencies: treatment

Phase 1 Therapy
- **Initial Treatment 1 and 2**
  Anti-infectious/causal, non-surgical therapy
- **FMT – "Full Mouth Therapy"**

- Adjunctive medicinal therapy – oral-systemic and topical

Phase 2 Therapy **Summaries of:**
Anti-infectious and corrective therapy
Periodontal surgery
- Access flap, regenerative and resective therapy
- Furcation treatment
Mucogingival plastic surgery

Phase 3 Therapy **Maintenance – Recall**
A must! – long term success, negative aspects?

"Alternative" Therapy? Dental Implants (Summary)

Left side:

Histologic section in polarized light; True regeneration of the periodontium following Guided Tissue Regeneration (GTR-surgery) *M. Hürzeler et al. 1997*

1 Dentin
2 *New acellular cement,* fibers
3 Periodontal fiber apparatus

Courtesy *P. Schüpbach*

Treatment Planning—Sequence of Treatment

In principle, the course of periodontitis therapy is similar for all forms of the disease (p. 209), and is administered in *stages* or *phases* of varying duration, depending upon the extent and severity of the disease.

However the *details* of individual therapy may be dramatically different. These details are dependent upon the type of disease, the patient's own desires, patient age, financial circumstances and, not least, the preference of the individual clinician! It is well known that "many roads lead to Rome"!

Pre-phase—Systemic Health, Oral Hygiene

"Phase 0" consists primarily of identifying the patient's *systemic health* (general medical history, p. 167; readiness for treatment, p. 212), as well as a comprehensive data collection, the establishment of a provisional diagnosis and a case presentation (current status, necessary treatment). During Phase 0, any emergency treatment is also rendered.

The establishment of optimum *oral hygiene* and securing the patient's willing *compliance* are extremely important for subsequent planning and the long-term result.

Professional supragingival plaque and calculus removal, the removal of iatrogenic irritants and plaque-retentive niches, as well as patient instruction in simple yet effective plaque-control will quickly improve the intraoral situation. This will convince and motivate the cooperative patient toward further and definitive participation in the comprehensive treatment program.

In a few (rare!) instances, it will be necessary to avoid systematic and comprehensive dental treatment completely (**X**), for example in the face of severe medical/systemic concerns or complications (cf. ASA, p. 212), but in worst cases also when home care by the patient is totally lacking, there is no regard for or appreciation of oral hygiene and oral health, and compliance is non-existent.

Phase 1—Causal, Antimicrobial, Anti-infectious

During this treatment phase, the findings, diagnosis and prognosis are verified. During the pre-phase, oral hygiene by the patient and the hygienist will have led to reductions in plaque and inflammation, therefore also to reduction of tissue swelling; it is reasonable to now establish a *definitive* diagnosis (and prognosis) based upon the important clinical findings (probing depths, attachment loss), and to formulate the definitive treatment plan.

While all of the pre-phase procedures are carried out with all patients, during Phase 1 the treatment modalities can differ. In some cases, *closed root planing,* with or without the concurrent use of medicaments (p. 287) may be performed, while in other cases the treatment moves directly into surgery (Phase 2).

In mild cases, above all with chronic periodontitis, *closed therapy* is frequently sufficient if the patient's compliance is good.

In more severe cases it may be indicated to move into *surgical-corrective therapy* immediately after an intensive pre-phase.

In most cases, however, open therapy will follow closed therapy: As a consequence, in such cases fewer sites (in fewer sextants) will have to be treated surgically. The resultant tissue loss (papillae, marginal gingiva) will be less post-operatively.

Whether the case is treated solely closed (**A**), solely open (**C**), or initially closed and subsequently open (**B**; p. 209) depends not only upon the pathomorphologic situation, but also upon the practice structure. The competent dental hygienist performs the entire *closed* phase of therapy (p. 314, Fig. 707).

Phase 2—Surgical, Corrective

Following Phase 1 therapy that includes closed, subgingival root debridement, a *reevaluation* must always be performed. If the treatment result is not satisfactory, individual root surfaces may again be treated with closed therapy (**a**). If deep pockets persist and if root fusion, grooves, furcation involvement etc. are present, these must be surgically addressed.

If the goal is to *correct* periodontal defects, following the pre-phase, surgical-corrective procedures are indicated. Tissue shrinkage should be avoided at all costs so that the surgical site will be optimally covered with gingival tissue following eventual application of restorative materials and/or membranes.

Most important is that the healing after surgical therapy must be continuously and professionally *monitored,* i.e., the operated area must be maintained supragingivally plaque-free as much as possible. The noble role of the dental hygienist!

Phase 3—Preventive, Anti-infectious, "Life Long"

After conclusion of active periodontitis therapy—regardless of the type of treatment—*check-up findings* are collected 2–3 months later. If the therapy is deemed to be successful, the patient should be started on a regular recall (organized maintenance therapy; p. 309).

However, if individual sites exhibit problems (residual pockets, bleeding), the sites must be re-treated either closed (**c**) or surgically (**b**).

In such situations, the use of topical slow-release medicaments may be indicated (p. 293).

**450 Course of Therapy—
Three Possibilities: A, B, C**

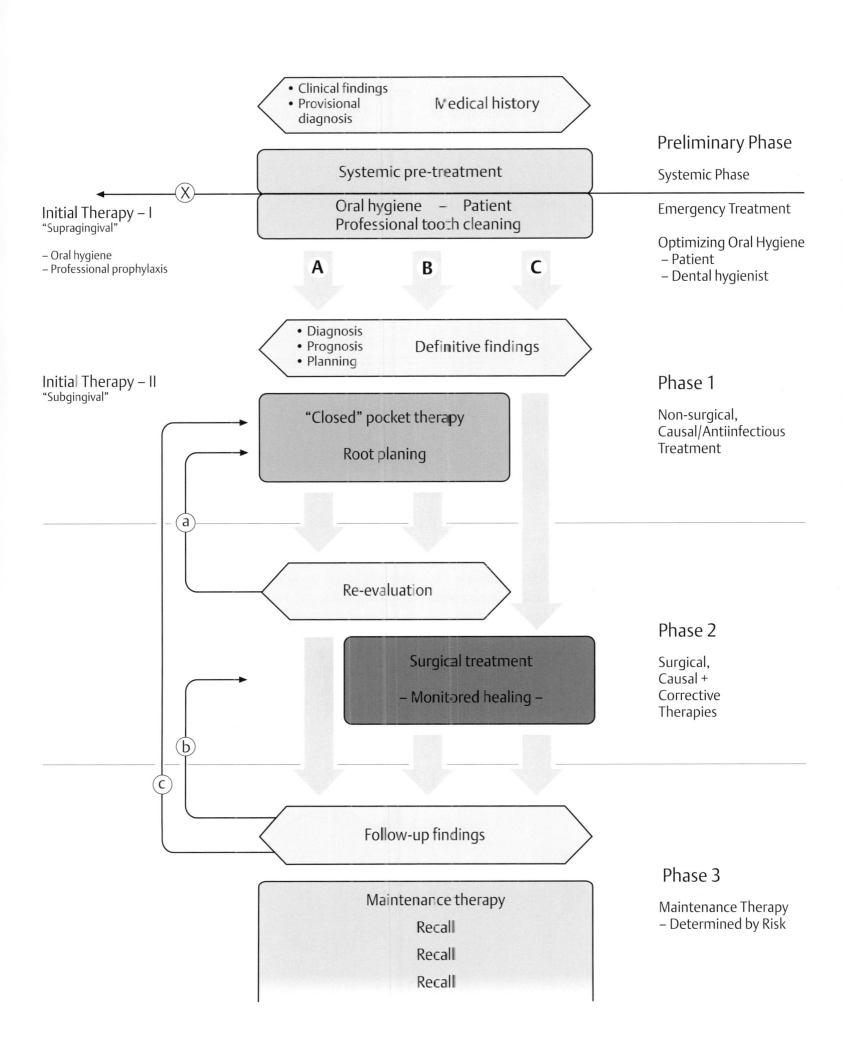

- Clinical findings
- Provisional diagnosis

Medical history

Preliminary Phase

Systemic pre-treatment

Systemic Phase

Oral hygiene   –   Patient
Professional tooth cleaning

Emergency Treatment

Initial Therapy – I
"Supragingival"

– Oral hygiene
– Professional prophylaxis

Optimizing Oral Hygiene
– Patient
– Dental hygienist

A   **B**   **C**

- Diagnosis
- Prognosis
- Planning

Definitive findings

Initial Therapy – II
"Subgingival"

Phase 1

"Closed" pocket therapy

Root planing

**Non-surgical,
Causal/Antiinfectious
Treatment**

(a)

Re-evaluation

Phase 2

Surgical treatment

– Monitored healing –

**Surgical,
Causal +
Corrective
Therapies**

(b)

(c)

Follow-up findings

Phase 3

Maintenance therapy

Recall

Recall

Recall

**Maintenance Therapy
– Determined by Risk**

General Course of Therapy—Individual Planning

In the preceding pages the basic treatment planning and the course of therapy for patients with gingivitis and/or peri-odontitis were presented. In general, such treatment is performed according to the "phase" plan (phases of therapy; pp. 208–9).

Treatment, healing times and "pauses" for consideration of the patient and his/her oral hygiene will differ dramatically. Nevertheless, following each and every phase of treatment, a *re-evaluation* of the case must be performed: The treatment result and the planned further procedures must be reconsidered, and adapted as necessary to the new situation.

Causal Therapy—Traditional Clinical Course

Phase 1 therapy consists of the exquisitely careful debridement of subgingival root surfaces in all periodontal pockets. For decades, this procedure has been performed *quadrant-by-quadrant* (Badersten et al. 1981, 1984; p. 280). The interval between individual appointments normally is one or two weeks. The quadrant scaling immediately follows the so-called "hygiene phase," during which the patient is educated and trained to perform adequate plaque control at home.

451 Quadrants—Sextants
Traditional mechanical/instrumental pocket treatment is usually performed at separate appointments for *quadrants* (**Q1–Q4**) or *sextants* (**S1–S6**); in mild cases, the left and right arch segments can be treated at one appointment.
The time required for each appointment will be determined by the severity of the case; appointments for such Phase 1 therapy are usually scheduled at 1–2 week intervals.

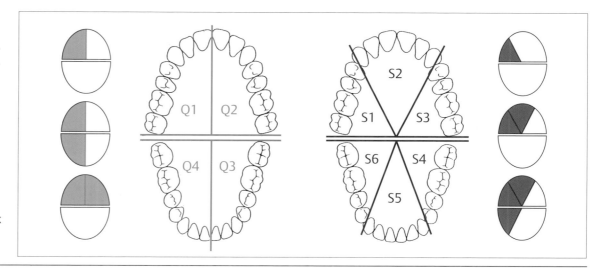

Causal Therapy—"Full Mouth Therapy" (FMT)

FMT represents an effort to synthesize all new knowledge from recent years. FMT is a consequential, anti-infectious approach, comprised of the following: Initial therapy includes an extended, systematic anti-microbial treatment, initially involving only supragingival pretreatment of the dentition (mechanical) and all oral niches (above all, the tongue). Only after achieving the prescribed clinical condition (p. 287), subgingival debridement (mechanically and with use of topical medicaments) is performed in the shortest possible time; in "extreme cases," within a 24-hour period. This procedure is appreciated by most patients!

During this short-term but intensive treatment, disinfection agents such as chlorhexidine (CHX; p. 235), betadine or even oxidizing NaOCl ("bleach") are used to rinse the mouth and the individual pockets. The goal is to prohibit re-colonization and re-infection of even shallow pockets (p. 256).

Because significantly better results have been achieved using this type of closed periodontitis therapy (p. 285), in contrast to the traditional "quadrant-by-quadrant" technique, it is very likely that the FMT method will become more widespread. The necessity for surgical intervention may be reduced and the comprehensive treatment of even advanced cases may become financially more feasible

452 "Full Mouth Therapy—FMT",
"Full Mouth Disinfection—FMD"
This new type of treatment using closed therapy is performed in the shortest possible time, preferably in only two appointments, e. g., for the left and the right sides.
Intensive pretreatment and optimum oral hygiene usually eliminate shallow pockets so that only the few remaining deeper pockets must be treated, using anesthesia (FMT, p. 281).

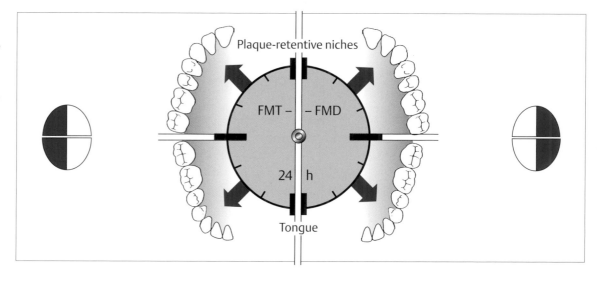

Systemic Pre-Phase

- **Systemic Problems**
- **Systemic Risks**

The purpose of the systemic pre-phase is to protect both the patient and the clinician by ascertaining any general systemic risks associated with the patient.

It is critically important that *infectious, above all viral diseases* (Herpes, Hepatitis B and C, HIV infection) be detected and/or diagnosed: Every patient may harbor such diseases! It is therefore necessary to employ the usual hygiene measures for all dental examinations and treatments, e.g., gloves, mask and protective eyewear.

Individuals with severe systemic diseases (see ASA Classification, p. 212) can seldom be treated periodontally under the rubric "comprehensive therapy." Usually these patients can only be treated with limited "emergency" measures, and with the participation of the patient's physician.

Special precautionary measures are indicated with patients who suffer from multiple maladies, and most particularly with patients who are susceptible to the *life-threatening* danger of infectious endocarditis (Reichart & Philipsen 1999).

With *non-life-threatening* diseases, dental therapy should be planned in collaboration with the physician or internist, who may prescribe appropriate medications (polypharmacy); these should be checked for possible drug interactions with other agents prescribed by the dentist, as well as the possibility of undesired adverse effects (cf., gingival hyperplasia; pp. 121–124).

Thanks to modern medicine, many of our patients lead the normal life of a *healthy* person. The possibility of injuring such patients during dental treatment must be ruled out (allergies, anticoagulants, hypertension, hypercholesterolemia).

Genetic and hereditary risks must be assessed, and decisions made concerning the individual patient's treatability or non-treatability (uncontrolled Diabetes mellitus; smokers).

This chapter presents the following discussions:

- The patient—ASA classification
- Cardiovascular diseases—"blood thinning"
- Bacteremia—prevention of infectious endocarditis
- Endocarditis prevention—antibiotics
- Diabetes mellitus—risk factor for periodontitis
- For the smoking risk factor—information, tobacco cessation program

Evaluation—Can the Patient be Safely Treated?

Before initiating any dental treatment, the relevant medical history provided by a "new" patient must be carefully checked, regardless of whether comprehensive therapy is anticipated or only an emergency procedure. Of particular importance are serious diseases or conditions, such as:

- Cardiovascular diseases
- Pulmonary diseases
- Renal diseases
- Endocrine diseases
- Compromised immune response
- Psychological/psychiatric conditions

Acute situations should be thoroughly discussed before treatment; these include allergies, anaphylactic reactions, but also patient fear of the treatment or even fear of the injection needle.

The dental team must be systematically prepared for emergency situations. Corresponding checklists, supplies and devices must be at hand (emergency kit, materials for cardiopulmonary resuscitation, and perhaps even a defibrillator).

The classification by the American Society of Anesthesiologists (ASA) helps to establish the physical status of a diseased patient (ASA Classes I–VI; Fig. 453)

453 ASA Classification of Patients—Health Status
Normally, only patients in Classes I and II are treated in the private dental practice, and in rare cases Class III. In the latter case, active collaboration and cooperation with the patient's treating physician is highly recommended.

ASA Class	Patient description — Classification criteria
I	Normal, *healthy* patient *without* systemic disease
II	Patient with *mild* systemic disease
III	Patient with *severe* systemic disease, which limits her/his activity but is not life-threatening
IV	Patient with a *severe* systemic disease that is constantly life-threatening
V	*Moribund* patient, who is not expected to live beyond 24 hours with or without operation
VI	*Brain-dead* patient whose organs may be harvested for transplant
E	Emergency patient — This category is re-defined, according to the clinical condition, in Grades I – IV (e. g., ASA III – E)

Medical Risk Factor—"Blood Thinning"

Patients with cardiac and circulatory diseases (post-myocardial infarction, Angina pectoris etc.) or other conditions (e. g., post-surgical condition, dialysis patients, thrombosis prophylaxis etc.) usually take *anticoagulants*:

- Short-term therapy: Heparin
- Long-term prophylaxis: Aspirin derivatives
- Long-term therapy: Cumarin derivatives
                         (e. g., Warfarin)

In order to avoid life-threatening hemorrhage, the patient's actual "Quick-time" (Cumarin) must be assessed. A Quick value of ≥ 30% usually does not affect dental or oral surgical

procedures, but values between 15 and 25 % demand consultation with the treating physician.

- The effect of blood-thinning medications is *enhanced* by non-steroidal anti-inflammatory agents such as salicylate, mefenamine acids, tetracycline, metronidazol and sulfonamides (Scully & Wolff 2002).
- Their effects will be *reduced* by barbiturates, glucocorticoids, alcohol, and foodstuffs with a high vitamin-K content.

The antidote for Cumarin is vitamin K; there is no antidote for the rapidly metabolized heparin. If necessary the patient may stop taking this medication for a short period of time.

454 Coagulation—
Tests of Blood Thinning
Because the results vary greatly, the old Quick-Test will be abandoned in the near future.
It will be replaced by the INR blood thinning test ("International normalized ratio") which provides constant values and ease of use by the patient!

Therapeutic bandwidth:
INR values of **2.5–4.5**, depending upon the risk status of the patient.

Coagulation test	INR	% Quick	Seconds
Measurement boundaries	1.2	70	13.2
	1.4	50	14.2
	1.6	40	15.6
	1.9	30	16.6
	2.1	25	17.4
	2.5	20	19.0
	3.0	16	20.8
Therapeutic band width	3.5	13	22.5
	4.0	11	24.0
	4.5	10	25.5
	5.0	9	26.9
Measurement boundaries	8.0	5	34.0

Bacteremia—Endocarditis Prophylaxis

Transient bacteremia is a natural, daily occurring situation (chewing, tooth brushing). In healthy persons, oral bacteria that enter the blood stream are efficiently eliminated by the host defense system.

Infectious endocarditis (IE) is a life-threatening disease, an infection of hemodynamically exposed defects (plaque formation on heart valves), usually elicited by oral microorganisms (streptococci).

Depending upon the virulence of the etiologic microbe and the resistance of the patient, various forms of IE can be differentiated (Müller 2001):

- *Acute, infectious forms*
  Sepsis, fever, endocardial destruction;
  death in less than 6 weeks
- *Acute/Subacute forms*
  Intermediate forms, often elicited by enterococci
- *Subacute forms*
  Slight fever; if untreated,
  death between 6 weeks and 3 months
- *Chronic forms*
  Symptoms the same as subacute;
  death in more than 3 months

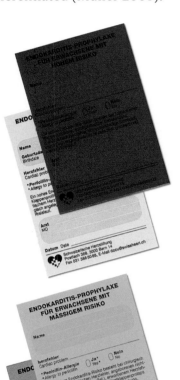

Indications for endocarditis prophylaxis
Heart failure and post-operative findings

High risk for endocarditis
- Condition following biological or mechanical heart valve replacement
- Condition following infectious endocarditis, in the absence of cardiac pathology

Moderate risk for endocarditis
- Inherited or genetic heart valve insufficiency
- Inherited cardiac defects, e. g.
  - Aortic isthmus stenosis
  - Ductus Botalli apertus
  - Ventricular septal defect
  - Sub- or supra-valvular aortic stenosis
  - Cyanotic vitium
- Condition following palliative operation for genetic heart failure
- Incompletely corrected genetic cardiac failure
  Hypertrophic, obstructive cardiomyopathy (HOCM)
- Mitral valve prolapse (MVP) with systolic sounds

No elevated risk of endocarditis
- Auricular septal defect
- Condition following successful closure of an auricular or ventricular septal defect
- Condition following successful coronary bypass surgery
- Mitral valve prolapse without systolic sounds
- Physiologic, functional or otherwise harmless heart sounds
- Previous Kawasaki disease without valvular dysfunction
- Previous rheumatic fever without valvular dysfunction
- Condition following implantation of a pacemaker
- Condition following surgery for aortic isthmus stenosis

455 Heart Diseases and Cardiac Defects—Indications for Endocarditis Prophylaxis
Within the new wording of the prophylaxis program from the AHA (American Heart Association; Dajani et al. 1997) the risk structure of the heart was newly categorized in three groups:
- **High Risk (red)**
- **Moderate Risk (green)**
- **Non-elevated Risk**

Of importance for the hygienist is that the presence of a cardiac pacemaker is not an indication for antibiotic, pre-treatment prophylaxis (but care must be exercised when electronic instruments such as ultrasonic scalers are employed).

Left: Individual patient cards from the Swiss Heart Foundation, listing guidelines and dosages for endocarditis prophylaxis.

- **High Risk**
  red → adults
  yellow → children
- **Moderate Risk**
  green → adult
  blue → children

Infectious Endocarditis (IE)

A wide variety of microorganisms such as bacteria, mycoplasm, fungi, rickettsia or chlamydia can elicit IE if they enter the bloodstream due to trauma or tissue manipulation. Regions of the cardiovascular system that experience slow blood circulation or a high level of turbulence are particularly susceptible to infections.

The most frequent source of microorganisms that elicit IE is the oral cavity. The primary pathogens are gram-positive streptococci (*viridans* type), especially *Streptococcus sanguis*.

In addition to *S. aureus* and *S. epidermis*, more and more often one also observes gram-negative bacteria from the oral cavity and the upper respiratory tract that elicit IE; for example, *A. actinomycetemcomitans, Hemophilus ssp., Cardiobacterium ssp., Eikenella corrodens, Kingella ssp., Capnocytophaga, Neisseria ssp.*

For the protection of IE-endangered patients, bacteriocidal antibiotics of the "penicillin type" (p. 214) are recommended. As early as 1983, J. Slots and others suggested that IE prophylaxis could also include metronidazol (p. 287).

Endocarditis Prophylaxis with Antibiotics

According to new guidelines from AHA (Dajani et al. 1997), the prophylactic dose of standard antibiotic (*Amoxicillin*) was reduced to 2 grams; in addition, no follow-up dose is now recommended; not all other Heart Associations agree.

It is comforting for hygienist to know that most of the, albeit rare, cases of endocarditis do not result from invasive, surgical treatments! Nevertheless: Oral, especially periodontal surgical procedures take place in a highly contaminated area. Expansive and/or deep surgical procedures have almost always been performed with antibiotic prophylaxis. For this reason, recommendations concerning which dental procedures require endocarditis prophylaxis were welcomed (Newman & Winkelhoff 2001).

456 Endocarditis Prophylaxis
The standard antibiotic for IE prophylaxis is *Amoxicillin*.

For patients who are allergic to this bacteriocidal broad spectrum penicillin, and/or those who cannot swallow pills, some alternatives are provided.

* Maximum children's dose, depending upon body weight; do not exceed the adult dose!
** Cephalosporine and penicillin must not be used with Type 1 hypersensitivity!

Endocarditis prophylaxis	–	AHA (American Heart Association)		
Patient	**Antibiotic**	**Dose**		**Ingestion before dental procedure**
		Adult	**Child***	
Standard prophylaxis	Amoxicillin	2g oral	50mg/kg oral	1h before
Unable to swallow pills	Ampicillin	2g i.m./i.v.	50mg/kg i.m./i.v.	30min before
Penicillin allergy	Clindamycin	600mg oral	20mg/kg oral	1h before
	Cephalexin** Cefradoxil**	2g oral	50mg/kg oral	1h before
	Azithromycin Clarithromycin	500mg oral	15mg/kg oral	1h before
Penicillin allergy *and*	Clindamycin	600mg i.v.	20mg/kg oral	30min before
unable to swallow pills	Cefalozin	1g i.m./i.v.	25mg/kg oral	30min before

Dental Procedures Carrying the Risk of Bacteremia

Bacteriemia will occur following all dental procedures that elicit *bleeding*. The endangered patient must be premedicated with the "one-shot" prophylaxis (AHA) before:

- Periodontal probing (Fig. 457 left).
- Calculus removal
- Suture removal, dressing change
- Intraligamentous anesthesia
- Tooth extraction, surgical tooth extraction
- Root tip resection

Bacteriemias of varying frequency and severity also occur after chewing hard foodstuffs (15–50%), during *tooth brushing* (5–25%), or during oral irrigation (25–40%; according to Neu 1994).

The percentage and number *anaerobic* species were approximately twice as high in patients with poor oral hygiene and advanced periodontal diseases in comparison to patients with good oral hygiene. Bacteriemia occurs in these patients also, but patients at risk for endocarditis should not abandon mechanical oral hygiene; rather, they should rinse 30 minutes beforehand with chlorhexidine.

457 Dental Procedures Requiring Antibiotic Endocarditis Prophylaxis (E-P)
For *single* procedures the prophylaxis measures suggested above are sufficient.

If, however, an extended phase of treatment is planned, a longer-lasting (adjunctive) medication must be considered, combined with an intensive intraoral antiseptic regimen (p. 287).

Dental procedures: E-P *recommended*
Professional tooth cleaning procedures if hemorrhage is anticipated
Periodontology – Probing, scaling and root planing, surgery, recall therapy, placing subgingival medicaments
Anesthesia – intraligamentous injection
Surgery – Tooth extraction, further procedures
Dental implants – Seating intraosseous implants
Endodontics – Canal instrumentation or surgery beyond the apex

E-P: *not recommended**
Local injection anesthesia (excluding intraligamentous)
Various: Rubber dam placement, suture removal, impression-taking, fluoride application, radiographs, adjustment of fixed orthodontic appliances Removal of highly mobile deciduous teeth
Operative and prosthetic dentistry – with or without retraction cords
Endodontics: Root canal treatment, post build-ups etc.
* E-P coverage if hemorrhage is anticipated

Diabetes mellitus (DM)—Risk Factor for Periodontitis

A new classification for Diabetes mellitus was presented in 1997 (WHO; American Diabetes Association):

- Diabetes mellitus Type 1 (formerly IDDM)
- Diabetes mellitus Type 2 (formerly NIDDM)
- Other diabetes with known etiologies
- Gestation Diabetes (pregnancy Diabetes)

Untreated, all forms of the disease are similar in the elevated blood sugar level and alterations in carbohydrate and lipid metabolism (DGP 2002/Risk factors).

- The less common DM Type 1 occurs due to the autoimmune-elicited destruction of insulin-producing β-cells of the pancreas. The consequence is acute insulin deficiency.
- DM Type 2 diseases are not primarily insulin-dependent (over eating, sedentary lifestyle!); Type 2 Diabetes today has achieved epidemic proportions. The number of cases is increasing rapidly, and is estimated at 150,000,000 cases worldwide.

DM today is frequently one component of the "metabolic syndrome," together with obesity, elevated blood lipid and high blood pressure ("Deadly Quartet"; Syndrome X).

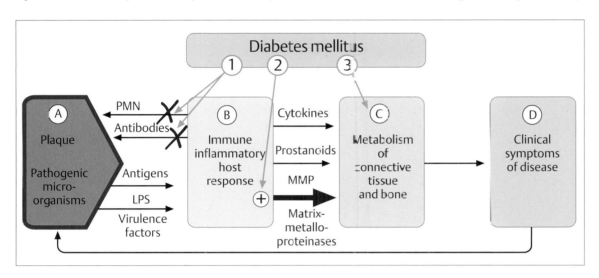

458 Risk Factor—DM
The effects of persistent hyperglycemia are many. Various target cells react inappropriately to glycosylated lipids and proteins (AGE, "advanced glycated endproducts"), mediated via the specific receptor RAGE.

1 Defective PMNs and antibodies
2 Macrophages with enhanced catabolic mechanisms
3 Altered extracellular matrix

Adapted from *R. Page 1998*

459 Differences in Host Response in Health, Type 1 Diabetes and Periodontitis Patients
The levels of the strong pro-inflammatory mediator prostaglandin E2 (PGE2; p. 49) differ massively.

In patients with Diabetes and periodontitis (**E**), an extreme over-production of PGE2 is observed, which complicates the disease picture.

Adapted from *G. Salvi et al. 1998*

Periodontitis Therapy for Diabetes Patients

An important first step is the meticulous anti-infectious initial therapy and the establishment of an optimum blood sugar level (internist). Persistence or progression of periodontitis can lead to elevated insulin resistance, and can increase the diabetic consequences:

- Retinopathy (vascular damage, p. 133; blindness)
- Nephropathy (renal high pressure as a consequence)
- Neuropathy
- Angiopathy (atherosclerosis—peripheral, heart, brain)
- Disturbances of wound healing
- Severity of periodontitis (the "sixth complication")

Periodontitis and Diabetes mellitus exhibit numerous reciprocal effects. Both can therefore be referred to as reciprocal risk factors. Chronic infection of the periodontal pocket (gram-negative microorganisms, lipopolysaccharide) elicit within the altered glycosylating cells of a diabetic an increase in excessive reactions of the defense cells, which is characterized by release of large amounts of pro-inflammatory, catabolic mediators (Grossi & Genco 1998). Diabetes and periodontitis should therefore be treated simultaneously, where necessary employing systemic antibiotic support (doxycycline) (Miller et al. 1992; Westfelt et al. 1996; Tervonen & Karjalainen 1997).

Smoking—An Alterable Most Important Risk Factor

Because of its numerous negative consequences for general systemic health, regular heavy smoking is one of the most dangerous addictions. It is also the most significant *alterable* risk factor for periodontal diseases.

In addition to *nicotine*, tobacco smoke contains up to 4,000 toxic, cancer-causing components. Therefore, a *tumor-screening* examination should be performed on all patients who smoke, including meticulous inspection of the entire oral cavity (Reichart 2002, Reichart & Philipsen 1999).

Pathogenesis: Nicotine and its by-products compromise the host response to infection, including within the periodontal tissues (Müller 2001):

- Reduced chemotaxis and phagocytosis by PMNs
- Reduced synthesis of immunoglobulins (IgG2)
- Stimulation of pro-inflammatory cytokines and additional mediators (IL-2, IL-6, PGE2)
- Elevated numbers of anaerobes in the subgingival region, including *T. forsythia*, *P. gingivalis*, and also members of the "orange complex" (Haffajee & Socransky 2001)
- Damage to fibroblasts (gingival and periodontal)

460 Risk Factor—Smoking
Where and how does tobacco smoking influence the pathogenesis of periodontal diseases?

1 Activity of PMNs, reduced secretion of immunoglobulins (IgG2)
2 Enhancement of subgingival anaerobic microorganisms
3 Influence on gingival, periodontal and osseous metabolism

Adapted from *R. Page & K. Kornman 1997*

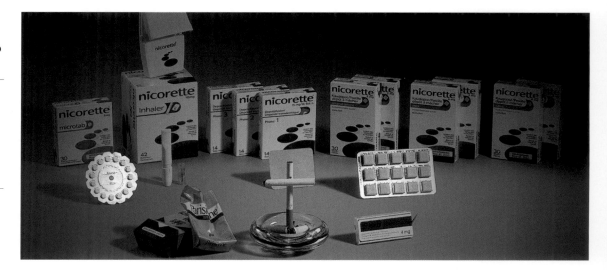

461 Smoking Cessation Using Nicotine Substitutes
"Nicorette" products; from left to right:

- Microtabs: Sublingual tablets
- Inhaler: Cartridges within a cigarette mouthpiece
- Transdermal patch: For 16 hours (5, 10 and 15 mg)
- Nicorette chewing gum

The Nicorette products are available in differing concentrations and in some instances different taste formulations.

Smoking Cessation

The dental hygienist sees the patient in recall at least twice per year and is therefore almost predestined to accompany the tobacco cessation process. Treatment results in smokers with aggressive periodontitis and poor oral hygiene are definitively poorer, on average, than in non-smokers. Caution is the watchword before regenerative procedures, e.g., filling bony defects, whether on natural teeth or dental implants. In the face of additional risk factors (oral hygiene, Diabetes, positive IL-1 polymorphism etc.) one is wise to avoid regenerative procedures of any kind (Tonetti et al. 1995, Müller et al. 2002, Jansson et al. 2002, Machtei et al. 2003).

If the smoking cessation program is to be effective, the time factor, and uncompromising patience, will play major roles. Motivational discussions about smoking cessation often follow the "five A's": Ask, Advise, Assess, Assist, Arrange (Ramseier 2003).

Cessation programs including the various forms of nicotine replacement substances (Fig. 461) have proven effective. Without nicotine, the medicament "Zyban" (bupropion) is effective.

Emergency Treatment

Many periodontitis patients are not aware of their disease, even though it may have been progressing over many years. Only when pain and acute inflammatory symptoms appear do such patients seek out a dentist or dental hygienist.

Such emergency cases must be treated immediately. However, to avoid life-threatening incidents, a succinct *general medical history* must be taken, with particular attention to any medicines the patient may be taking (anticoagulants!) and an assessment of the necessity for infection prophylaxis (endocarditis, HIV etc.), as well as allergies and previous significant incidents.

Next, a clinical and radiographic examination should be performed for emergency patients; despite the pain, this is absolutely necessary before any treatment.

Included in the category "periodontal emergency situations and treatments" are:

- Initial topical medicinal and mechanical treatment for acute NUG
- Treatment of acute, suppurating pockets
- Opening periodontal abscesses
- Immediate extraction of hopelessly mobile teeth that cannot be maintained
- Acute, combined endodontic-periodontal problems
- Treatment of periodontal trauma following accidents

Acute ulcerative gingivoperiodontitis (acute NUG/NUP) is painful and progresses very rapidly. Careful instrumentation and application of topical agents generally bring relief within a few hours and a reduction of the acute situation.
Caution: Ulceration may be a symptom of HIV-seropositivity (opportunistic infection).

Active suppurating pockets generally are not painful if drainage is established at the gingival margin (exception: abscess). Such pockets represent an exacerbating inflammatory process, which leads to rapid attachment loss. They must be treated immediately with application of rinsing solutions or ointments; mechanical cleansing must also be initiated.

Periodontal abscesses are usually very painful. They must be drained immediately. This can usually be accomplished via probing from the gingival sulcus.
In the case of molars with deep pockets or furcation involve-

ment, an abscess that penetrates the bone may develop subperiosteally. These cannot always be reached via the gingival margin, and must be drained by means of an incision.

Immediate extraction should be reserved for teeth that cannot be maintained or are highly mobile or which cause the patient undue discomfort. In the case of anterior teeth, for esthetic reasons, extractions should be avoided when possible, or an immediate temporary should be prepared.

Acute, endodontic/periodontal processes have a more favorable prognosis if the primary problem is of endodontic origin. The root canal should always be treated first, subsequently the pocket.

Periodontal trauma due to accident usually requires immediate splinting (following any necessary reimplantation or repositioning of the tooth).

462 Emergency Situation: Acute Necrotizing Ulcerative Gingivitis (NUG)
The severe pain in the acute stage permits only a very careful peripheral attempt at cleansing. Treatment of this acute condition involved gentle debridement with 3 % hydrogen peroxide, and application of a disinfecting ointment containing anti-inflammatory and analgesic ingredients. The patient was told to rinse at home with a chlorhexidine solution.

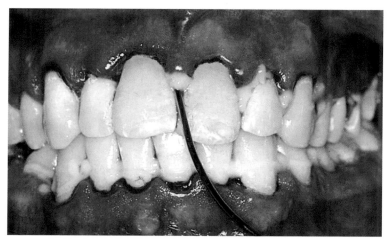

Acute "necrotizing ulcerative gingivitis" (NUG)

463 After Emergency Treatment—Subacute Stage
Several days after gentle topical application of the medicaments and careful mechanical debridement, the signs of active NUG—especially the pain –subsided. Treatment by means of systematic subgingival scaling can now proceed. A gingivoplasty may be indicated subsequently in the normal course of treatment.

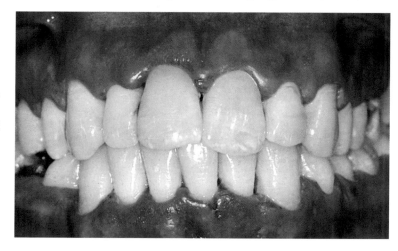

464 Emergency Situation—Localized Acute Pocket
Tooth 31 is vital and should be maintained despite the 10 mm pocket. Very little pus has formed; drainage via the gingival margin appears possible. The tooth is slightly percussion sensitive. Prior to systematic mechanical treatment, the tooth is treated on an emergency basis with topical application of a medicament, and the pocket is disinfected.

Right: Note the deep defect on the distal of tooth 31.

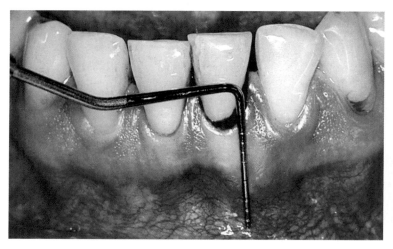
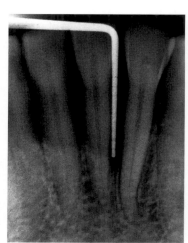

"Acute pocket"—acute pocket inflammation

465 Emergency Treatment Using Local Medicament, and Follow-up
As an emergency measure the pocket was first rinsed thoroughly with chlorhexidine solution and then filled with achromycin ointment (3 %). Once the acute symptoms subside, a thorough root planing can be performed.
Right: Eight weeks after the emergency therapy, the gingiva has regained its resiliency and has shrunk somewhat. Probing depth is now only ca. 3 mm.

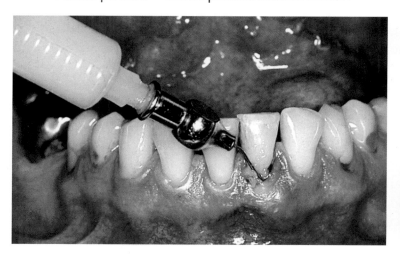
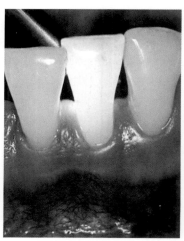

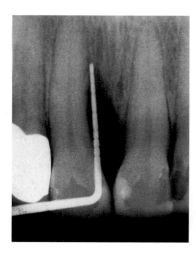
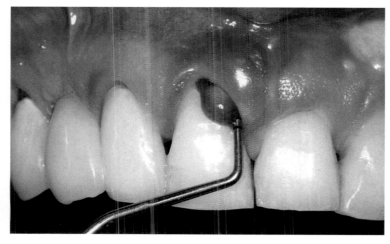

466 Emergency Situation: Pocket Abscess—Drainage After Probing From the Gingival Margin
Originating from a deep pocket mesial to tooth 11, a periodontal abscess has formed. Copious pus exudes when the pocket is probed.

Left: The radiograph depicts the periodontal probe inserted to the base of the osseous defect.

Pocket abscess

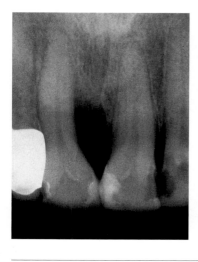
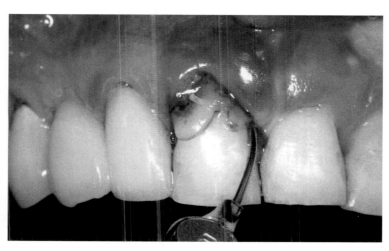

467 Emergency Treatment Using Topical Medicament— Radiographic Follow-up
The abscess has opened via the gingival margin. The pocket is first thoroughly rinsed, then filled with an antibiotic-containing ointment. Once the acute symptoms have subsided, definitive therapy can be undertaken.

Left: Radiograph 6 months after definitive therapy: New bone formation is apparent.

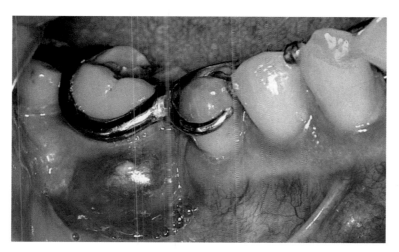

468 Emergency Situation: Periodontal Abscess Anticipates Drainage Through the Gingiva
Originating from the deep, one-wall infrabony pocket mesial to the tipped but vital tooth 47, an abscess has developed. The buccal gingiva is distended as the abscess is about to penetrate through the mucosa.
Tooth 47 is an abutment for a removable partial denture that is ill-fitting, but the patient wants to retain the partial denture.

Periodontal abscess

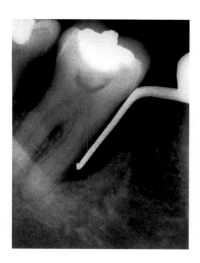
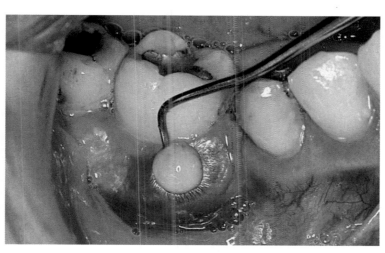

469 Abscess—Drainage
As soon as the mucosa was touched the abscess opened and copious pus exuded.

Left: In the radiograph one observes the deep mesial periodontal pocket with a hoe scaler *in situ*. Since the furcation appears not to be involved, it is possible to consider maintaining this tooth. The ensuing treatment included mechanical debridement and topical application of medicaments.

470 Emergency Situation in the Posterior Segment: Hopeless Molar (37)

Pus exudes spontaneously from the deep distal pocket and the buccal furcation of tooth 37.

The tooth is vital, highly mobile and painful to the slightest touch.

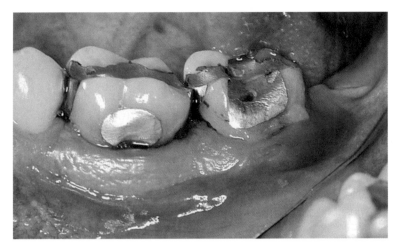

Abscess—distal pocket/furcation

471 Radiograph of 37 Before Immediate Extraction

The periodontal probe can be inserted almost to the root apex in the deep buccal pocket. Without clinical probing, such a defect at this location would be almost impossible to detect. The shape of the furcation is very unfavorable in terms of treatment; the two roots appear to fuse apically.

Right: Highly infiltrated granulation tissue remains attached to the root after extraction.

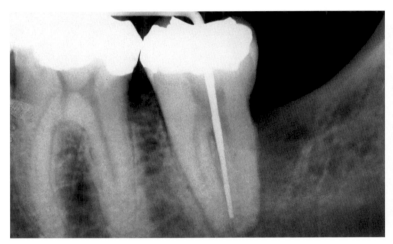
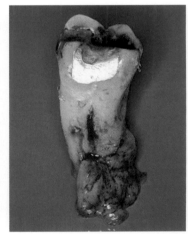

472 Emergency Situation in the Anterior Area: Painful Tooth 11 is Hopeless—Fistula

A fistula emanating from the deep pocket has developed. The non-vital tooth is highly mobile and sensitive to percussion. This tooth cannot be saved; it was extracted immediately.

Right: The radiograph reveals that a probe can be carefully inserted far beyond the apex (endo-perio problem).

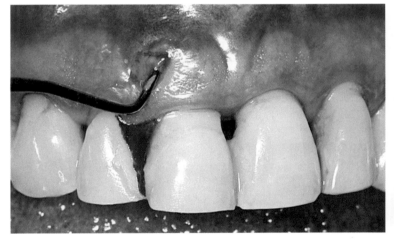
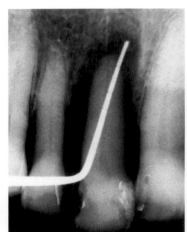

Acute perio-endo problem—fistula

473 Immediate Extraction— Immediate Temporary

An immediate temporary is necessary for esthetics. Following extraction the root was severed and the crown was used as a temporary. A wire and acid-etched resin secured the crown to the adjacent teeth. This type of temporary can usually be maintained until definitive reconstruction.

Right: Radiographic view of the temporary replacement consisting of the patient's own tooth crown.

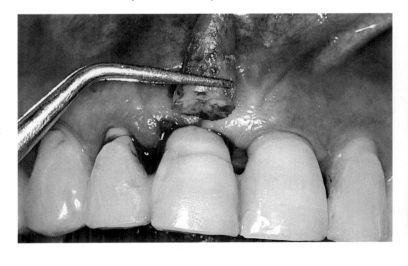
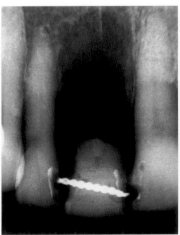

Phase 1 Therapy

**Causal, Antimicrobial,
Non-surgical Therapy**

Primary prevention—the *early* prevention of disease—is initially the responsibility of parents. Using simple, non-traumatic tooth brushing methods, the small child is gently guided down the path of personal hygiene and especially oral hygiene, hopefully with the support of his/her role models: Mother, father and perhaps older siblings. It should become a habit that the results of a child's own efforts in oral hygiene be observed, lauded and, when necessary, modified.

In *healthy* individuals, prophylactic measures are usually short, painless and require little time. Nevertheless, they prevent dental caries and gingival diseases!

If disease occurs over the course of time, e.g., initial gingivitis in the specialty of periodontology, a brief description of the cause (bacterial biofilm), and its professional removal, as well as renewed instruction in plaque control by the patient (tooth brushing, oral hygiene), healthy conditions can be again established—*secondary prevention.*

If true pockets have formed and attachment has been lost, it is necessary to intervene as early as possible for such cases of early *periodontitis*. Using the simple measures of closed, causal therapy (debridement, root planing) such cases can be *cured*. Only a few years ago, predictable treatment success was only possible in pockets of 4–6 mm; but today it is possible to achieve predictable success even in pockets of 8 mm and more with the help of new and improved procedures ("After Five" curettes, disinfectants, modified timing, and other equipment innovations).

Nevertheless, anatomical relationships such as furcation involvement, grooves, narrow bony craters, and the regeneration of tissue defects oftentimes make it necessary still today to employ a multifaceted, often complicated corrective (surgical) technique with open therapy (Phase 2 therapy/surgery; p.295) following Phase 1 (closed, subgingival) treatments.

This chapter, "Phase 1 Therapy," will unfold as follows:

- Case presentation – Motivation toward self-help
- Initial treatment 1 – Oral hygiene by the patient
  – Creation of hygienic relationships by the dental team
- Initial treatment 2 – Traditional closed pocket treatment
  – FMT—"full mouth therapy"

Case Presentation—Motivation—Information

The maintenance or reinstatement of periodontal health (freedom from inflammation, full function) is possible even in terms of esthetics assuming certain prerequisites. But this can only be accomplished through the *cooperative* interaction between the patient and the hygienist: The patient must be interested in maintaining the health of the oral cavity, and must be *interested* in a proposed treatment, and must be *motivated* to participate (compliance).

The patient should first be informed about the causal relationships that led to the disease process. The dental hygienist has numerous possibilities to demonstrate to the patient soft tissue alterations elicited by inflammation, and the responsible etiologic factors (Roulet & Zimmer 2003).

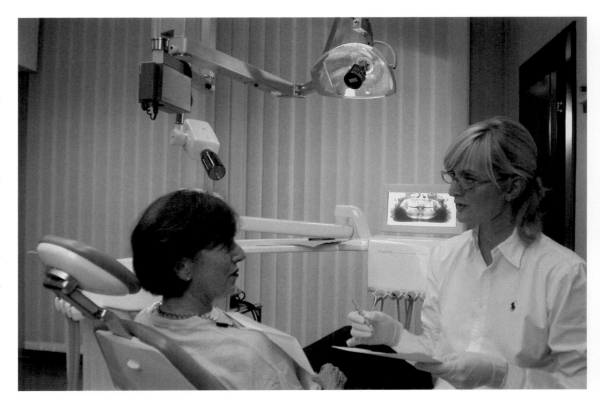

474 Motivation and Information During the Case Presentation
During the very first appointment, during the discussion of medical history and the collection of diagnostic data (by the dental hygienist), the patient will want to be informed as much as possible about his/her oral condition. This is an opportunity to motivate the patient and solicit compliance, because "without compliance, a good result will not be achieved."
A primary goal of the case presentation is to convince the patient of the many possibilities for bringing the treatment to a successful conclusion.

Oral Hygiene Instruction Aids

The hygienist must consider and take seriously the fact that the patient's own case is what interests the patient most. Panoramic radiograph on the light box, easily visible clinical findings such as recession, plaque-retentive areas, bleeding on probing, gingival erythema and swelling etc. are easy to demonstrate and explain to the patient who holds a mirror.

At subsequent appointments, the interested patient can again be informed and motivated, for example through use of disclosing agents (p. 224) to visualize plaque at the gingival margin or in the interdental spaces. Dental plaque microbial "vitality" can also be used for patient motivation by means of microscopic enlargement ("Plakoscope", cf. p. 180); an inexpensive TV camera and monitor can dramatically depict plaque vitality for the patient.

Additionally, other instructional materials such as brochures, tooth models, and high-tech instruments such as digital intraoral cameras can be used to transmit to the patient the necessary information about health and disease.

It has been reported and demonstrated many times that a flood of new information often overloads or exceeds the patient's available memory, and the patient is soon no longer capable remembering all of the details. It has therefore proven to be helpful to give the patient small but informative take-home brochures or pamphlets, to be read and studied as follow-up to the information the patient heard as he/she sat in the treatment chair.

Initial Treatment 1—
• Oral Hygiene by the Patient

The patient's oral hygiene (plaque control) remains today the primary supportive pillar of peri-odontal *prophylaxis*. It also supports *treatment*, and has great significance for *maintenance* of the treatment results.

Without continuous compliance by the patient, periodontal treatment by the dentist and the dental hygienist will be less successful and the success will be of shorter duration. Oral hygiene by the patient means, above all, reduction of the amount of plaque and pathogenic microorganisms in the oral cavity. Gingival massage with the toothbrush is of secondary importance, with perhaps some "psychological" effect.

In special indications, mechanical plaque control can be enhanced or supported for a limited peri-od of time by topical medicaments (disinfection agents such as chlorhexidine).

This chapter will describe:

- Plaque disclosing agents, revealing the plaque
- Manual toothbrushes
- Toothbrushing techniques, systems
- Electric toothbrushes
- Interdental hygiene—interdental hygiene aids
- Dentifrices
- Chemical plaque control—CHX, additional products
- Irrigators—of value?
- Halitosis, bad breath—oral hygiene
- Possibilities, successes and limitations of oral hygiene

Toothbrushes of all kinds are important aids for mechanical plaque removal. They reach, however, only the *facial, oral* and *occlusal* tooth surfaces.

The initial lesions of gingivitis and periodontitis, as well as dental caries, usually occur in the *interdental region*. Therefore, the toothbrush must be enhanced by additional hygiene aids that can ensure cleansing of the interdental area.

There is no single oral hygiene method that is right for every patient. The type and severity of the periodontal disease, the morphological situation (crowding, spacing, gingival phenotype etc.) as well as the patient's own manual dexterity determine the required hygiene aids and the cleaning techniques. During the course of periodontitis therapy, the techniques may have to be changed or adapted to the new morphological situation (longer teeth, open interdental spaces, exposed dentin).

The patient must be informed about his/her daily oral hygiene, its frequency, time spent and amount of force to be applied. In most cases, *once per day* is sufficient for a thorough and systematic plaque removal (disruption of the developing biofilm; Lang et al. 1973).

In the final analysis, though, it is not the hygiene aids, the technique or the time spent that is the determining factor, rather the result: *Freedom from plaque*. This parameter as well as the health of the of the gingiva (BOP) must be checked at regular intervals.

Motivation—Gingival Bleeding

Since 1980, the clinical symptom "bleeding on probing" has assumed the foreground in patient motivation, replacing plaque disclosure. The profession realized that it is not the amount or expanse of plaque or its depiction in a microscope that was most meaningful to patients, rather it was the reaction of the patient's own tissues to the microbial irritation that held the highest motivational value.

Each person exhibits very *different individual reactions* to the biofilm, its constituents and especially the microbial

metabolites. Thus, even with identical amounts of plaque, quite different levels of pathogenic danger may be present.

Using the PBI (Saxer & Mühlemann 1975, Mühlemann 1978) or BOP (Ainamo & Bay 1975, p. 69) the severity of gingival inflammation can be numerically portrayed. If the gingival bleeding index decreases during initial treatment (1), as depicted by repeated clinical recording of the index, this provides visible evidence of success while simultaneously giving further motivation to the patient.

Bleeding on Probing as a Motivating Factor

475 Initial Condition: Moderate Periodontitis
The patient can clearly see the severe hemorrhage as the hygienist performs the bleeding index (PBI or BOP).

Right: As a second step, *disclosing the plaque* reveals the cause of the disease. The next steps include initial oral hygiene instruction and professional, supragingival prophylaxis.

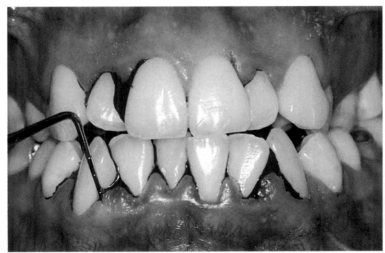
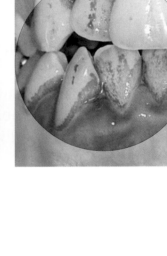

476 Clinical Situation: Two Weeks Later
Following professional prophylaxis and repeated OHI, the patient can readily see the return to health as indicated by the minimal bleeding during recording of the PBI data.
The patient is motivated by this success to further intensive cooperation and compliance.

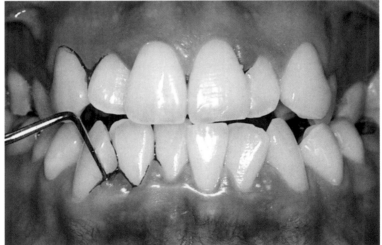

477 Clinical View at 4 Weeks
The virtual absence of bleeding (inflammation) and the dramatic plaque reduction convinces the patient definitively of the logic of this treatment.

Right: The minimum plaque accumulations demonstrate the correlation: Less plaque = less gingivitis.
Additional oral hygiene instruction is now targeted toward those sites that are not completely plaque-free, e. g., interdental areas.

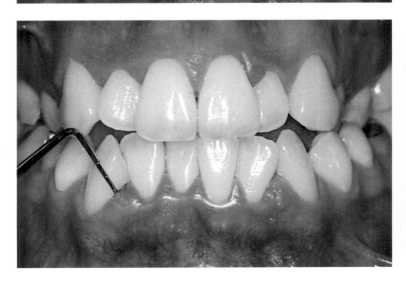
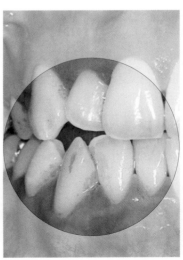

Plaque Disclosing Agents

Frequently during the case presentation, when motivation is being emphasized using the bleeding index, the patient will pose questions concerning the *cause* of periodontal disease. Now—right now!—is the prime time for demonstration of microbial plaque, the most important etiologic factor in gingivitis and periodontitis.

Using non-toxic food coloring agents, the adherent plaque on tooth surfaces and gingiva can be selectively stained. The patient watches in a mirror as the clearly visible plaque is revealed and then scraped off using a probe.

Patients are further impressed to hear that only 0.001 grams of plaque contain ca. 300,000,000 bacteria. The necessity and possibility for plaque removal via oral hygiene measures becomes visible to the patient, and the initial toothbrushing instruction session falls on fertile soil.

One disadvantage of plaque disclosing agents that remain in the mouth for some time can be avoided by using the Plaklite system (Fig. 480). A solution that is virtually invisible in daylight clearly reveals accumulated plaque bacteria when illuminated with blue or UV light.

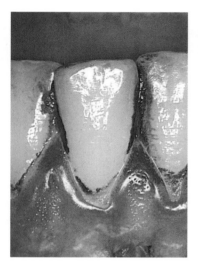 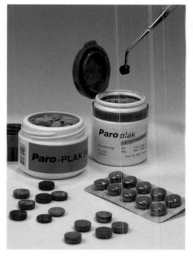 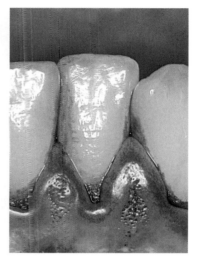

478 Red and Violet Disclosing Agents
Left: Classic red staining by erythrosin. This procedure is still permitted by the FDA.

Middle: Plaque disclosing agents for the patient (tablets) and for the clinician (solutions, pellets).

Right: Differential disclosing agents that stain "fresh" plaque *light violet*, and old, "mature," plaque a *darker violet* color.

Erythrosin	Patent Blue	Phloxin B	Na⁺-Fluorescein
Tetraiodofluorescein sodium	CI 42090	CI 45410	Fluorescein disodium salt
C. I. Acid Red 51	FD+C Blue No. 1	C. I. Acid Red 92	Soluble fluorescein
CI 45430	Brilliant blue	Tetrachloro-tetrabromo-fluorescein	
E 127	E 133		
Do not use if patient is iodine-sensitive!			

479 Details of Four Plaque Disclosing Agents
(adapted from Roulet & Zimmer 2003)
Older, deeply-staining agents such as basic fuschsin, malachite green and other "histologic stains," which are depicted in some illustrations in this *Atlas*, are no longer used in clinical practice because of their potentially injurious side effects or toxicity.

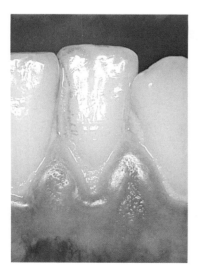 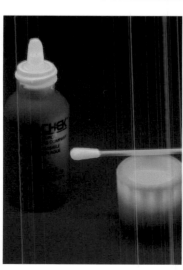 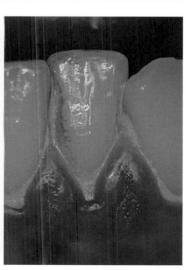

480 Fluorescent Disclosing Agents, Blue or UV Light
In normal room lighting, plaque disclosed with 0.75 % Na-fluorescein solution appears light yellow (left), but glows intensively yellow-green under blue light (right).

The disclosing products are available from Vivadent, Lactona, Clairol and International Pharmaceutical Co. (IPC) and others.

A disadvantage of this technique is the requirement of a special light source or a filter mirror.

Toothbrushes

For centuries, the toothbrush has served to remove food debris and plaque from all *facial, oral* and *occlusal* tooth surfaces. Today the toothbrush remains indispensable, but it does not provide adequate interdental hygiene. In addition, when used with excessive force it has the potential to injure even healthy gingiva.

There is no ideal toothbrush (shape, size, handle) but in periodontics more and more brushes with softer, flexible bristles have found acceptance. Rounded bristle tips are the standard today.

Worthy of consideration also is the fact that toothbrushes are always used with toothpastes (p. 234). It seems only reasonable that these two components should be "synchronized" for each individual patient (König 2002) and this must be accomplished by the dental hygienist. This should replace the often wildly extravagant commercial claims with *facts*, and permit targeted recommendations for each individual patient.

481 "The Best Brush"
Patients always ask: "What's the best toothbrush"? Who wins gold, silver or nothing?
Fact: There is no "best" brush!

For the hygienist it is important to know the commercially available brushes, but more important to know the needs of the individual patient, in order to properly advise.

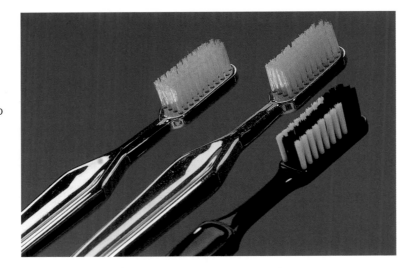

482 ADA Type and New Trends
New brushes and their efficacy are standardized according to ADA guidelines after *in vitro* testing. Clinical tests with human subjects are more costly and provide limited data. The ADA "norm" (left) is a four-row brush, multi-tufted. At right today's trend, the Oral-B "Cross Action."

Right: Rounded bristle tips are today's standard.

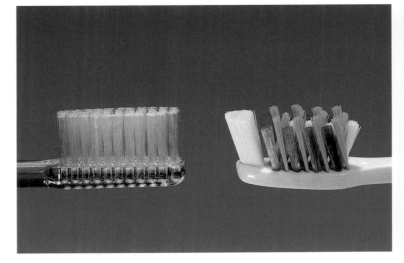
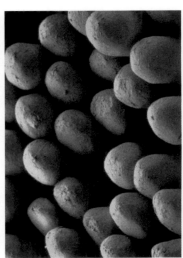

483 Toothpaste and Toothbrush: One Goal
The role of the toothbrush is generally overvalued! Only in combination with a dentifrice is it effective; the toothbrush is really only a carrier. Its positive effects (gingival massage?) are insignificant. Its negative effects, especially with hard bristles, can be grave: Damage or injury to gingiva and mucosa can lead to gingival recession or aphthous ulcers.

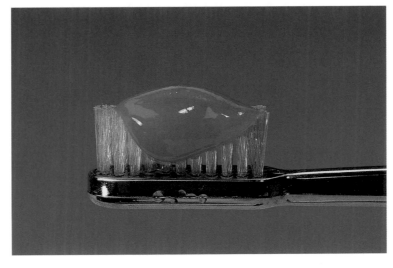

Oral hygiene devices have become a huge worldwide market. The industry has done and will continue to do everything in its power to persuade consumers of the efficacy of its product, using brilliant colors and bizarre shapes! Using the latest generation of high-tech machines, it has been possible to create exceptional types of bristle arrangements—parallel or crossed, variously colored bristles, flat plane or irregular, straight or round brush heads etc.

The question that remains, however, is whether any of this is actually *useful* for patients!

It is up to dental hygienists and dentists not to *react* but rather to *act*! Guidelines for good toothbrushes need to be defined, for example, for periodontitis patients with thin gingiva, recession, large interdental spaces etc. Worthy of thought: A motivated patient brushes daily for 60, 70 or 80 years! Long-term freedom from injury is more important than momentary efficiency.

It seems that a start has been made: Superfine bristles—they clean just as well as hard bristles—and unconventional 3-headed brushes are being widely discussed.

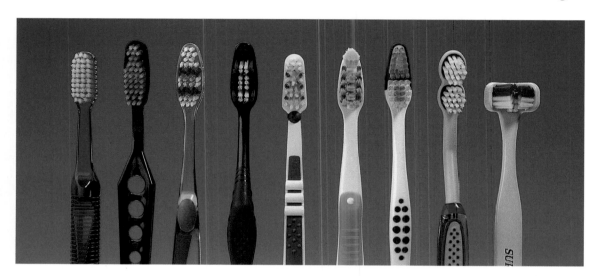

484 Modern Toothbrushes—Frontal View
How is one to evaluate the enormous differences in shape, bristle array, handle etc.?

The best that a toothbrush can offer is its ability to effectively clean the teeth, while preventing damage or injury to gingiva or teeth, and help reduce bad breath.

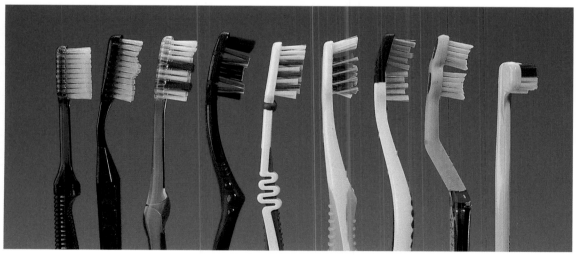

485 Modern Toothbrushes—Lateral View
This figure corresponds to Fig. 484. From left to right...

- **Elmex**   Supersoft
- **Paro**   Future
- **Elmex**   Inter X medium
- **Trisa**   FlexHead soft
- **Dr. Best**   X-aktiv Flex
- **Oral-B**   Cross Action
- **Colgate**   Navigator medium
- **Mentadent** Insider soft-medium
- **Superbrush** Junior

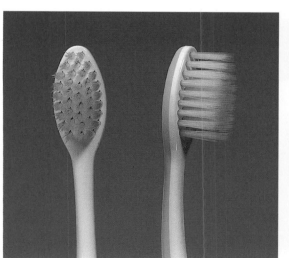 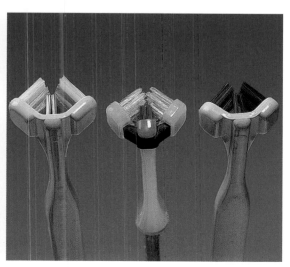

486 Meridol and Superbrush—New Developments; Progress?
Left: The Meridol brush has superfine, flexible bristles, designed to absorb excessive force.

Right: The three brush heads simultaneously clean vestibular, occlusal and oral tooth surfaces. Using a light vibratory movement, teeth are cleaned one-by-one. This design was superior to other brushes in clinical trials (middle: head of the Nais electric toothbrush. cf. p. 230).

Toothbrushing Technique

Innumerable toothbrush movements have been recommended over time, and then abandoned: Rolling, vibrating, circular, vertical and horizontal (Jepsen 1998). More important than the technique is the *efficiency* of cleaning, a *systematic* procedure and that *no damage* is caused.

Dental hygienists have recognized again and again that most patients, despite instruction, seem to be satisfied with an apparently "genetically determined" *horizontal scrubbing technique.*

The most frequently recommended "modified Bass technique" (Bass 1954) is depicted below.

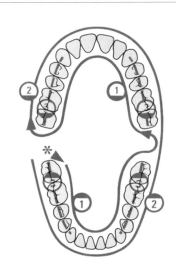

487 Systematic Toothbrushing
The sequence depicted has been shown to be effective (start: right, posterior*)

1 **Oral Surfaces** mandible/maxilla, and all distal surfaces at the end of each arch.
2 **Facial Surfaces** mandible/maxilla
3 **Occlusal Surfaces** mandible/maxilla

4 **Interdental Spaces,** using special hygiene aids

Modified Bass Technique
488 Placement of the Toothbrush
Toothbrush bristles positioned perpendicular to the tooth long axis will not effectively clean the interdental spaces.

Right: Instead of the "original" Bass technique, which used a two-row brush, today the "sulcus cleansing technique" is performed with the more common three- or four-row brushes. This combination should provide improved cleaning.

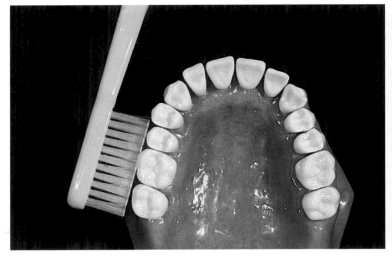

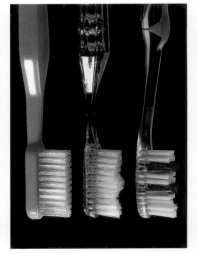

489 45° Angle of the Bristles—Occlusal View
When the brush is applied at a 45° angle to the teeth and then rotated toward the occlusal plane, the bristles slip easily into the interdental areas and gingiva sulci *without* excessive force. With the brush in this position, *small rotatory* or *vibratory* movements will effectively remove plaque.

Problem zone: Angular arch form in the canine regions.

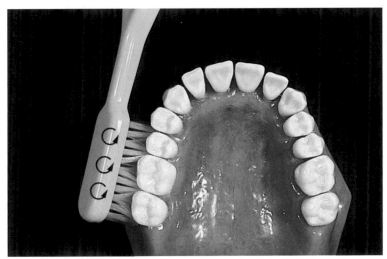

490 45 Degree Angle—Distal Surfaces
Viewed from the distal, the position of the bristles in the Bass technique becomes obvious.

Right: Distal surfaces will not be effectively cleaned by hard bristle brushes; extremely flexible toothbrush bristles may provide effective distal cleaning.
Dental floss is not recommended for such surfaces, which often exhibit concavities and/or furcations. Single-tuft brushes are more effective (right).

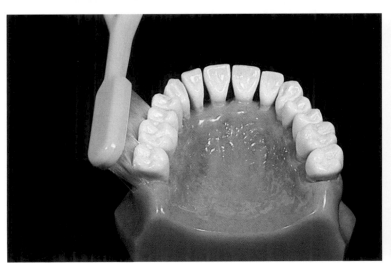

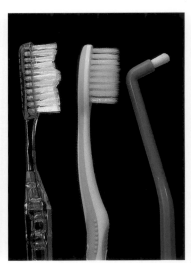

The Solo Technique—A Different Way to Brush Your Teeth

In 2000, Jiri Sedelmayer described the unreasonableness of the usual toothbrushing methods of many individuals: "Among other things, areas that scarcely need cleaning, such as prominent tooth surfaces and gingiva, are often injured. Notorious plaque-retentive areas, above all the interdental spaces, gingival sulcus and oral-distal tooth surfaces are regularly cleaned by only a disappearing few."

Sedelmayer was in fact correct, and in the same breath suggested a new technique, an alternative to the usual scrubbing, at least for individuals who are prepared to devote adequate time for their oral health.

The problem with classical toothbrushes is that when they are used with the recommended non-traumatic slight pressure, the niches are not achieved; with heavier force, however, prominent tooth surfaces and gingiva are so abused that true long-term damage is the consequence (recession, wedge-shaped defects etc; p. 316; Lussi et al 1993).

Using a soft, round, single-tuft brush with light force, the technique cleans tooth-by-tooth, above all the lingual aspects perfectly, including marginally and deep into the interdental space. However, other special hygiene aids are also necessary.

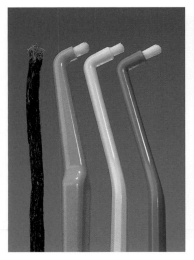

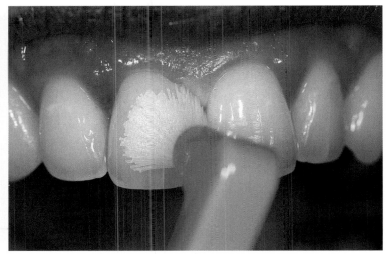

491 "Solo" Technique—Begin at Mesial of Tooth 11
The round, single-tuft brush is applied to the tooth surface with light force, and the bristles splay out. The mesial sulcus of tooth 11 is cleaned using minimal circular movements.

Left: An example of "solo" brushes, beginning (left) with the ages-old chewed twig!
Round "solo" brushes are commercially available from TePe, Curaden, Tandex etc.

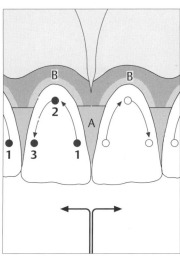

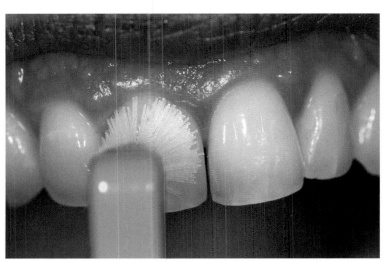

492 Continuing Along the Gingival Margin...
The gingival margin and gingival sulcus are effectively de-plaqued, using the patient's own sense of feel.

Left: Simple schematic—initiate tooth cleansing "from the middle toward the side" (e. g., tooth 11):
1 **Mesial**
2 **Marginal**
3 **Distal**

A **Papilla**
B **Gingival Margin**

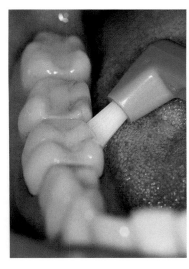

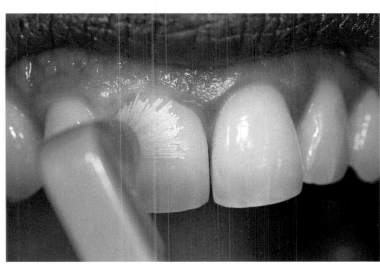

493 ... and Continuing Distally
The brush is guided distally and angled so that it achieves maximum contact with distal tooth surfaces, sulci and the papillary region.
This procedure is repeated for each tooth.

Left: What the classical brushes almost never accomplish: Perfect cleaning of the ligual marginal surfaces and interdental areas in the posterior segment of the mandible.

Electric Toothbrushes

Comparative clinical studies have shown that the efficiency in plaque removal of the newest electric toothbrushes is at least as good as that achieved with manual toothbrushes. Various products offer primarily advantages for persons with reduced manual dexterity, or the handicapped, but also offer an alternative to the hand toothbrush for highly motivated individuals. Preferred today are electric brushes with round heads, and sonically active toothbrushes, the latter because of their additional hydrodynamic activity (van de Weijden et al. 1996, Zimmer et al. 2000, Warren et al. 2001).

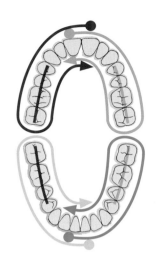

494 Effective Cleaning with Electric Toothbrushes
One can use the same system described for manual toothbrushes (Fig. 487) for the "quadrant system" built into some electric brushes. This provides 30 seconds of brushing per quadrant (see below; Q1-Q4).

Q1 —— Quadrant 1
Q2 —— Quadrant 2
Q3 —— Quadrant 3
O4 —— Quadrant 4

495 A "Collection" of Some Commercially Available Electric Toothbrushes
(from left to right)

- Interplak
- RotaDent
- Philips Sonicare
- Braun Oral-B
- Waterpik
- Ultra sonex
- Roventa
- Nais
- Oralgiene

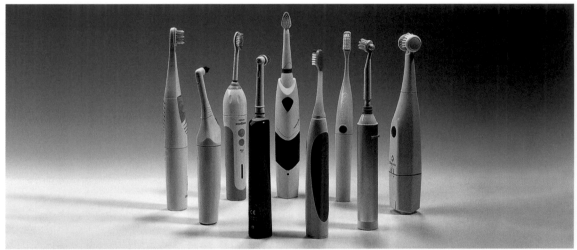

496 Brush Heads
The choice of a brush head is as important as the choice of the electric brush itself. With the high frequency brushes, there is a potential danger of gingival trauma. Brushes whose bristle movement stops when excessive force is applied should be recommended (e. g., Sonicare).

Each patient should be informed and instructed in the proper use of the electric toothbrush.

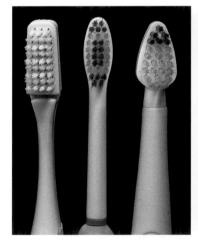
Sonic brushes

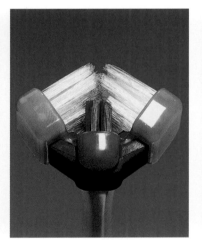
Three-head brush

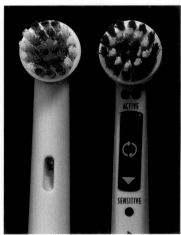
Round brush heads

497 Current Trends ...
... include primarily sonic or combined sonic-ultrasonic toothbrushes, e. g., the Ultrasonex, Sonicare and Waterpik (*left*), the Nais electric toothbrush (*middle*; with its "normal" and three-unit head). The hydrodynamic effects of these brushes removes plaque even where the bristles cannot physically reach.
Brushes with round, rotating or oscillating heads are today mature products of high efficiency (Braun Oral-B, 5th generation and Trisa, *right*).

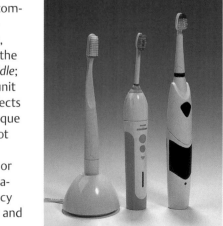

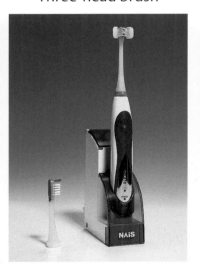

Interdental Hygiene

Gingivitis and periodontitis are usually more pronounced in the interdental area than on oral or facial aspects. Dental caries also occurs more frequently in the interdental region than on oral or facial smooth surfaces. Therefore, interdental hygiene, *which cannot be achieved with the toothbrush*, is of critical importance for periodontitis patients. The most appropriate interdental hygiene aids must be selected for each individual patient. The selection from the numerous commercially available devices depends for the most part on the morphological situation of the interdental spaces.

Dental Floss

The use of dental floss is indicated for healthy patients, and for gingivitis and mild periodontitis cases, as well as for patients with crowded teeth. It is well known, however, that the acceptance of dental floss (floss, tape, super floss) is quite low for most patients, especially males! Alternative interdental hygiene aids should be recommended even if these are less efficient than floss if patients will at least use them daily.

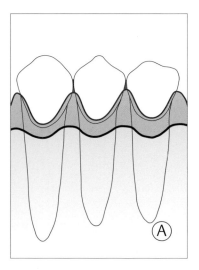

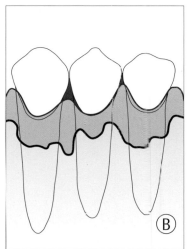

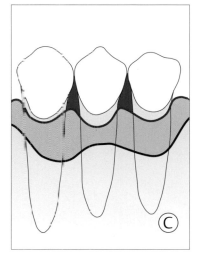

498 Morphology (schematic) of the Periodontium

A Healthy
B Periodontitis
C Treated, Healed Periodontitis

These three situations require differing techniques and various hygiene aids for interdental plaque control.
The diagrams portray the course of the alveolar bone, the gingival margin and the expanse of the interdental spaces (red).

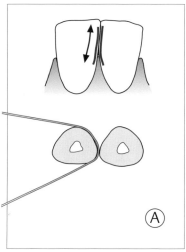

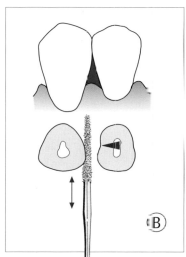

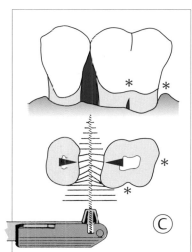

499 Size of the Interdental Space and Oral Hygiene Aids
The choice of a hygiene aid for interdental plaque control depends primarily upon the size of the interdental space.

A Dental Floss
for narrow interdental spaces
B "Tooth Sticks"
for slightly open interdental spaces
C Interdental Brushes
for widely open interdental spaces, root concavities and grooves

Toothpicks, Interdental Brushes

Toothpicks or *interdental brushes* are indicated for plaque removal if the interdental spaces are open, e.g., following completion of periodontitis therapy, as well as for patients who accept dental floss but seldom actually use it.
The newest "toothpicks" are no longer simply wooden throw-away articles, rather they are adorned with tiny hair-like bristles, they are elastic, multi-use, fine plastic files ("Brush Sticks"). Some patients become passionate about these devices!

With expansive areas of exposed root surface, especially in the molar regions, one often observes more or less severe grooves which can only be cleaned using *interdental brushes.*
These devices should be used without dentifrice except in special cases and then only short-term. The abrasive in dentifrice would rapidly abrade exposed dentin in the interdental space.
These devices can also be regularly used to apply fluoride or chlorhexidine gel into the interdental space to prevent caries or the recolonization of residual pockets.

Dental Floss

500 Choices: Floss, Tape, Ultra- and Superfloss

Today's dental floss, with filaments of nylon, kevlar etc., is strong enough to traverse even the tightest contact points. For splinted teeth, bridges etc., various threading devices are available (e. g., Eez Thru, Butler). Both waxed and unwaxed dental floss can be recommended.

Right: **Dental Tape** (Colgate)

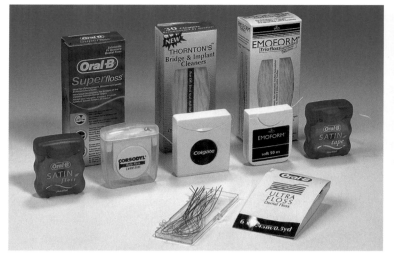
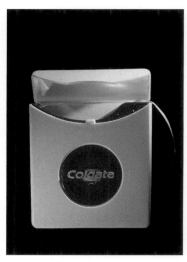

501 Use of Dental Floss

To avoid injury to the papillae, the dental tape is carefully maneuvered through the contact point using a sawing motion. Cleaning of both proximal surfaces is accomplished with up and down movements (double arrow) into the sulcus with the floss stretched tightly.

When the floss "sings" the tooth surface is clean.

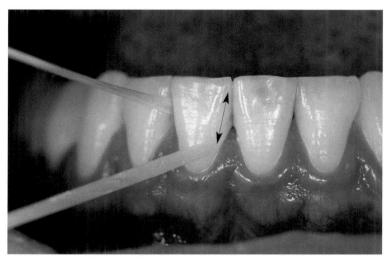

"Tooth Sticks"

502 Selection

The traditional wood interdental cleaners exhibit a triangular profile. The various manufactures use either hard or soft wood (birch, balsa, linden). Some products are impregnated with various substances (fluoride, CHX, mint, nicotine!).

Right: The new acrylic **"Brush Stick"** (Esro) cleans very effectively.

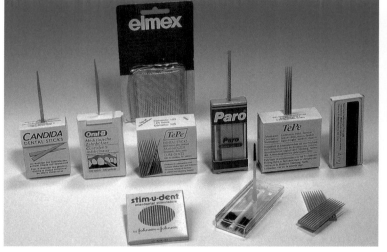
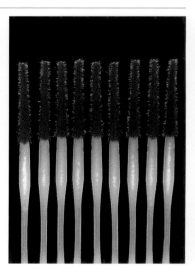

503 Clinical Use of "Brush Sticks"

The red, felt-like tip is guided into the interdental space at a slight angle. Plaque removal is accomplished by horizontal back and forth movements (double arrow). If the interdental spaces are large, the brush stick is first pressed against the proximal surface of one tooth, and then the adjacent tooth. Concavities can be cleaned very well using the blunt end of the Brush Stick!

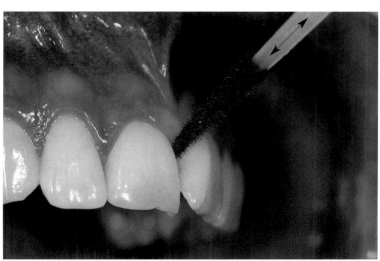

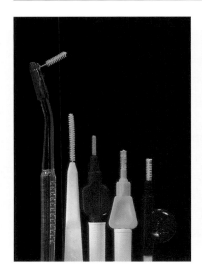

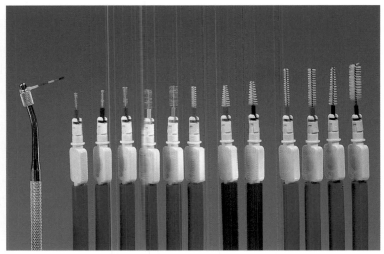

Interdental Brushes

504 Selection
Numerous companies offer inter-dental brushes. Excellent products include various bristle lengths, strength and diameter, with handpieces or separate holders (pictured is the assortment from *Curaprox*; at left, the coded measurement probe for the choice of brush type).
Left:
Oral-B (with handpiece),
Top Caredent, TePe, Oral Prevent, Paro (*Esro*).

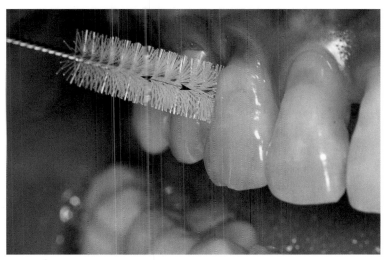

505 Use of a Large Interdental Brush
Appropriate interdental brushes are available today for the smallest to the largest interdental spaces. They represent the ideal cleaning tool, especially for periodontitis patients. The brush is inserted obliquely into the interdental space, from apical. Cleaning is performed with a back and forth motion (double arrow).

The trend today is toward long, flexible (soft) bristles.

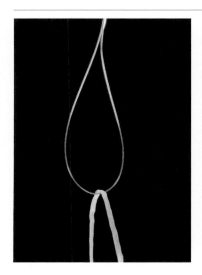

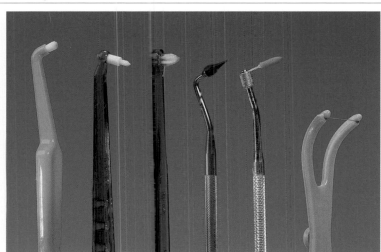

Additional Hygiene Aids

506 Hygiene Aids for Special Problems

- **Round Solo Brush** (p. 229)
- **Pointed, Single-Tuft Brush,** e. g., for the furcation entrance
- **Stimulators** Massage in the area of the interdental papillae
- **Soft-Foam Attachment** (Oral-B) Cleaning for titanium implants
- **"Fork"** for dental floss

Left: **Threader** for floss and tape.

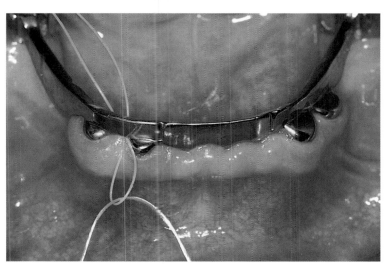

507 Threading Dental Tape
With fixed splints, bridges and bar constructions, the dental floss cannot be applied from the occlusal, but must be inserted. In such cases this can be accomplished using a threading sling (e. g., Butler).

The threader is particularly helpful for patients with limited manual dexterity, and also for interdental spaces for which the superfloss threader is too "soft."

Dentifrice

A dentifrice is an integral component of daily home care to enhance oral hygiene. Dentifrices effectively double the efficiency of mechanical *plaque removal* and therefore help to prevent oral diseases such as caries and gingival inflammation (*active principle of prevention*).

The most important component of any dentifrice is the abrasive substance. Manufacturers use many different abrasives, which vary not only with regard to their chemical composition (phosphates, carbonates, silica, alumina etc.), but also in particle size and shape (rounded, angular). These differences determine the polishing effect of the product, as wells as the abrasiveness of the dentifrice on dentin (measured *in vitro* as the RDA value: "Radioactive/relative dentin abrasion").

The non-mechanical components of dentifrices include their chemical ingredients (*passive principle of prevention*): These ingredients prevent caries (fluorides), treat hypersensitive exposed dentin (K- and Sr-salts; fluoride; p. 318), possess disinfecting properties (Triclosan), and serve to whiten stained teeth (H_2O_2; carbamide): All in one tube!

508 Dentifrices—"World Selection"
From the enormous number of products on the market, the dental hygienist must select only a few, and must know the advantages and disadvantages of each in order to provide proper information during oral hygiene instruction.

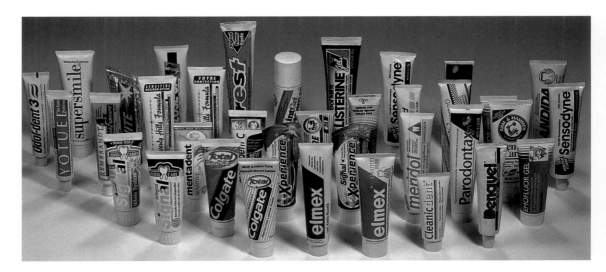

509 Damaging Toothpaste? Damaging Technique?
Left: Healthy dentition. How will it look in 40 years?

Middle: Loss of enamel is minimal after a single toothbrushing (**A**), but this is not the case with fruit acids and chelators from foodstuffs (grapefruit; **B**/yellow). Toothbrushing after consumption of acidic foods is yet worse (**C**).

Right: This patient brushed with a scrubbing technique for 50 years, while also consuming acidic foods!

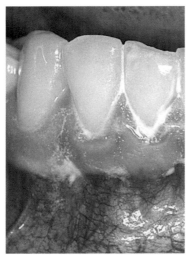
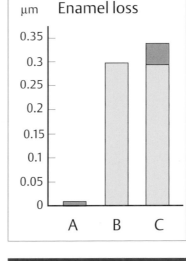
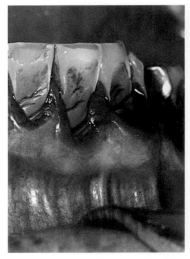

510 Types of Dentifrices

- **"Whitening" Dentifrices** (left)
- **Normal Fluoride Dentifrices** (middle)
- **Dentifrices for Tooth Neck Sensitivity** (right)

Does long-term use of whitening dentifrices cause tooth damage? Must exposed dentin be cleaned using mildly abrasive dentifrice?

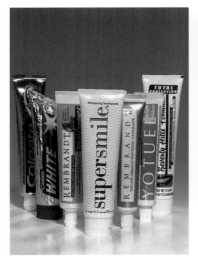
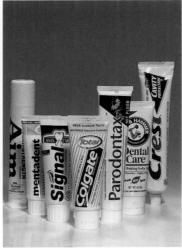
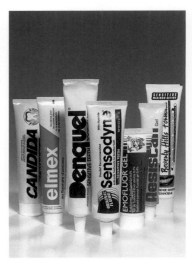

Chemical Plaque Control—"Soft Chemo" Prevention

Purely mechanical plaque control is effective up to a certain point, but excessively robust toothbrushing can injure the gingiva and damage tooth structure. Optimum personal oral hygiene can only be achieved through the use of certain supportive antimicrobial agents, which may be included as ingredients in dentifrices or mouthwash. These chemical ingredients must not interact with other substances within a dentifrice and should exhibit high substantivity (AAP 1994, Brecx et al. 1997, Cummins 1997). The substantivity of plaque-inhibitory substances depends upon:

- Pharmacokinetics
- Concentration and dose
- Effectiveness over time
- Site of application

A therapeutically effective "soft chemo" substance should affect at least an 80 % plaque reduction. Until today, this level of effectiveness has been achieved only by the bis-biguanide chlorhexidine (CHX). For this reason, CHX in all of its commercially available forms remains today the substance of choice.

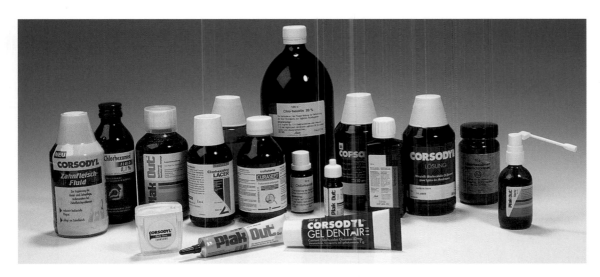

Chemical plaque control – Disinfection agents, "soft chemo"

Chemical classification	Examples	Effect	Products
Bisbiguanides	• Chlorhexidine (CHX)	• Antimicrobial	Mouthwashes, gels, dentifrices, throat spray
Quaternary ammonium substances	• Cetylpyridium chloride • Benzalconium chloride	• Antimicrobial	Mouthwashes
Phenols and essential oils	• Thymol, menthol, eucalyptus oil • Triclosan	• Antimicrobial • Antimicrobial, anti-inflammatory	Mouthwashes, dentifrices
Metal ions	• Tin, zinc • Strontium, calcium	• Antimicrobial, desensitizing	Mouthwashes, dentifrices
Halogens – Fluorides – Iodine	• Sodium fluoride, sodium monofluoro-phosphate • Stannous fluoride • Amine fluoride • Providone (PVP) iodine	• Caries inhibitory (antimicrobial), desensitizing • antimicrobial	Dentifrices, gels, mouthwashes, varnish Rinsing solutions
Amine alcohols	• Delmopinol	• Inhibits biofilm formation	No product yet available
Oxygen-splitting ligands	• Hydrogen peroxide • Sodium perborate • Sodium percarbonate	• Antimicrobial	Mouthwashes
Plant products	• Sanguinarin	• Antimicrobial	Mouthwashes, dentifrices
Enzymes	• Glucose oxidase • Amylglucose oxidase	• Antimicrobial	Dentifrice

511 CHX Digluconate Products
In Europe and elsewhere, but not in the USA, various CHX mouthwashes, gels, sprays etc. are available for patients, in concentrations of
- **0.06–0.12 %**
- **0.1–0.2 %**
- **10 %** (concentrate; PlakOut)

For clinical use, concentrations up to **20 %** CHX are available, as well as **CHX-HCl** in powder form. Diluted or dissolved, this provides a cost-effective disinfectant, and can also be used as the cooling solution for ultrasonic instruments.

512 Agents for Chemical Plaque Control—"Soft Chemo"
CHX in all its available forms is the most potent agent for *supragingival* plaque control.

Most of the additional disinfection products listed in this table work as *antimicrobials*, and in appropriate concentrations are *bacteriocidal*.

While CHX represents the second generation of effective plaque inhibitors, the aminoalcohols (e. g., delmopinol) represent the third generation. These are not bacteriocidal, rather they inhibit the formation of biofilm. This new group evolved from the newest research on biofilm formation (p. 24).

Note: Plaque reduction is not synonymous with inflammation reduction. Therefore, in this table no specific *inflammation-reducing* products are listed.

Irrigators

The supragingival efficacy of mouthwashes containing caries-preventive (fluorides) or antiseptic ingredients (e.g., chlorhexidine) is well acknowledged. Mouthwashes and also the use of intraoral irrigators represent only adjuncts to mechanical oral hygiene.

The pulsating, hydrodynamic forces produced by irrigators can rinse away food debris from interdental spaces and plaque-retentive areas, but *do not remove* plaque biofilm (Hugoson 1978). Irrigation solutions have always contained aromatics, and later also disinfective ingredients. The use of

chlorhexidine in sub-optimum concentrations (e.g., 0.06%) led to improved plaque inhibition and an anti-inflammatory effect (Lang and Räber 1981, Flemmig et al. 1990).

In contrast, the success of pulsating irrigators with the common tips is limited in the subgingival area, and in periodontal pockets (Mazza et al. 1981, Wennström et al. 1987). With special tips, the pulsating stream penetrates more deeply, but biofilm is not removed (Flemmig 1993, reported up to 90% penetration during pocket rinsing).

513 Mouthrinsing—Irrigators

A Mouthrinsing—no solution enters the pocket (< 5%).

B Single or multiple sprays—about half of the pocket depth is penetrated (ca. 50%).

C Special tips (PikPocket)—the solution is forced deeply into the pocket (ca. 90%).

Modified from *Flemmig 1993*

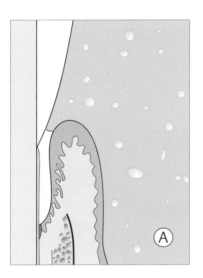
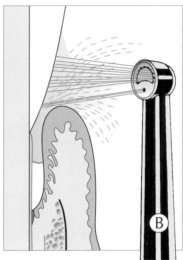
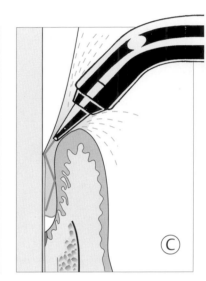

514 Oral Irrigator—Waterpik
The "mother of all oral irrigators."

Waterpik represents the first technically simple oral irrigator. Contemporary models feature an off/on button on the handle, as well as pressure regulation. In this case, CHX was added to the rinsing solution; the toothbrush in the foreground reminds that the irrigator should be used *after* toothbrushing.

Right: Normal tip (left) and special tip (PikPocket).

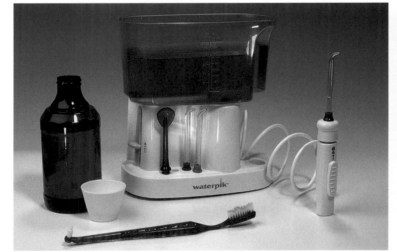
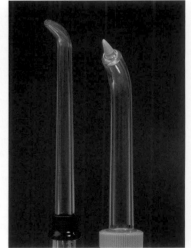

515 "Professional Care Center"—Braun Oral-B
The well-known *Braun electric toothbrush* offers a large assortment of brushes, including the "Interspace" brush, and the special *oral irrigator* (Oral-B Oxyjet) in a combined unit.

Right: In combination with a special attachment, this device produces fine *micro air bubbles* in the water stream. It is claimed that this effectively attacks plaque bacteria and removes food deposits from between the teeth.

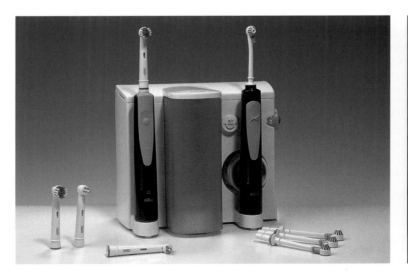
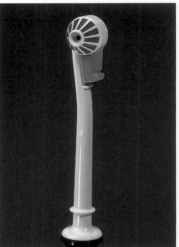

Oral Hygiene for Halitosis—Tongue Cleansing

It has been estimated that half of all people suffer from episodic or permanent halitosis. A myriad of factors could be responsible for this pathologic *Foetor ex ore*—systemic, oronasal and oral, associated with a large and diverse number of volatile molecules.

In the absence of systemic diseases, 9 out of 10 cases of halitosis originate from the tonsils and the tongue, particularly the posterior dorsal tongue surface (Stassinakis 2002).

Gram-negative anaerobic microorganisms from the periodontal pocket may also contribute to halitosis, primarily by way of their metabolites, not only their lipopolysaccharides but also short-chain fatty acids such as butyric acid and propionic acid. Breakdown products of the host defense response may also play a role in halitosis. Clinically, it is relatively easy to measure volatile sulfur compounds such as hydrogen sulfide (H_2S) and thiol (mercaptans; v. Steenberghe and Rosenberg 1996, Loesche and Kazor 2002).

The most important step to reduce halitosis appears to be improved oral hygiene, especially cleansing of the tongue (Saxer 2000, 2002; Seemann et al. 2001).

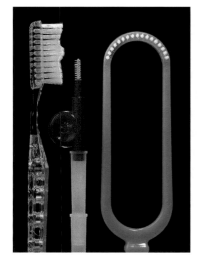

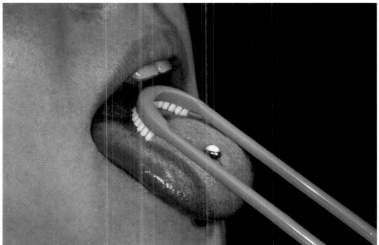

516 Tongue Cleansing
Special scrapers are available for cleaning the tongue. Patients should be informed that it is most important to clean the *posterior* portion of the tongue dorsum. An initial gag reflex usually subsides quickly.
Note: This procedure not only reduces halitosis, it also removes a large *reservoir* of periodontopathic bacteria.

Left: Combo for oral hygiene: Toothbrush, interdental brush, and the tongue brush.

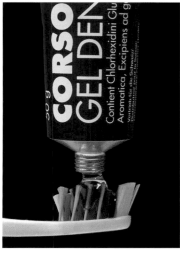

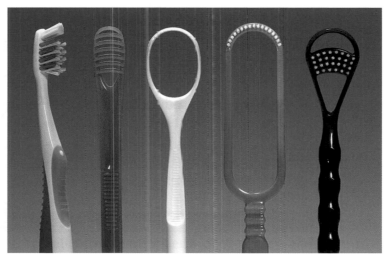

517 Tongue Scrapers
In addition to the normal toothbrush, which can also be used for tongue cleaning, a variety of tongue scrapers is commercially available: Scraper, tongue brush and combinations.

Left: In addition to mechanical cleaning, antiseptics may also be used; e. g., 1 % chlorhexidine gel. The toothbrush is loaded with gel.

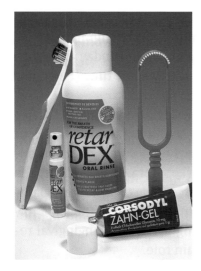

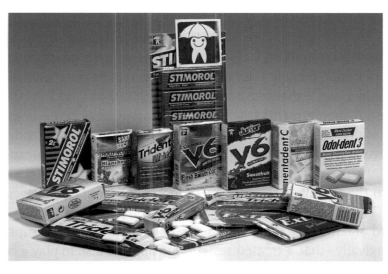

518 Additional Options on the Road Toward "Full Mouth" Cleansing
Chewing *sugar-free* gum increases saliva flow (enamel remineralization), massages the gingiva and may remove some bacteria that are then swallowed.

Left: Articles for oral hygiene—mechanical: toothbrush, tongue scraper; chemical: antimicrobial sprays, gels and mouthwashes (e. g., retarDEX, Esro).

Supragingival Tooth Cleaning—Power-driven Instruments …

The removal of all stains, deposits and concrements comprises the first phase initial therapy. It is also an important preventive measure in the healthy periodontium, and the most significant post-operative measure following completion of periodontitis therapy. Thorough tooth cleaning is performed during each recall appointment (maintenance phase, p. 309).

The prevention/treatment/maintenance therapy trio "without end" is the sole responsibility of the dental hygienist. It also demands rationalization, standardization and work simplification, as well innovation in the development of new instruments (ultrasonic devices, Air-Scaler etc.).

Difficult-to-remove stains resulting from medicaments (e.g., chlorhexidine), tobacco, beverages (tea, wine) and foodstuffs as well as dental plaque can be removed using instruments that provide a water-powder spray (e.g., Cavitron-Jet). The powder that is used in the water spray must be minimally abrasive for dentin and restorative materials (Iselin et al. 1989). Furthermore, the spray should never be directed perpendicular to the tooth surfaces, and should

520 Powder-Water Spray Device (Cavitron-Jet)
The powdered abrasive consists primarily of sodium bicarbonate ($NaHCO_3$) which can remove tough deposits and stains when used with a water spray.
The water-powder spray requires use of a high-speed evacuator.

Right:

"Jet Shield"

This "mini-evacuator" is affixed directly to the working end of the Cavitron-Jet.

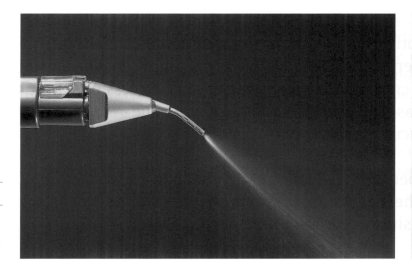
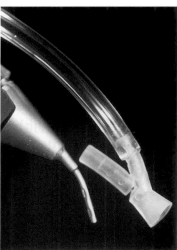

521 Stabilized Power System (SPS) with Ultrasonic Scaler Tips (Cavitron Thru Flow Inserts—TFI)
In modern instruments, the water coolant is directed through the instrument tip in a groove on the instrument head. Ultrasonic scalers work at between 25,000–50,000 cycles per second, with very small amplitudes.

Right: Various ultrasonic scaler tips; from left to right:

TFI-1000, TFI-9, TFI-1, TFI-7.

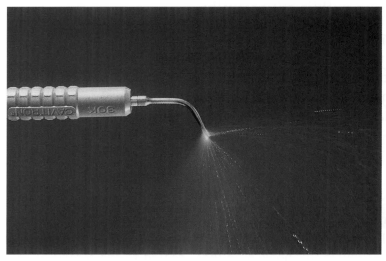
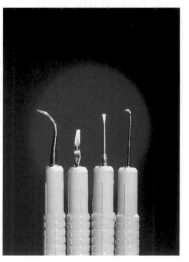

522 Air-Scaler (Titan-S, "Sonic Scaler")
The air-scaler has a regulable frequency of maximum 6,000 Hz and thus is considerably slower than an ultrasonic instrument. The motion of the tip of the instrument is between 0.08–0.20 mm; relatively slow.

Right: Three tips for the Titan-S device.
Additional manufacturers:

- KaVo
- Satelec, and Others

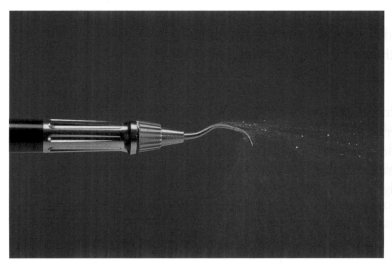
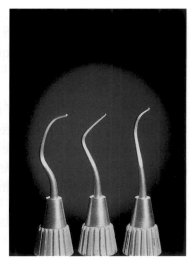

... and their Use

usually be used only on enamel, with constant movement of the tip. Such devices do not guarantee perfect cleaning in interdental spaces or niches. The spray with normal abrasive powder should not be directed into pockets. With the new, "mild," minimally abrasive agents and fine tips, effective cleansing can be achieved, in certain circumstances, even subgingivally (e.g., glycine powder from Espe, with the EMS Airflow Handy 2; p.282; Petersilka et al. 2002).

After the removal of soft deposits, calculus becomes visible. Calculus is an excellent substrate for plaque accumulation and must be completely removed. Numerous power-driven instruments are available: Ultrasonic apparatus (e.g., Cavitron) as well as Air-Scaler that can be attached to the air-water supply of the dental unit (e.g., Titan-S, Satelec; Sonicflex KaVo etc.; Hermann et al. 1995).

However, the most important and most precise means for removal of concrements remains: hand instruments (p.242).

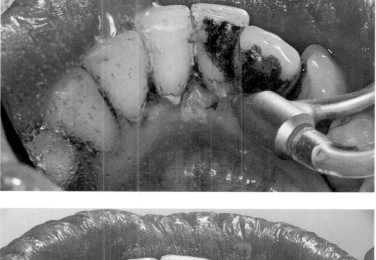

523 Removal of Soft Deposits and Stains
Tough deposits, plaque and stains from tobacco, tea, wine or chlorhexidine can be removed from accessible enamel surfaces using the powder-water device. Cleaning in interdental areas, however, is insufficient. The stream should be directed onto the tooth surface at an angle of 45°. A high speed evacuator is used to retrieve the reflected solution.

Caution: Highly abrasive on cementum, dentin and restorations!

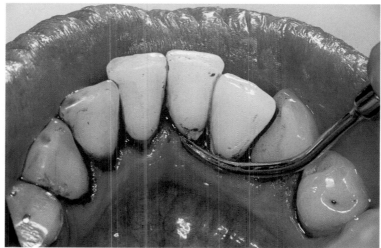

524 Removal of Hard, Supragingival Concrements with an Ultrasonic Device
Following removal of soft debris and plaque, remaining calculus is completely removed using the ultrasonic device. In narrow, poorly accessible sites and niches, fine ultrasonic tips or hand instruments must be used afterwards.

Caution: Overheating, cracks in enamel and porcelain!

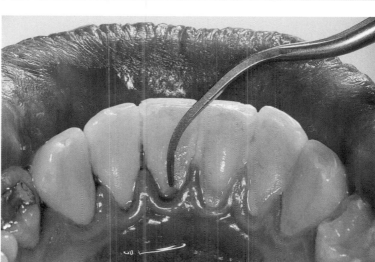

525 Removal of Hard Supragingival Concrements Using the Air-Scaler
This instrument, which attaches to the turbine handpiece air-water orifice, permits removal of concrements in a manner similar to the ultrasonic instrument; however, the sensitivity is improved and the frequency can be regulated. Less pressure is necessary, and rinsing is continuous. This simplifies therapy, improves visibility and permits more efficient performance.

Pictured is the Titan-S scaler.

Supragingival Tooth Cleaning—Hand Instruments, Prophy Pastes ...

In addition to ultrasonic devices, hand scalers and curettes remain the most important instruments for periodontal therapy and prophylaxis. For the removal of soft deposits and stains, hand instruments are enhanced by the use of brushes, rubber cups and polishing strips along with cleaning and polishing pastes.

It is not the manufacturer that is critical for successful treatment, rather the shape of the instrument, especially its de-gree of sharpness, and above all the manual dexterity of the dental hygienist (scaling technique)!

For the removal of supragingival deposits, *chisels*, straight and angled *scalers* and also *lingual scalers* are effective. In premolar and molar segments, also on difficult-to-reach areas, grooves and depressions on the crown, as well as exposed root surfaces, the removal of supragingival concrements may require *curettes* in addition to scalers, usually without anesthesia.

526 Scalers
For supragingival calculus removal and for concrements that are located only a few millimeters below the gingival margin, sharp-edged, pointed scalers in various shapes are indicated:

- **Zerfing Chisel** ZI 10 (white)
- **Zbinden Scaler** ZI 11, 11 R+L (blue), straight and paired
- **Lingual Scaler** ZI 12 (black)

Right: Working end of the Zerfing chisel (45° sharpening angle!) and the lingual scaler.

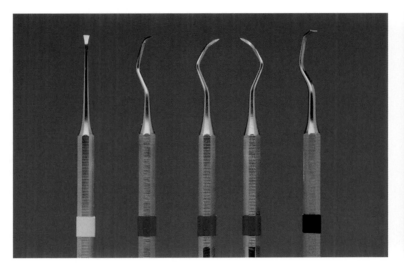
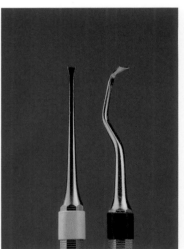

527 Curettes
For difficult-to-reach areas and for subgingival accretions, the scaler armamentarium must be enhanced by curettes:

- **Universal Curettes** ZI 15 (yellow) 1.2 mm wide
- **Anterior Curettes** GX 4 (orange), Deppeler
- **Posterior Curettes** M 23 A (red); both are ca. 0.95 mm wide; Deppeler

Right: Working ends of a pair of universal curettes.

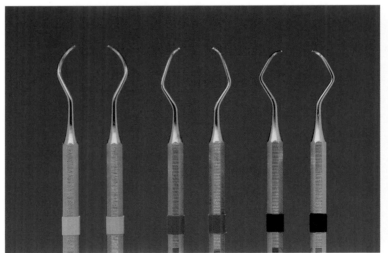
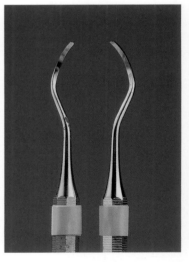

528 Standardized Prophy Pastes—RDA
Prophy pastes are available according to abrasiveness. The standardization is achieved on the basis of dentin abrasion, measured by radioactivity. All are fluoride-containing:

RDA Value	Abrasiveness	Color
• 40	mild	yellow
• 120	normal	red
• 170	moderate	green
• 250	heavy	blue

Right: Finger cups with color-coded prophy pastes.

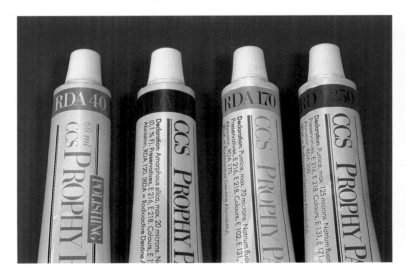
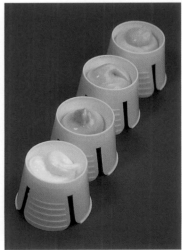

... and Their Use

For the first phase of initial therapy, the classical universal curettes are indicated. The slender *Gracey curettes* which are sharpened on only one edge, are used almost exclusively for subgingival scaling and root planing in periodontitis patients (p. 259). Today, ultrasonic and sonic devices are being used more and more often, in addition to hand instruments.

If supragingival calculus is covered with thick soft deposits, these should be removed with brushes and coarse prophy paste before mechanical debridement.

Whenever calculus is removed, the teeth should be polished afterwards with a rubber cup and polishing paste. This polish of the teeth and any exposed root surfaces is performed with fluoride-containing prophy pastes, which are classified according to their *dentin abrasiveness* (radioactive dentin abrasion = RDA; p. 234).

Contact points and the interdental areas can be cleaned using fine polishing strips (see p. 244).

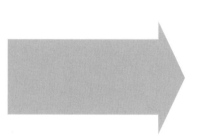

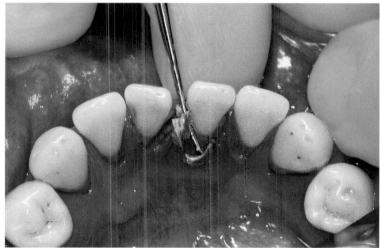

529 Supragingival Calculus Removal
The Zerfing chisel is the only instrument that is used in the anterior segment with a *pushing* motion.
Straight and angled scalers and/or ultrasonic devices are then used for removal of any remaining calculus.
The lingual scaler (Fig. 526, right) smoothes the narrow lingual surface of mandibular anterior teeth.

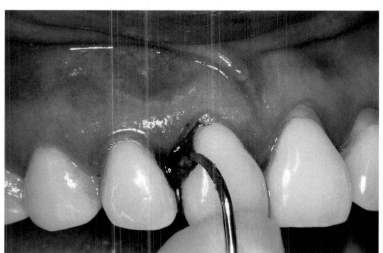

530 Subgingival Calculus Removal
The largest masses of subgingival accretions are located only a few mm apical to the gingival margin. These should be removed during gross debridement, without anesthesia, using scalers and curettes or ultrasonic devices, as necessary.

Gingival bleeding will occur even during very careful scaling, as the ulcerated pocket epithelium is injured.

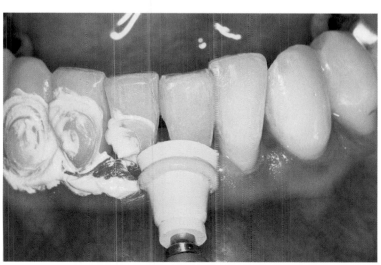

531 Polishing with Rubber Cup and Prophy Paste
Each time scaling is preformed, the teeth must be polished, otherwise rough surfaces will enhance re-accumulation of plaque bacteria.
Rubber cups and polishing paste are ideal for this procedure (RCP technique, "rubber cup and paste"), because they are kinder to the gingival margin than are rotating brushes. The rubber cup can be used near shallow pockets to achieve polishing 1–2 mm beneath the gingival margin.

Creating of Conditions that Enhance Oral Hygiene—Removal of Iatrogenic Irritants

Concurrent with mechanical removal of plaque and calculus, all imperfect dental restorations are corrected with the goal of creating smooth supra- and subgingival tooth surfaces as well as impeccable transitions areas between natural tooth surfaces and the margins of restorations and crowns. Only when this is done will it be possible for the patient to maintain efficient plaque control: *Creation of hygiene capability.*

The most important iatrogenic irritants, which must be removed or corrected, include:

- Rough, poorly contoured restorations
- Overhangs of restoration margins
- Open crown margins located subgingivally
- Improperly contoured bridge pontics
- Depressible clasps, prosthesis saddles etc., which can injure the periodontium directly.

532 Instruments for Recontouring and Polishing Old Restorations
High-speed handpiece with variously-shaped, fine, flame-shaped diamond burs.

Right:

- Round stone
- Round bur
- Flame-shaped, fine diamond bur
- Rubber tip polisher (Shofu "brownie")

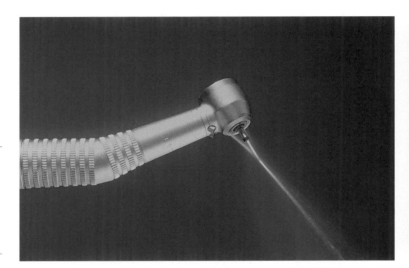
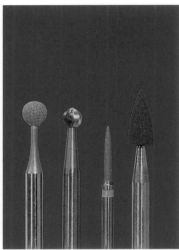

533 Mechanical Files
Handpiece with prophylaxis head (EVA system; KaVo). 0.4–1.5 mm length. Regulable speed, up to 10,000 rpm.

Right:

- **Proxoshape Set** (Intensiv) Diamond coating coarseness: 75 µm, 40 µm (yellow), 15 µm (red)

Possibility to remove restoration overhangs even in relatively narrow interdental spaces.

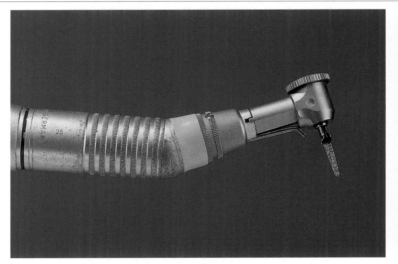
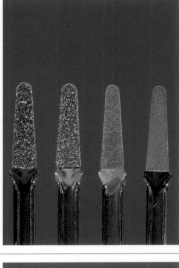

534 Manual Filing
A strip holder simplifies the removal of restoration overhangs and polishing in areas of narrow interdental spaces, and also protects the cheeks, tongue and lips. Pictured:

- **LM Holder; Steel Strips** (Horico)

Right: **MEBA Separator**
Extremely narrow contact points are not always accessible even for the finest strips. The separator can provide access.

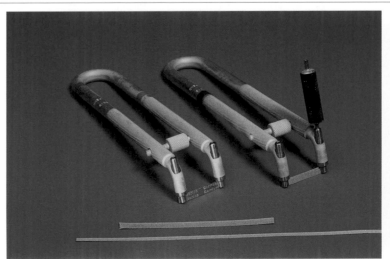
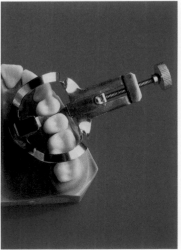
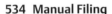

More important than direct irritation, however, is the fact that even minor imperfections of dental restorative work represent plaque-retentive areas. The result at such locations is gingival inflammation and, over the long term, possibly periodontal destruction (Lange et al. 1983, Iselin et al. 1985).

The finishing and polishing of all restoration surfaces can be performed with fine diamonds (water cooling), round burs and finishing disks.

Interdental amalgam overhangs can be removed with flame-shaped diamonds and periodontal files or with the Proxoshape files (EVA system).

Metal and plastic strips, either hand-held or in an appropriate holder, are also useful in the marginal/proximal regions for smoothing restoration margins. Old restorations exhibiting overhangs or cracks *should be replaced*, because secondary caries is common beneath defective restorations!

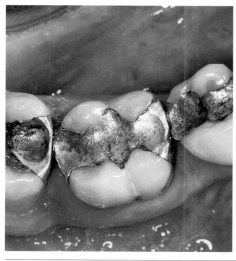

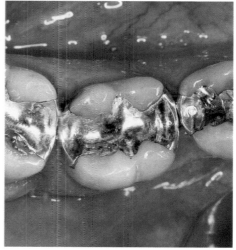

535 Old Amalgam Restorations Before and After Recontouring
Left: The rough, discolored surface of old restorations enhances plaque accumulation. Even though the occlusal surfaces do not have any direct contact with the marginal periodontal tissues, polishing the restorations leads to a reduction in the bacterial load in the oral cavity. Functional contacts in centric occlusion and lateral occlusion must be maintained.

Right: Contoured and polished old amalgam restorations.

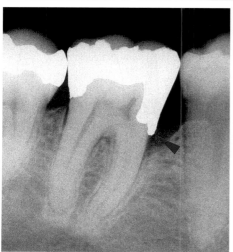

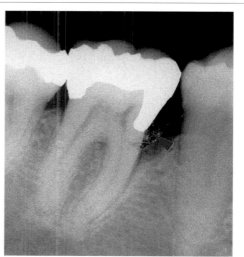

536 Amalgam Overhang Before and After Removal
Left: Tooth 46 exhibits a pronounced marginal overhang on the mesial aspect (massive plaque accumulation, arrow). A deep bony pocket is also located near this iatrogenic niche.

Right: The proximal overhang was removed and the restoration was polished. The margin is now perfect, discouraging any further plaque accumulation. If there is suspicion of caries, the restoration should be replaced.

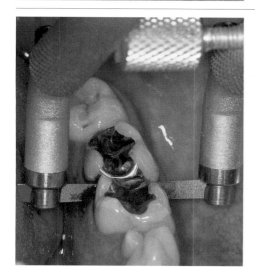

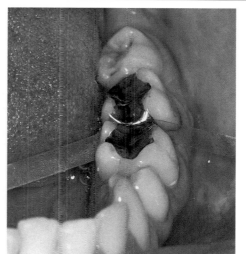

537 Smoothing the Proximal Restoration Surface Using Strips
Left: LM strip holder with diamond-coated steel strip during smoothing of the distal surface of tooth 36. The contact area must be protected.

Right: The interdental surface of the restoration is finally polished using fine, very mildly abrasive linen strips, which can also be used in the contact area.
Goal: Smooth proximal surfaces make possible perfect interdental hygiene with dental floss.

Reduction of Natural Plaque-retentive Areas—Crowding: Morphologic Odontoplasty

Crowding is one of the few tooth position anomalies that may play an indirect role in the initiation and progression of gingivitis/periodontitis. In such cases, occlusal/functional factors play no role. Crowded teeth create niches for plaque accumulation, and simultaneously render the patient's oral hygiene more difficult.

Extensive orthodontic treatment involving selective tooth extraction, is often not possible due to the large technical, temporal and financial considerations, especially in adults.

Careful *morphologic odontoplasty* may represent an alternative to orthodontics in cases of tooth crowding; the procedure can also improve the esthetics. Odontoplasty is performed using fine diamonds, *exclusively in enamel*. Following the procedure, tooth surfaces must be polished and treated with fluoride.

544 Crowding—
Plaque-Retention Factor
In this case of severe anterior crowding in the mandible, one observes severe gingivitis and plaque accumulation on those tooth surfaces that do not benefit from *self-cleansing* by the lip and tongue. This situation can be significantly improved by minor odontoplasty.

Right: View from the occlusal aspect. Tooth 31, in its severely labioverted position, is never touched by the tongue.

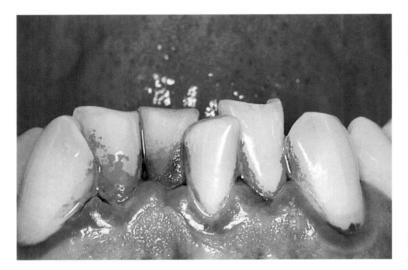
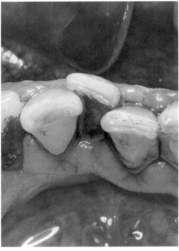

545 Odontoplasty—
Morphologic Grinding
Minor esthetic odontoplasty was performed on the incisal edges, while retaining all occlusal contacts in centric (red). The black surfaces will be selectively and morphologically smoothed, to decrease the niches.

The extremely narrow contact surfaces are polished using abrasive strips so that the interdental areas become accessible for dental floss.

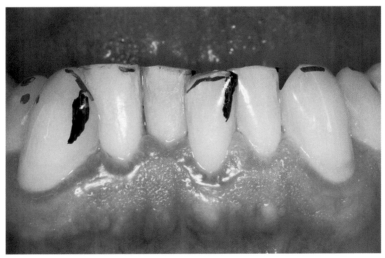

546 Clinical View Following
Odontoplasty and Prophylaxis
The plaque-retentive areas are no longer so expansive. Disclosing agent reveals only minor plaque accumulation. Interdental hygiene with floss is now possible.
This minor odontoplastic treatment and optimization of oral hygiene by the patient led to significant reduction of gingival inflammation.

Right: Even in the lingual area, the clinical situation is improved. Mild marginal inflammation persists.

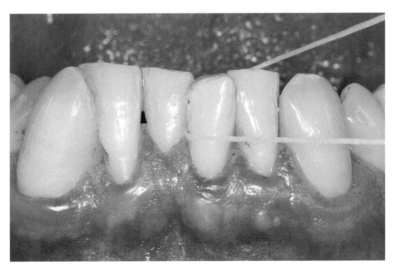
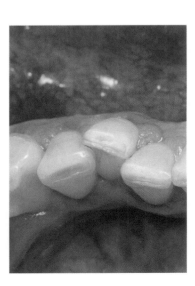

Treatment of Plaque-elicited Gingivitis

Clinical Procedure, Step-by-Step

The treatment for gingivitis ("gingival disease," classified as Type I A; p. 328) is identical to the "initial treatment 1" (hygiene phase) performed collaboratively between the patient and the hygienist. It includes motivation, information, oral hygiene instruction and check-up, as well as professional supragingival plaque and calculus removal (*debridement*).

When performed throughout the entire dentition, this treatment can be extremely time-consuming. It will be demonstrated here in the mandibular anterior segment. The 30-year-old female exhibited a moderate, plaque-induced gingivitis. There was *no* attachment loss, but pseudopockets to 4 mm were noted. The patient had never received comprehensive oral hygiene instruction. OHI was therefore provided simultaneously with *professional tooth cleaning* procedures.

Initial findings (mandibular anterior):

PI: 72%   BOP: 69%   TM: 0–1 (p. 174)

The clinical appearance and radiographs are depicted below.

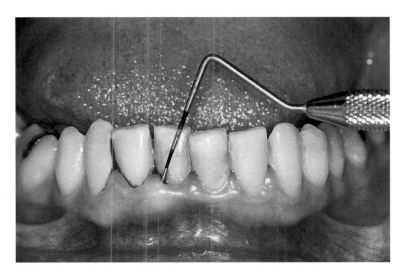

547 Initial Findings— Moderate Gingivitis
The gingivae are swollen by edema, especially in the papillary area. Profuse hemorrhage occurs immediately after gentle probing, particularly in interdental areas. The patient's generally mediocre oral hygiene is enhanced in the mandibular anterior area by mild crowding, which favors plaque accumulation.
The width of the attached gingival is normal.

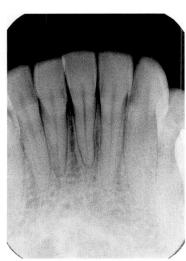

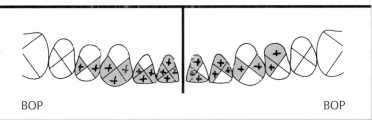

BOP   BOP

548 Bleeding Index (BOP) and Plaque Index (PI or PCR)

BOP: On 22 of the 32 measured sites (mesial, facial, distal, oral) bleeding occurs after gentle periodontal probing (Indices, p. 68).

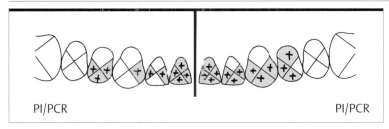

PI/PCR   PI/PCR

PI/PCR: Plaque was detectable on 23 of the 32 examined tooth surfaces (8 teeth: 34–44).

Left: Radiographic findings. There is no radiographic evidence of bone loss.

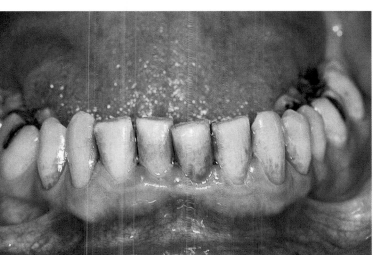

549 Stained Plaque
On almost all teeth, there is more or less pronounced plaque accumulation, particularly in the marginal and interdental regions.

Plaque and Calculus Removal in the Mandibular Anterior Area; Lingual View

550 Initial Condition
A plaque-induced gingivitis with supragingival calculus is shown from the lingual aspect.
Oral hygiene instruction (toothbrush) was given at the first appointment.
Interdental hygiene (using dental floss) was demonstrated at the next appointment.

Right: Gingivitis, facial view.

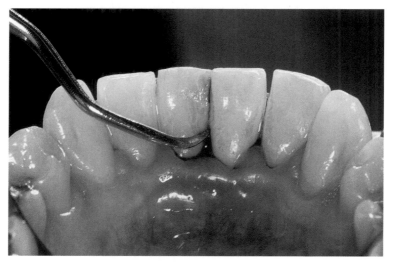
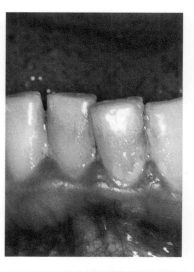

551 Debridement Using the Ultrasonic Scaler
Power-driven devices are particularly indicated for the initial removal of soft and hard supragingival deposits (gross debridement).

Right: Historical (left) and modern ultrasonic instruments with internal cooling (middle; Dentsply Cavitron) or sonic scaler (e. g., KaVo Sonicflex, right).

Caution: These create aerosols; barriers are indicated.

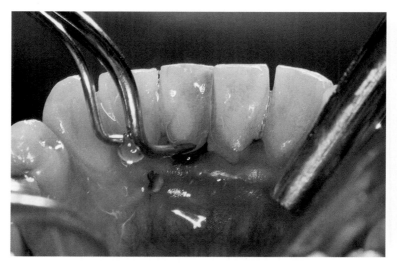
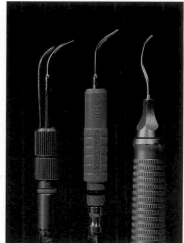

552 Scaling—Tooth Cleaning Supragingivally Using Hand Instruments
After use of power scalers, it is imperative that hand instruments (scalers and curettes) be systematically employed for fine debridement.
Less important than the particular instrument used is the result:
A perfectly clean tooth.

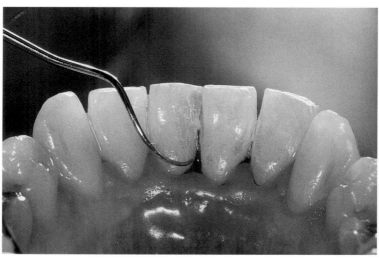

553 Checking with a Pointed Explorer
The smoothness of the tooth and root surface is checked with a very fine explorer.

Right: Fine, pointed explorers:

- **EXD5**
- **EXD3CH**
- **EXS3A**
  All instruments from Hu-Friedy Co.

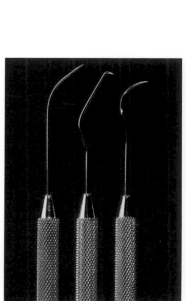

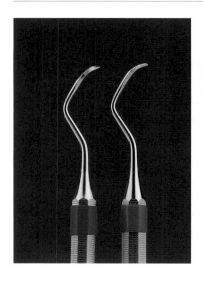
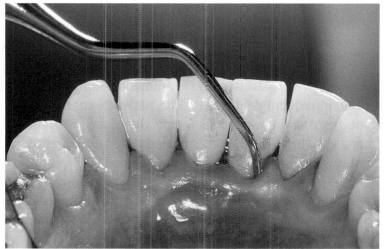

554 Subgingival Cleaning with Universal Curettes
Even in gingivitis therapy, fine curettes are applicable. Their rounded ends injure gingiva only slightly when they are used subgingivally in pseudopockets with a horizontal stroke.

Left: Instruments:

- **Scaler M23**
- **Curette M23A**
  (Deppeler Co.)

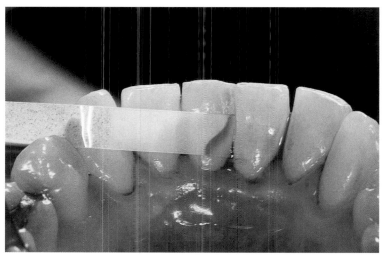

555 Plaque Removal And Preliminary Polishing in the Interdental Area—Strip with Mild Abrasiveness
Following mechanical therapy of the oral and facial tooth surfaces, the proximal surfaces and the contact areas are cleaned with strips incorporating fine abrasives.

For polishing, dental tape or smooth, uncoated strips may be used with a fluoride-containing prophy paste (p. 232).

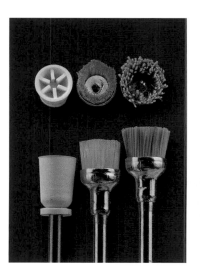
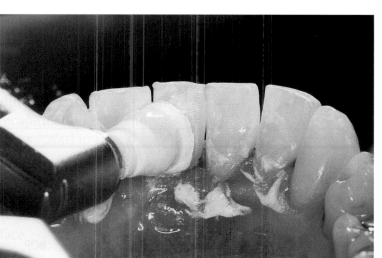

556 Polishing with a Rubber Cup and Paste—RCP Method
Using the RCP method, tooth surfaces are carefully treated. Soft deposits (plaque!) should be removed exclusively with RCP, because repeated *mechanical* scaling (e. g., during recall visits) could enhance the formation of recession and wedge-shaped defects.

Left: Depending upon the tenacity of the deposits (stains), rubber cups or soft-hard brushes can be employed.

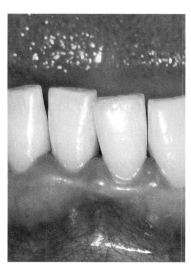
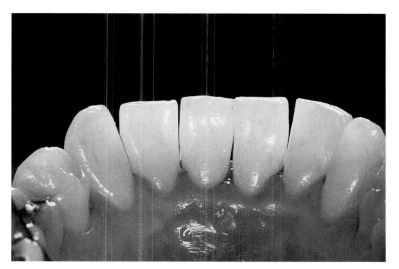

557 Mandibular Anterior Area Immediately After Treatment
Plaque and calculus have been removed. The time for these procedures was ca. 15 min. Even with very careful mechanical treatment of the tooth surfaces, minute trauma to the gingiva cannot be avoided. Such minor injuries heal within a few days.

Left: View from the facial, immediately following plaque and calculus removal.

Non-surgical, Anti-infectious Therapy—Goals of Treatment

The goal of traditional, non-surgical therapy is the elimination of the microorganisms responsible for periodontal destruction, from the pocket and surrounding tissues. The creation of a clean tooth and a clean, biologically compatible root surface that is as smooth as possible, and the removal of diseased or infected tissues are essential to therapy (Frank 1980, Saglie et al. 1982, Allenspach-Petrsilka & Guggenheim 1983, O'Leary 1986, Adriaens et al. 1988, Petersilka et al. 2002).

Removal of the pocket epithelium and portions of the infected connective tissues was a matter of controversy until recently; current research results clearly demonstrate the possibility of bacterial colonization of pocket epithelial cells (intracellular) and of connective tissue components. The most frequently encountered colonizers are *A. actinomycetemcomitans, P. gingivalis, T. denticola* and, in addition to the acknowledged pathogens, also *Streptococcus constellatus* (Socransky & Haffajee 2002).

Today's question? Should the pocket epithelium be removed in addition to removal of biofilm from the soft tissue pocket wall?

562 Principles of Conservative Pocket Therapy
This stained histologic section through a gingival pocket (HE, 20x) will be used to illustrate *root planing* (*debridement*) and *soft tissue curettage*.
Soft tissue curettage (**2**) is never used alone. True "causal" therapy includes the elimination of microorganisms wherever they have become organized as a biofilm.
It is imperative that the root surface be thoroughly debrided (**1**).

1 Scaling and Root Planing
The unilaterally sharp Gracey curette (**1**) removes plaque, calculus, endotoxin-containing cementum and sometimes dentin from the root surface. The arrow indicates the direction toward which the curette tip is pulled.

2 Gingival Curettage
A Gracey curette sharpened on its other edge (**2**) is used to remove pocket epithelium and remaining (apical) junctional epithelium, as well as the infiltrated connective tissue.

Oral Epithelium (Keratinized)

Pocket Epithelium

Pocket

Calculus (Plaque-Covered)

Ulcerated Pocket Epithelium

Inflammatory Infiltrate

Subepithelial Connective Tissue

Junctional Epithelium

Cementum

Dentin

563 Subgingival Biofilm at the Base of a Pocket
Histologic section, plaque stained with toluidin blue and methylene blue, modified.
Of special interest is the biofilm formation on the soft tissue wall.

1 *Biofilm/plaque on the root surface*
2 *Biofilm attached to the soft tissue wall: "red complex?"*
D Dentin
C Cementum
ICT Infiltrated connective tissue

Courtesy *M. Listgarten*

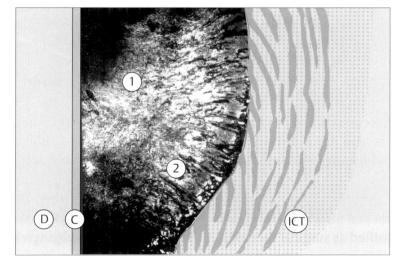

Antimicrobial Therapy—Combating the Reservoir

The answer to the question posed on the previous page would be: *Yes.* However, the AAP (2002) in its "Academy Statement Regarding Gingival Curettage," concluded that soft tissue curettage has *no* additional effect beyond scaling and root planing.

In any case, it is most important that purely mechanical therapy as a means to achieve the ultimate goal—periodontal healing—should be enhanced by the use of all antimicrobially effective measures.

The initial question concerns the bacterial reservoirs in the ecosystem represented by the oral cavity. The diagram below (Fig. 564) demonstrates the possible niches, the plaque-retentive areas in which periodontopathic microorganisms may be harbored.

Such microorganisms can rapidly contaminate (re-colonize) a freshly-treated pocket, and thus compromise the treatment results. Therefore, such bacterial reservoirs must also be "treated," especially in highly susceptible patients.

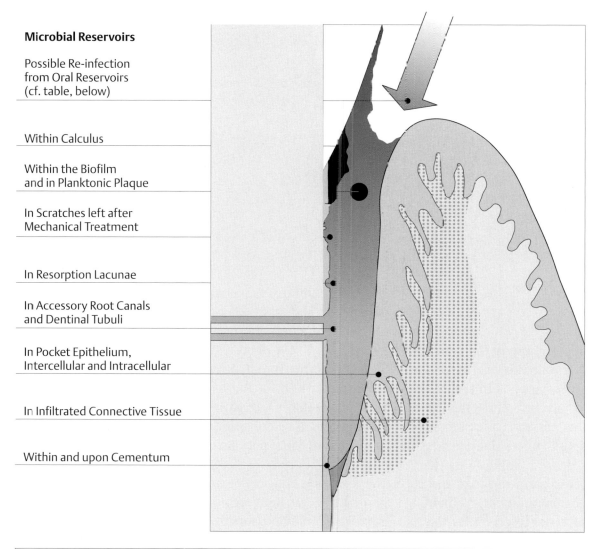

Microbial Reservoirs

Possible Re-infection from Oral Reservoirs (cf. table, below)

Within Calculus

Within the Biofilm and in Planktonic Plaque

In Scratches left after Mechanical Treatment

In Resorption Lacunae

In Accessory Root Canals and Dentinal Tubuli

In Pocket Epithelium, Intercellular and Intracellular

In Infiltrated Connective Tissue

Within and upon Cementum

564 Oral Microbial Reservoirs
Increases in plaque accumulation occur wherever microorganisms find a secure and undisturbed niche with good nutritive sources. Clusters of microbial colonies are always found in the small scratches that remain following root surface debridement, as well as the deep crypts in tonsils and on the dorsal surface of the tongue; many such clusters harbor the well-acknowledged periodontopathic anaerobes. Even a 0.5 mm thick biofilm provides oxygen-free (anaerobic) conditions for these microbes.

Modified from *P. Adriaens 1995*

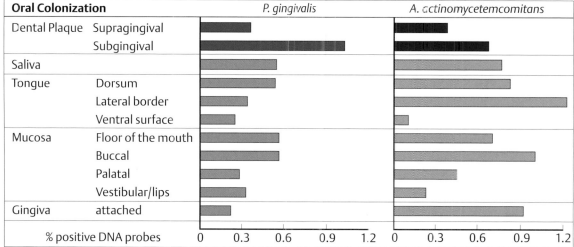

Oral Colonization		P. gingivalis	A. actinomycetemcomitans
Dental Plaque	Supragingival		
	Subgingival		
Saliva			
Tongue	Dorsum		
	Lateral border		
	Ventral surface		
Mucosa	Floor of the mouth		
	Buccal		
	Palatal		
	Vestibular/lips		
Gingiva	attached		
% positive DNA probes		0 0.3 0.6 0.9 1.2	0 0.3 0.6 0.9 1.2

565 *P. gingivalis* and *A. actinomycetemcomitans* in the Oral Reservoirs
Occurrence of the two species in 24 patients.
The presence and relative concentrations support the thorough cleaning of the tongue surface (pp. 237 and 281), and not only for patients with halitosis.

Modified from *Socransky et al. 1999*

Root Planing—With or without Curettage?

The primary goals in pocket treatment are removal of the biofilm and thorough debridement of the root surfaces.

Following elimination of non-adherent and adherent plaque, all subgingival calculus is removed. The superficial layers of the root cementum contain endotoxin. This lipopolysaccharide (LPS) from gram-negative bacteria can inhibit connective tissue regeneration and reestablishment of the periodontal ligament to the root surfaces. For this reason, root planing should be performed into "healthy" (hard) cementum or dentin layers.

After the root surface is thoroughly planed, the "peeling out" of the pocket epithelium and infiltrated connective tissue can be accomplished. If the curettes used for root planing are sharp on both edges (universal curettes), some soft tissue curettage will be accomplished inadvertently while the hard tooth structure is being planed.

The goals of these procedures include elimination of infection within the pocket and the pocket epithelium, and the ultimate healing of the periodontal lesion.

566 Root Planing and Curettage—Principles

A Cleaning the Root and the Pocket
The root surface is treated (**1**), and the plaque (**P**) is removed from the pocket.

B Original Pocket
With calculus, adherent plaque and non-adherent microorganisms.

C Soft Tissue Curettage
In addition, but never as the sole therapy, pocket epithelium/infiltrate (**2**) and junctional epithelium (**3**) are removed.

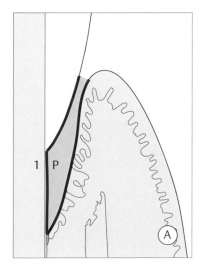 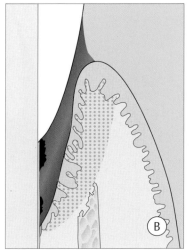 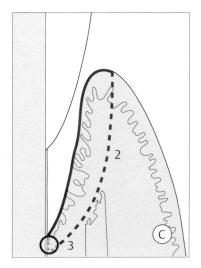

Effects of Subgingival Debridement— Pocket Healing or Recolonization?

The goal of closed anti-infectious therapy is the complete healing of all periodontal pockets, but this goal is seldom achieved. Access and vision are severely limited during closed instrumentation. Almost always, here and there, residual pockets of varying depths persist (Badersten 1984; p. 280). The so-called "critical depth" of residual pockets is 4–5 mm. Such pockets offer anaerobic conditions, which provide the well-known pathogenic, gram-negative anaerobic microorganisms a favorable environment. Remaining deeper pockets can serve as a bacterial reservoir for the re-

colonization of residual pockets. Patients who harbor residual pockets should be maintained in a strict recall schedule to control or eliminate such pockets.

Subgingival instrumentation (debridement) normally removes about 90 % of the bacteria from a pocket, including both "favorable" and pathogenic flora: The processes of healing and recolonization are in competition with each other, and residual pockets usually persist.

The favorable effect of closed pocket treatment is that the non-pathogenic flora recolonizes the pocket faster than the pathogenic microorganisms (Fig. 567; Petersilka et al. 2002).

567 Pocket Instrumentation— Schematic of Residual Pockets

A Untreated Pocket
Non-pathogenic (blue) and pathogenic (red) pocket flora.

B Following Instrumentation
The pocket flora is dramatically reduced.

C Recolonization + Shift
The percentage composition of the "blue" (non-pathogenic) has increased; in many cases, these and/or the host response will keep the "red" (pathogens) in check.

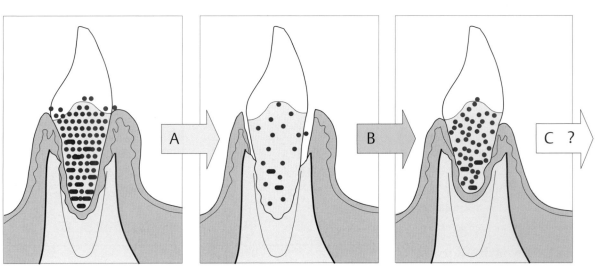

Closed Therapy—Indication, Instrumentation

It has been stated many times: Periodontal diseases should be prevented, or, failing prevention, should be diagnosed and treated early on.

Standard methods for the treatment of mild and moderate periodontitis include closed, non-surgical, anti-infectious pocket treatment (scaling and root planing). This approach is effective, tissue-friendly (minimal recession), less hemorrhagic, and routinely results in favorable treatment results. Perhaps even more important today, it is *affordable* for the (informed) patient.

With a technically adept and highly educated dental hygienist, closed therapy is the *definitive* therapy for uncomplicated cases, and represents the initial therapeutic approach for complex, advanced cases.

Contraindications for this approach are rare (patients on anticoagulant medications, risks for focal infection, systemic diseases).

Antimicrobial Approach

– Mechanical

+

– Chemical

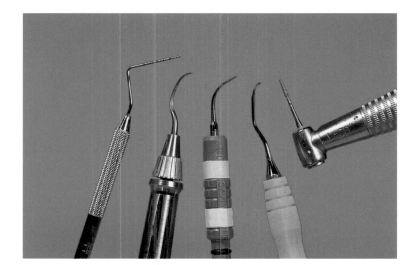

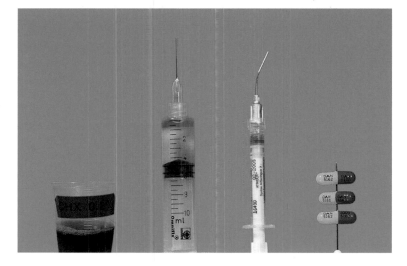

568 Instrumentarium for Mechanical/Anti-infectious "Closed" Therapy
These types of instruments are required for all patient treatments:

- **Periodontal probe**
- **Sonic scaler**—supragingival
- **Ultrasonic device**—pockets—subgingival
- **Curettes**—scaling, polishing
- **Motor-driven special instruments**—furcations, grooves, etc.

569 Chemical/Pharmacologic Adjunctive Therapy
The paradigm shift toward anti-infectious/antimicrobial therapy includes disinfectants and antibiotics more and more as co-therapeutic agents, above all for the treatment of aggressive cases.

- **Disinfectant Agents**
  FMT (pp. 235, 283)
- **Local CRD**
  "Controlled release drugs" (p. 292)
- **Systemic Antibiotics**
  (p. 288)

Conclusions

The goals of subgingival scaling are simple:
- Complete removal of biofilm and calculus
- Root planing (to reduce new plaque formation)
- Creation of a bioacceptable root surface (chemical conditioning with various substances, following mechanical treatment).

Subgingival scaling is a technically difficult endeavor, because it is performed without direct vision. Even the experienced hygienist will not always effectively treat all root surfaces, nor completely remove all plaque and calculus from all surfaces.

Today, the question is: How can we *improve* the "gold standard" of closed causal therapy and subgingival scaling?
Most recently, in addition to the classical, mechanical instrumentation, topical antimicrobial agents have been successfully employed (disinfectants, antibiotics); however, such adjunctive measures will only be helpful when used in combination with thorough scaling and root planing! Systemic antibiotics may often be indicated in severe, aggressive cases (p. 287).
A new television technique may bring "light and vision" into the periodontal pocket! The Dental View device can dramatically reduce the amount of "missed" subgingival calculus.

Hand Instruments for Scaling and Root Planing—Curettes

For the removal of large subgingival calculus deposits, curettes are indicated, in addition to sonic and ultrasonic devices (p. 259). For root planing and soft tissue curettage, curettes are the instruments of choice.

Numerous manufacturers offer a myriad of hand instruments, which may vary with regard to quality (e. g., steel) and design. In this *Atlas*, we do not make recommendations concerning specific manufacturers or instrument sets, because it is acknowledged that every "school" as well as each and every hygienist has its/her/his favorite instruments.

Most important is that a set of curettes must provide effective approaches to all root surfaces, while providing the proper angle of application of the blade to the root surface (ca. 80°). Curettes must be sharpened before each use (p. 268).

It is important to note the difference between universal curettes, which have two cutting edges, and Gracey curettes, which have only one cutting edge. Gracey curettes are primarily indicated for debridement and root planing, and less often for soft tissue curettage.

570 Curettes
(Deppeler Co.)

- **Universal Curettes, ZI 15**
  Yellow; for initial gross debridement
- **Anterior Curettes, GX 4**
  Orange; for anterior teeth and canines, and sometimes premolars
- **Posterior Curettes, M 23 A**
  Red; for premolars and molars

Right: Working end of the paired posterior curettes, M 23A.

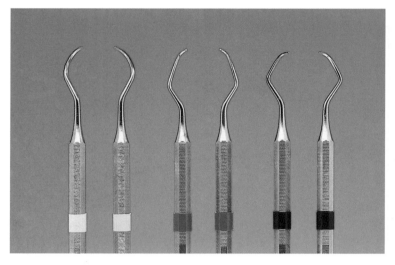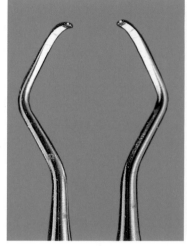

571 Minimum Gracey Set
In most clinical cases, a set consisting of four double-ended Gracey instruments is sufficient. Depicted here are color-coded curettes with soft grips (ADEC, Deppeler).

- **Gracey 5/6**   yellow
- **Gracey 7/8**   gray
- **Gracey 11/12** red
- **Gracey 13/14** blue

Right: Double-bend shank and working end of the paired Gracey curettes 13/14.

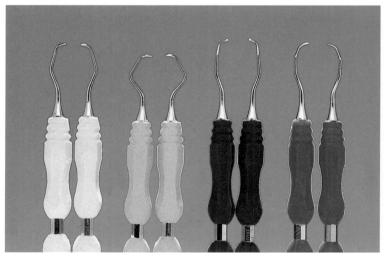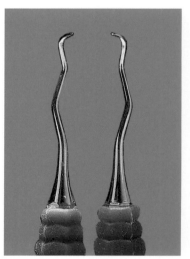

572 Complete Set of Gracey Curettes: 7 Double-ended Instruments
(Hu-Friedy Co.)

- **Gracey 1/2**
- **Gracey 3/4**
- **Gracey 5/6***
- **Gracey 7/8***
- **Gracey 9/10**
- **Gracey 11/12***
- **Gracey 13/14***

* These four (double-ended) instruments comprise the minimum set (Fig. 571).

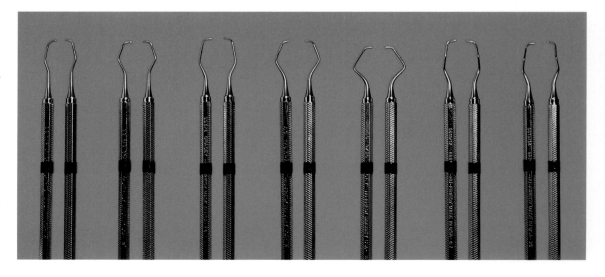

Powered Instruments for Debridement

In addition to the classical hand instruments, powered devices are finding increasing use in practice today for supra- and subgingival periodontal debridement. Included are:

- Ultrasonic devices (20–50,000 Hz)
- Sonic devices (up to 6,000 Hz)
- Motor-driven devices incorporating diamond-coated tips.

The goal, with both hand instruments and powered devices, is to create biologically acceptable root surfaces. Calculus must be completely eliminated, but without creating root surface roughness; rough root surfaces are more quickly colonized by bacteria than smooth surfaces. If used properly, curettes and ultrasonic devices can achieve relatively smooth surfaces; on the other hand, sonic and motor-driven devices more often elicit roughness (Römhild 1986; Schwarz et al. 1989; Ritz et al 1991; Axelsson 1993; Kocher & Plagmann 1997). Rough but clean tooth surfaces, especially in the region of the gingival margin, should always be given the "finishing touch" with curettes to ensure smoothness, and to inhibit or delay re-infection of the pocket.

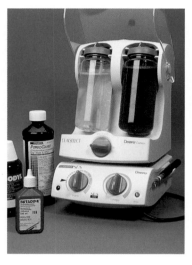

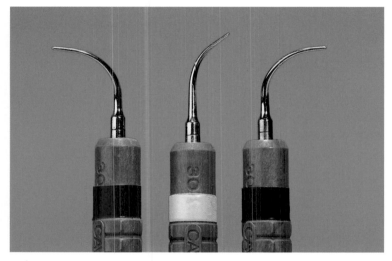

573 Ultrasonic Devices
Ultrasonic devices function in direct contact with the tooth surface according to the principles of cavitation and acoustic microstreaming. Examples:

- **Dentsply**
  Pictured: Slimline attachments
- **EMS**
- **Satelec**

Left: **Dual Select** (Dentsply). With this attachment, one can select water or one of two antimicrobial cooling solutions.

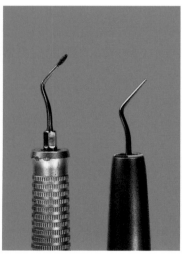

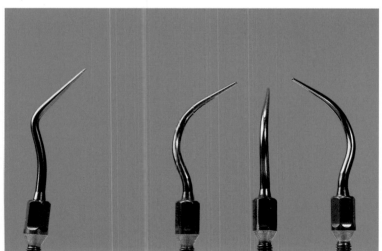

**574 Sonic Devices—
KaVo Sonicscaler—Insert No. 8 with Elongated Tip**
No. 60, 61 and 62 are special tips for subgingival application.

Examples of sonic devices:
- **Sonicscaler, KaVo**
- Airscaler, Titan-S
- **Siroson, Siemens**

Left: Working tips—overview. Diamond-coated tips for working in furcations.

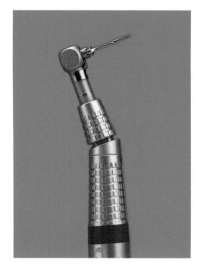

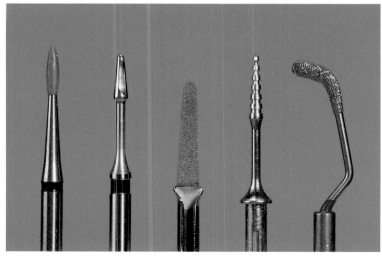

575 Additional Motor-driven Instruments for Subgingival Application

- **Perioset—Diamonds**
  (Intensive SA)
- **Scalex Tips** (Rotex)
- **EVA-System—Proxoshape**
  (Instensiv SA)
- **Peri-O-Tor** (Dentatus)
- **Perioplaner, Periopolisher**
  (Mikrona)

Left: Handpiece with the Peri-O-Tor attachment.

Gracey Curettes—Areas of Use

Complete Set

For closed ("blind") subgingival scaling and root planing, special instruments are indicated that are adaptable to the most varied root shapes. As early as the 1930's, Dr. C.H. Gracey, a dentist, together with an instrument maker by the name of Hugo Friedman (Hu-Friedy!), conceptualized a set of instruments that "…gives every dentist the possibility to treat even the deepest and least accessible periodontal pockets simply and without traumatic stretching of the gin-

giva. In addition, these curettes make it possible to completely remove all subgingival calculus, and to perfectly clean and plane every root surface, which will enhance subsequent tissue adaptation and re-attachment."

Numerous modifications of the instruments led finally to the Gracey curettes of today. The use of these instruments has been described in detail (Pattison & Pattison 1979, Hellwege 2002).

Anterior Teeth to the Premolars
Figs. 576–582 demonstrate the systematic use of the original Gracey curettes (GRA) in quadrant 2 (maxillary left).

576 Gracey 1/2—Incisors, Canines
The primary area of use for this paired instrument is the *facial* root surfaces of incisors and canines.

Right: **GRA 1/2**
Medium length shank, mild angulation

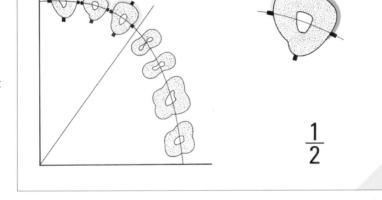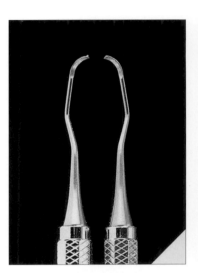

577 Gracey 3/4—Incisors, Canines
Primary use is the same as with GRA 1/2, but because of the more severe angulation, the 3/4 is particularly indicated for *palatal* and *lingual* surfaces.

Right: **GRA 3/4**
Shorter shank, sharper angulation.

The cutting edge of these paired instruments is the "outer" edge, along the *convex* curvature of the working tip.

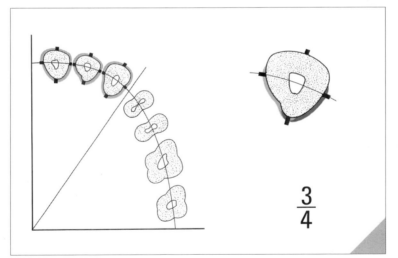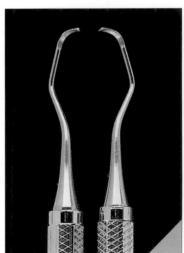

578 Gracey 5/6*—Anterior Teeth and Premolars
The area of use corresponds for the most part to that of an anterior universal curette.
This Gracey curette with its long, straight shank can be used in virtually all areas of the dentition where deep pockets exist.

Right: **GRA 5/6**

Longer shank, slight angulation.
* *The four double-ended instruments marked with an asterisk comprise the minimum Gracey set (cf. Figs. 571 and 587).*

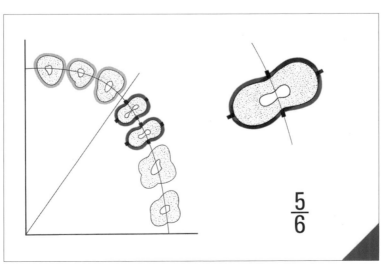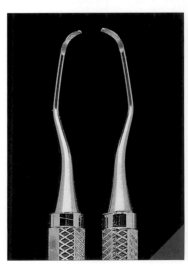

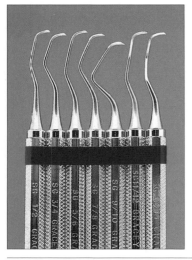
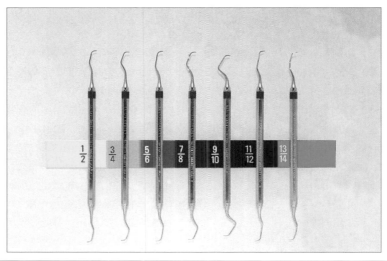

579 Complete Gracey Curette Set
(original Hu-Friedy Co.)

GRA	1/2	yellow
GRA	3/4	orange
GRA	5/6*	red
GRA	7/8*	magenta
GRA	9/10	purple
GRA	11/12*	violet
GRA	13/14*	blue

(Color-coding valid for this double page.)

Left: The seven different working ends of the complete Gracey set.

Posterior Area

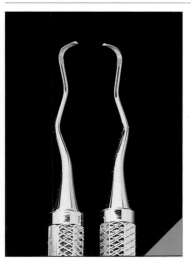
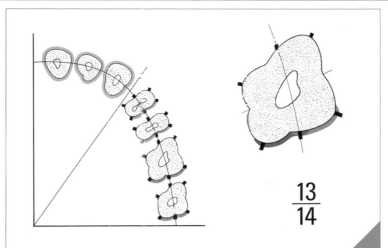

580 Gracey 13/14*— Molars, Premolars—Distal
First, for example, all *distal surfaces* are cleaned, from the facial (buccal) aspect and then from the oral (palatal/lingual) aspect. The *line angles* are indicated by short bars. This is the transition from one tooth (root) surface to another, where the use of individual instruments changes.

Left: **GRA 13/14***
Triple-bend shank.

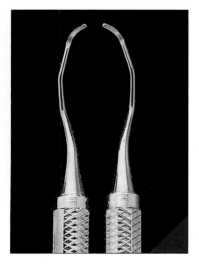
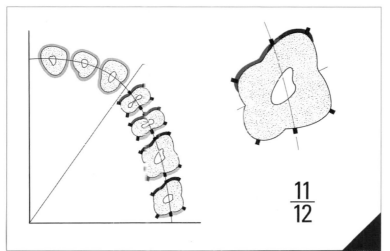

581 Gracey 11/12*— Molars, Premolars—Mesial
This instrument, with its sharp convex cutting edge, is indicated for treatment of all *mesial surfaces* from the buccal aspect, and the other end for mesial surfaces from the oral aspect.
Like the GRA 13/14, the GRA 11/12 is particularly well suited for multirooted premolars as well as in furcations and depressions.

Left: **GRA 11/12***
Longer shaft with several mild angulations.

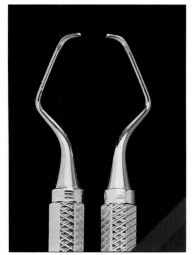
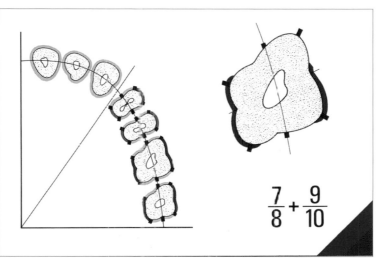
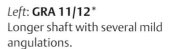

582 Gracey 7/8* and 9/10— Molars and Premolars— Facial and Oral Surfaces
Due to the rather severe angulation of the longer shank, both instruments, in addition to their primary indication on buccal and oral surfaces in the posterior area, are also useful in deep depressions and furcations. The angulation permits axial, oblique and horizontal strokes.

Left: **GRA 7/8***
Medium length, severely angled shaft.

Hand Instruments for Special Problems—Curettes

Closed debridement, whether as definitive treatment for mild periodontitis or as initial therapy prior to surgical intervention, is a demanding task that often includes scaling and root planing of poorly-accessible, irregular root surfaces in deep pockets and involved furcations, even in patients with minimal mouth opening capacity. These difficulties will also be encountered when mechanical debridement is performed in tandem with antimicrobial irrigation ("full mouth therapy," p. 281).

Problems and problem areas include:
- Deep, narrow pockets, e.g., on anterior teeth
- Distal pockets
- Patients with minimum mouth opening
- Substantial furcation involvement
- Dental implants in periodontitis-susceptible patients

Caution: Manufacturers offer hundreds of different hand instruments! The hygienist is wise to limit the number of instruments to only those that are necessary for successful treatment!

583 Special Gracey Curettes
Several special variations of the classic Gracey curettes are available for use in demanding situations (exemple: 11/12; Hu-Friedy):

- **Type SGR** "rigid": Incorporating a wider and more rigid shaft and working end
- **Type SG** "normal": With an elastic shaft
- **Type SRPG** "after 5": Elongated shaft for depths up to 8 mm
- **Type SAS**: Longer, finer working end; anterior teeth

Right: Comparative view.

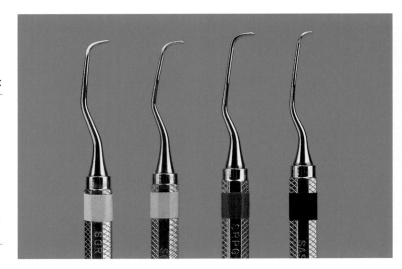 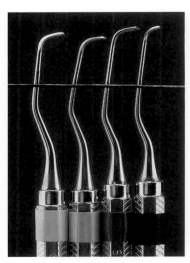

584 Enhanced Angulation
Gracey curettes 11/12 (mesial) and 13/14 (distal) require that the patient open wider for treatment of second and third molars. Depicted is the 13/14 (blue collar) with normal angulation of the shaft; the new number 17/18 (blue/yellow) can be used even with minimum mouth opening.

Right: Different angulation of the working end of numbers 13/14 and 17/18 for the distal aspect.

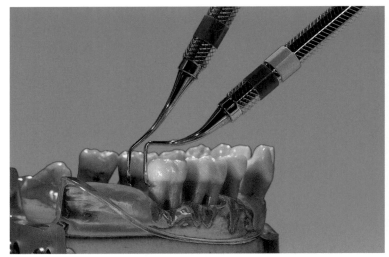 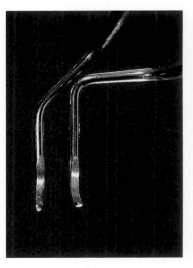

585 Plastic Instruments
For the treatment of the surfaces of titanium dental implants, the clinician must employ instruments that will not damage the fixture surfaces. Especially in cases of *mucositis* and also *peri-implantitis*, the accessible titanium surfaces should be cleaned using only *plastic* scalers.

Left: Curette tips (Hu-Friedy); *right,* probe (Deppeler) and carbon fiber curette (HaWe).

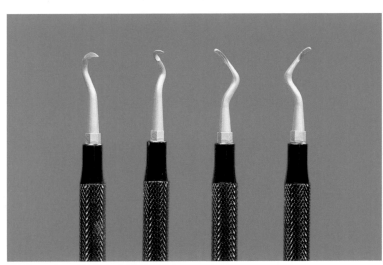 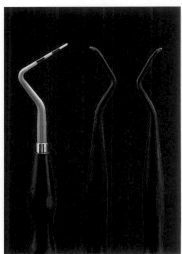

Practical Scaling Technique with Gracey Curettes—Systematic Approach

Minimum Gracey Set

An introduction to the scaling technique using Gracey curettes is simplified by limiting the instrument set to four double-ended instruments (p. 258, Fig. 571). Color-coded handles simplify their assignment to certain tooth surfaces. In addition to an adequate armamentarium, certain prerequisites must be fulfilled in order to optimally perform the technically difficult scaling procedures, such as patient position, operatory arrangement, and operator position (Wolf 1987):

- Positioning of the patient and the hygienist
- Operatory lighting
- Sharp instruments and selecting proper cutting edge
- Secure stroke (modified pen grasp and fulcrum)
- Precise knowledge of all probing depths
- Systematic procedure, step-by-step
- Detecting roughness

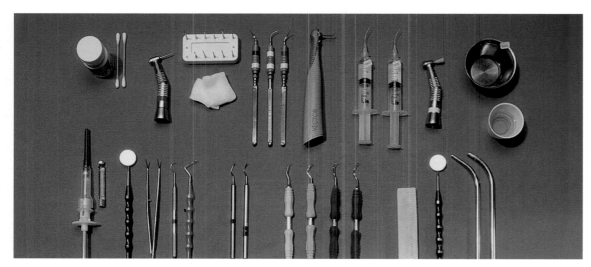

586 Basic Instrumentarium for Scaling—Complete

Above:
- Ultrasonic tips
- PerioSet diamonds
- Rinsing solution

Below:
- Anesthesia
- Mirror, forceps, pointed probe
- Periodontal probe
- Scaler, universal curettes
- **Minimum Gracey set**
- Sterile sharpening stone etc.

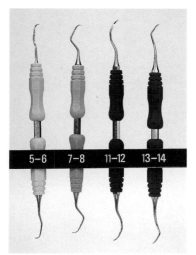

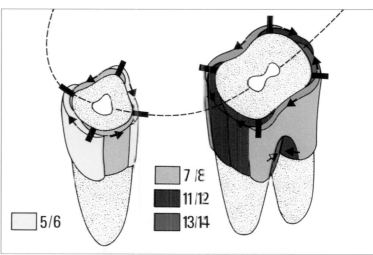

587 Minimum Gracey set: Areas of Use, Color Codes

- **Gracey 5/6**   yellow
  anteriors/canines
- **Gracey 7/8**   gray
  premolars and molars,
  buccal and oral
- **Gracey 11/12**   red
  molars and premolars,
  mesial, furcations
- **Gracey Gracey 13/14**   blue
  molars and premolars,
  distal, furcations

Left: Minimum color-coded set.

Checklist—Scaling Technique

Operatory: Light, power, water, air, instrumentarium

Clinician: Eye protection, mask, gloves

Treatment technique: Operator position, instrument selection, fulcrum, direct or indirect vision (mirror). Patient's periodontal data, including probing depths and radiographs.

The following pages, 264–267, demonstrate the systematic use of the minimum Gracey set in the maxillary left quadrant.

5–6

Anterior Region, Facial

588 Scaling on Distobuccal Surfaces—Tooth 22
Patient's head: Reclined position, head inclined to the right

Hygienist: ca. 9 o'clock position
Rest position/fulcrum: Intraoral, indirect, upon the thumb of the left hand
Vision of the operator: Direct

Right: GRA 5/6, working ends.

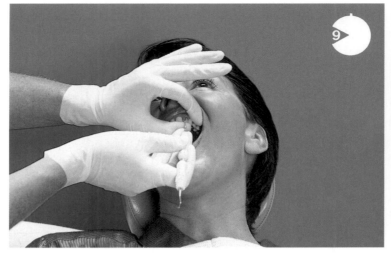
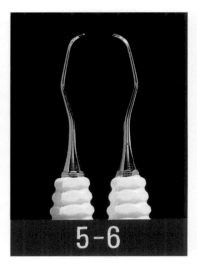

589 Model Situation
This indirect, intraoral rest position permits the fulcrum point of the working hand (4th finger) to be placed nearest to the root surface being treated.

Right: The cutting edge of the instrument cleans all distobuccal root surfaces, then the mesiobuccal surfaces are treated with the other blade of the double-ended Gracey 5/6 curette. Instrument changes are made at the indicated markings.

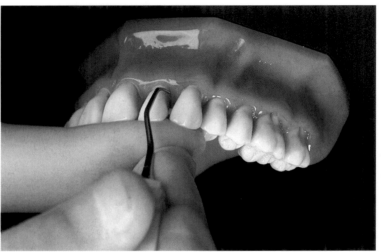
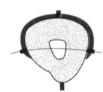

Anterior Region, Palatal

590 Scaling on Distopalatal Surfaces—Tooth 22
Patient's head: Extended to the right and dorsally

Hygienist: ca. 11 o'clock position
Rest position/fulcrum: Intraoral, directly on tooth 21
Vision: Indirect (mirror)

Right: Parallel, 3–4 mm working strokes from the palatal toward the interdental area.

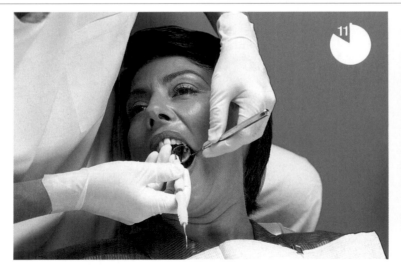
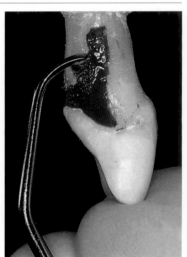

591 Model Situation
The mouth mirror permits indirect vision and insures proper lighting of the working field. Observe the modified pen grasp.

Right: Mesiopalatal and distopalatal root surfaces are approached using alternate ends of the 5/6 Gracey curette.

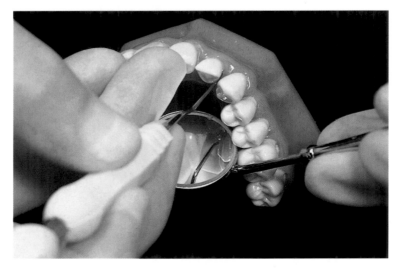
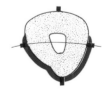

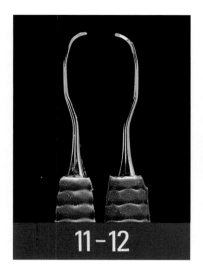

11–12

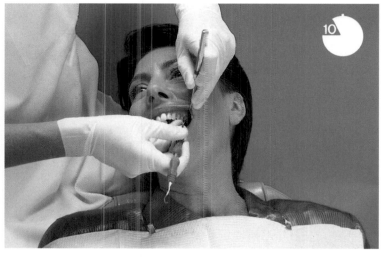

10

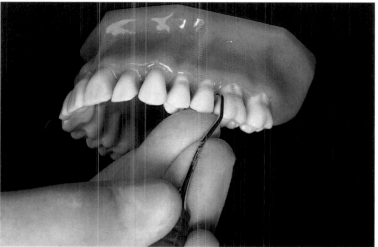

Posterior Segment—Mesial

592 Scaling on Mesial Surfaces, from the Buccal—Tooth 26
Patient's head: Inclined slightly to the right

Hygienist: ca. 10 o'clock position
Rest position: Intraoral, directly on the adjacent tooth
Vision: Direct

Left: Two working ends of the double-ended GRA 11/12 curette.

593 Model Situation
The ring finger establishes a fulcrum for the working hand, as near as possible to the mesial surface of tooth 26. The working strokes for subgingival scaling are initiated by a rotating movement of the *forearm* around the fulcrum.

Left: Section through tooth 26. GRA 11/12 is used from the buccal approach to scale the mesial surfaces from the mesiobuccal line angle, under the contact area, toward the palatal, including the mesial furcation.

Posterior Segment—Mesial

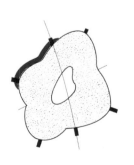

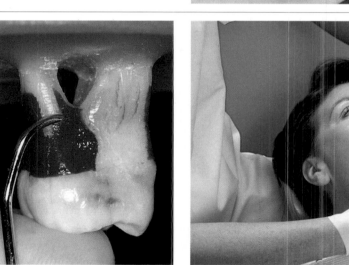

8

594 Scaling on Mesial Surfaces from the Palatal—Tooth 26
Patient's head: Inclined to the left and back

Hygienist: ca. 8 o'clock position
Rest position: Extraoral on the mandible or intraoral on the opposing arch. Guidance by the left thumb.
Vision: Direct

Left: Entrance to the mesial furcation can only be achieved from the palatal approach.

595 Model Situation
The left thumb guides and stabilizes the curette. Only light pressure is necessary for scaling the root surface if the instrument is properly sharpened.

Left: Section through tooth 26. The working area for the Gracey curette 11/12 is from the palatal approach.

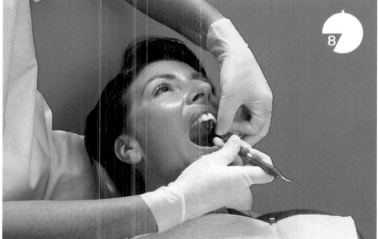

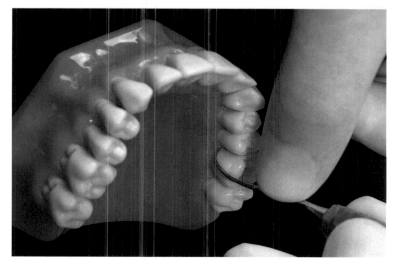

13–14

Posterior Segment—Distal

596 Scaling on Distal Surfaces from the Buccal—Tooth 26
Patient's head: Inclined far to the right

Hygienist: ca. 10 o'clock position
Rest position: Intraoral, directly upon the adjacent tooth
Vision: Direct; mirror retracts the cheek.

Right: GRA 13/14 working ends.

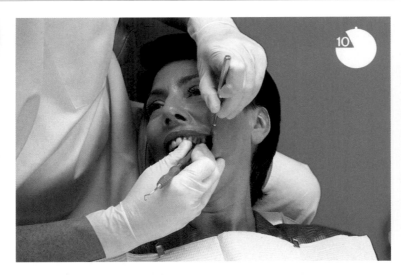

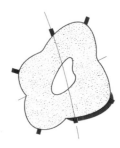

597 Model Situation
The rest position is with the ring finger on tooth 25, very near the working (distal) area of tooth 26. The shank portion immediately adjacent to the curette blade must be parallel to this tooth surface.

Right: Section through tooth 26. Contact points and the four line angles are depicted. From the buccal approach, the GRA 13/14 is indicated for the distal surface, from the distobuccal line angle to the contact area.

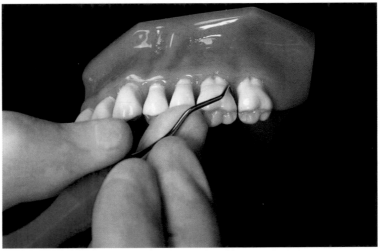

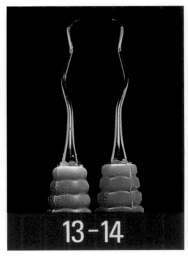

Posterior Segment—Distal

598 Scaling on Distal Surfaces from the Palatal—Tooth 26
Patient's head: Inclined to the left

Hygienist: ca. 9 o'clock position
Rest position: Intraoral, indirect, on the back of the first finger of the left hand. This finger also serves to guide the instrument and apply pressure to it.
Vision: Direct

Right: The palatal root is treated from the palatal toward the contact area and the distal furcation.

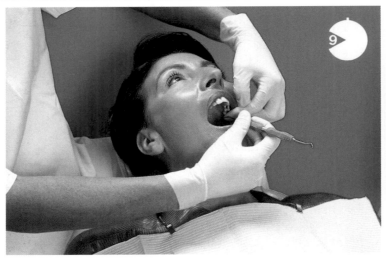

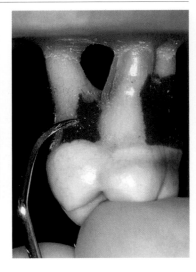

599 Model Situation
The first finger of the left hand serves two functions:
• Fulcrum for the working hand
• Guidance and lateral pressure for the curette

Right: Beginning on the palatal surface, the GRA 13/14 curette scales the distal surface of tooth 26 from the line angle, across and into the furcation region, then under the contact area.

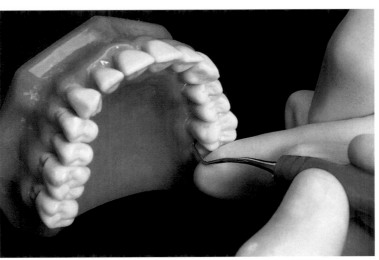

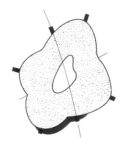

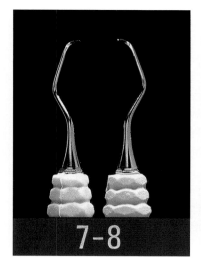

7-8

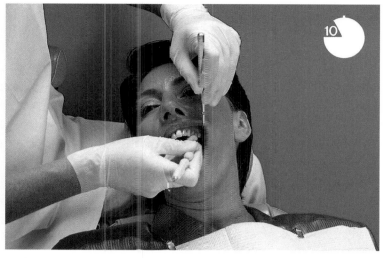

Posterior Area—Buccal

600 Scaling the Buccal Surfaces—Tooth 26
Patient's head: Tilted slightly toward the operator

Hygienist: ca. 10 o'clock position
Rest position: Intraoral, directly on the adjacent tooth
Vision: Direct

Left: Working ends of the GRA 7/8 curette

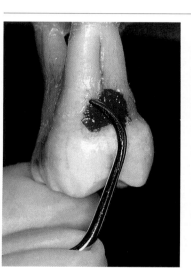

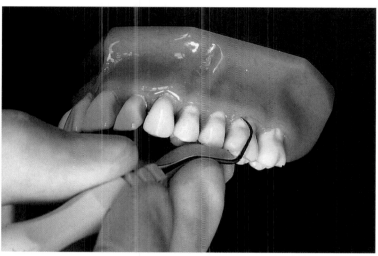

601 Model Situation
In addition to axial strokes, the buccal molar surfaces are often treated using oblique or horizontal strokes. The modified pen grasp is obvious, with the middle finger in the first curve of the instrument shank.

Left: The indentation represents the entrance to the buccal furcation. *Note*: Mesial and distal sections of the exposed roots near the furcation are treated using the GRA 11/12 (mesial) and 13/14 (distal).

Posterior Area—Palatal

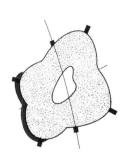

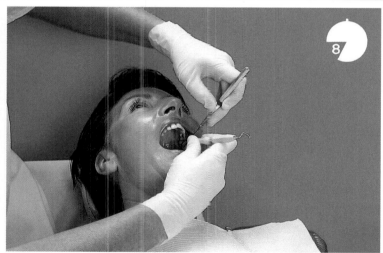

602 Scaling the Palatal Surfaces—Tooth 26
Patient's head: Tilted toward the left, away from the operator

Hygienist: ca. 8 o'clock position
Rest position: Intraoral, directly upon the occlusal surfaces
Vision: Direct

Left: The palatal root segments are basically round in shape, however, shallow grooves do occur and these may present difficulties during scaling.

603 Model Situation
Rest position (fulcrum) directly on the occlusal surface of tooth 26.

Left: GRA 7/8 curette is used to scale the palatal surfaces from the distopalatal to the mesiopalatal line angles. In this area, there are no furcations, but often grooves.

After scaling this final (palatal) posterior tooth surface, systematic treatment of the maxillary left quadrant is complete. The pockets are then rinsed and any bleeding is staunched.

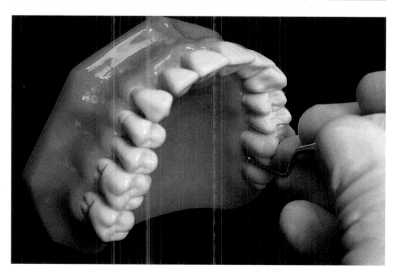

Instrument Sharpening

The curette is a universal instrument that serves both non-surgical as well as surgical periodontitis therapy. The curette is used for scaling, subgingival debridement, root planing, and curettage of the gingival soft tissues.

Knowledge of its characteristics and maintenance of its functions are therefore of great significance. Instruments that have become dull must be re-sharpened; no degree of manual dexterity or force can compensate for the disadvantage of a dull instrument. Dull instruments lack "bite"; calculus is burnished rather than removed.

The systematic sharpening of curettes may be accomplished before, during or after patient treatment. Especially the small, slender curettes quickly become dull during scaling because of contact with enamel or metal restorations. Such instruments must be re-sharpened during the treatment appointment, using a sterile, mildly abrasive sharpening stone (Fig. 606).

A curette that has been sharpened 10–15 times becomes thin and may break; it must be replaced.

604 Curette—Nomenclature (Example: Gracey Curette 13/14)
I   Handle
II   Shank
III Working End with Cutting Edge (Blade)

Right: Section through the working end (Gracey curette).

A Cutting Edge
The convex edge is sharp; the other edge is blunt (blue dot).
B Face
C Side
D Back

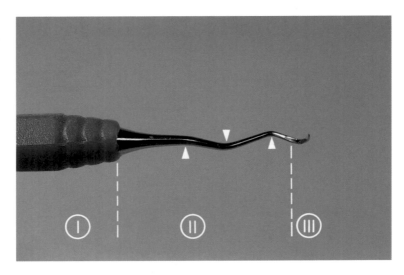
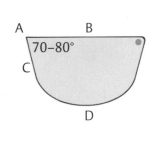

605 Differences Between Universal (A) and Gracey (B) Curettes
1 The face (B; Fig. 604) of the working end forms a 90° (universal) or 70° (Gracey) angle to the shank.
2 Both edges of the working end (universal curette) are sharpened; but only the convex (lower) edge of the Gracey curette.
3 Only in Gracey curettes is the working end arched over the surface as well as over the edge.

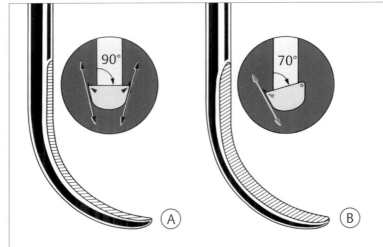

606 Sharpening Stones—Sharpening Oil

C "Carborundum"
SiC/Silicium carbide; artificial; gross, highly abrasive
I "India"
Al_2O_3, aluminum oxide, artificial, course grained, abrasive
A "Arkansas"
Al_2O_3, aluminum oxide, natural, average-to-fine grained, mildly abrasive

Right: Acid-free mineral oil (SSO; Hu-Friedy).

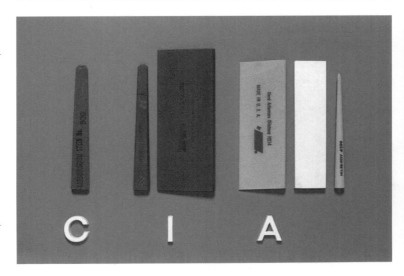
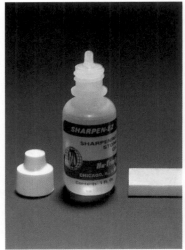

Manual Sharpening of Hand Instruments

Even though powered devices (sonic and ultrasonic) are widely used today, scalers and curettes still command a prominent role for all treatment techniques including both closed and open therapy, surgical procedures, and for prophylaxis (professional tooth cleaning), alone or in combinations.

Efficient and thorough scaling and planing, particularly on infected root surfaces, can *de facto* only be optimally performed with sharp instruments (Bengel 1998, Christan 2002).

Years of experience have clearly demonstrated that "free-hand" instrument sharpening is only rarely successful in providing perfectly shaped and sharp hand instruments. Thus, for manual sharpening and re-sharpening, sharpening *aids* are necessary. On the basis of years of experience, dental hygienist C.M. Kramer (1989, 1999) developed the two sharpening stations depicted below. The basic principles include precise positioning of the instrument (the "horizontal, facial side") and the predetermined sharpening angles on the jig (template), with separate settings for scalers and curettes.

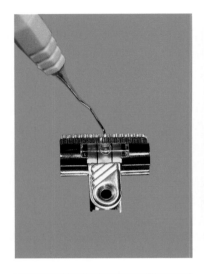

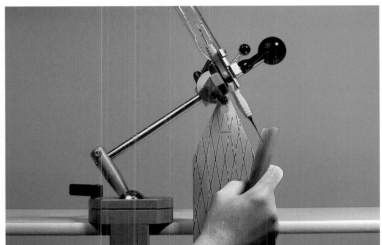

607 Instrument Sharpening with the Kramer Sharpening Station
The vise-like holder with the large ball joint permits positioning of the instrument in any conceivable position.

Left: Initially, the special clip is used to grasp the working end. The instrument face must be always positioned *horizontally*, and then the sharpening procedure can begin. The sharpening stone is held parallel to the guiding lines on the front of the station.

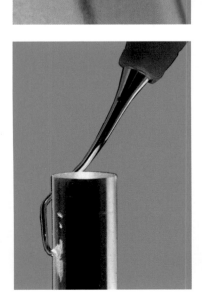

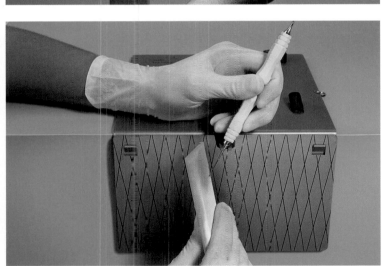

608 A Simplified Version— Kramer "Mini" Sharpening Holder
The above sharpening station is ideal for individuals with little experience, and is optimal for sharpening numerous instruments.
The advantage of the mini-sharpening station is that dull instruments can be sharpened at chairside.
The diamond-shaped lines on the vertical portion of the station insure that the scaler/curette is presented to the stone at the proper angle.

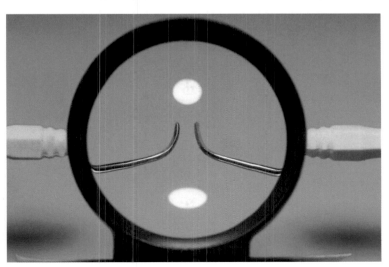

609 Tests for Sharpness: Light Reflection Test and Scratch Test
Manual sharpening (cf. Fig. 608, left) is performed with an oiled Arkansas stone.
The metal removal is clearly visible; it remains suspended in the oil and can be easily removed.
The final test for sharpness of the cutting edge: Dull edges do not reflect light, but sharp edges do.

Left: Acrylic rod (PST, Hu-Friedy) tests the sharpness of the instrument, which removes acrylic chips.

Automated Sharpening

The biggest problem during free-hand sharpening is the difficulty of maintaining the angle of the sharpening stone to the instrument tip, and maintaining this angle during the entire sharpening procedure. It demands manual dexterity, knowledge of the individual instrument's characteristics and … practice (Römhild & Renggli 1990, Pöschke 1990).

The primary goal of mechanical instrument sharpening includes not only simplification of the sharpening procedure, but also the elimination of the above-mentioned difficulties. This is possible using the "PerioStar" (Mikrona Co., 1990).

The main advantages of the PerioStar 2000 include:
- The device precisely holds the shank of the instrument, and permits fixation in any position.
- A special clip permits the horizontal positioning of the facial surface (the only "approximation").
- The adjustable sharpening module with its mounted sharpening wheel; when properly positioned, sharpening is performed with a secured angle of 72° for scalers and 78° for curettes.

Commercially available today is a simplified variant, the PerioStar 3000 (HaWe Neos; see below).

610 PerioStar 2000 (Left) and PerioStar 3000 (Right)
These commercially available devices are provided with various sharpening stones, sharpening pastes, as well as an acrylic rod for testing sharpness.

Right: Sharpening stones and the diamond-coated block for removing grooves and scratches from the sharpening stone.
Sharpening stones in fine, medium and coarse abrasiveness are available (coded with white, red and blue dots).

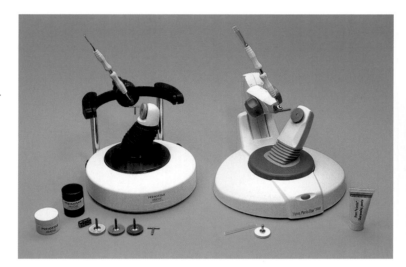
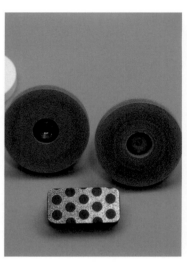

611 Adjusting and Sharpening—Gracey Curette 5/6 and PerioStar 3000
The mildly fluorescing rod of the chip—it sits upon the facial surface of the curette blade—is oriented horizontally with the instrument. The abrasive element is then brought to bear upon the instrument tip.

Right: The lubricated sharpening disk in action. Clearly visible is the precision holding device.

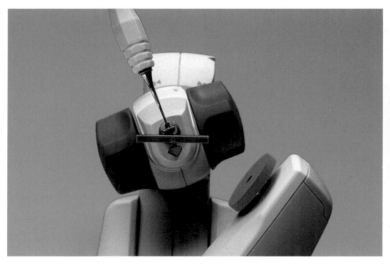
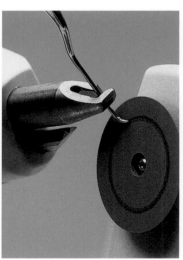

612 Overview—Adjusting and Sharpening with the PerioStar 2000
The sharpening disk can be adjusted with the dark *rotating table* (below) appropriately onto the curette tip for sharpening: The sharpening angle relative to the "face" is automatically established and reduced to 55°!

Right: Sharpening in progress—Note the precise holding mechanism to insure that the instrument is maintained at the most proximal portion of the shank.

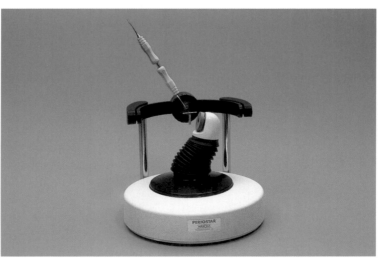
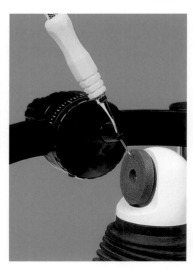

Subgingival Debridement—Closed Root Cleaning

Step-by-Step Clinical Procedure

Indications and prerequisites for closed therapy were described previously (p. 253).

The procedure is performed without direct vision. Treatment of a single tooth with moderately deep pockets may require 4–10 min, because of working "blind," and dependent upon the individual root anatomy/morphology. Ultrasonic instruments and hand curettes can be used in combination. In the case described here, the maxillary right quadrant is treated using Gracey curettes and a closed technique. In the other quadrants, following closed therapy, several sites required "open" therapy (p. 277).

The 29-year-old patient suffered from aggressive periodontitis (Type III), with localized deep pockets and pronounced gingivitis. A microbiologic examination revealed high levels of *Aa* and *Pi*.

Initial findings (values for Quadrant 1):
   PI: 61%   BOP: 86%   TM: 0–2 (p. 174)
   The clinical picture, probing depths and radiographic findings are shown in Figs. 613–615.

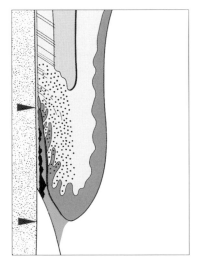
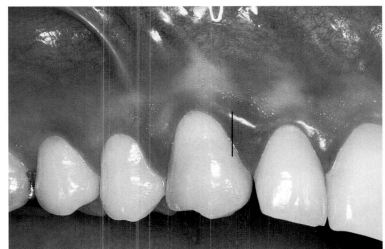

613 Initial Condition—Before Creation of Hygienic Relationships
Especially in the papillary areas, the gingiva is edematous and erythematous. Virtually no stippling.

Left: The schematic depicts the histologic situation on the mesiofacial aspect of tooth 13. In the cervical area, calculus and adherent plaque (blue) cover the root surface, and apically elevated levels of gram-negative microorganisms (red). The gingival connective tissue is infiltrated.

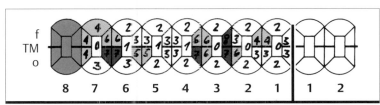
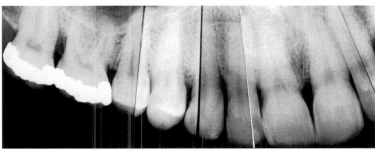

614 Clinical and Radiographic Findings
Probing Depths and Tooth Mobility (TM)
Probing depths up to 8 mm were measured. The very deep pocket on the mesiofacial of tooth 13 resulted from both attachment loss and swelling of the papilla.

Radiographic Findings
The radiograph clearly reveals the massive bone loss that was anticipated by the clinical pocket measurements.

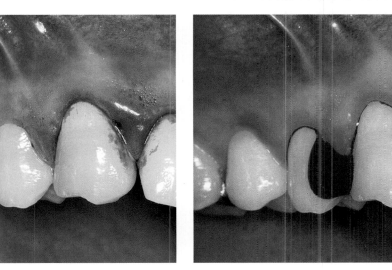
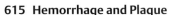

615 Hemorrhage and Plaque
After probing the pockets around teeth 13 and 14, copious hemorrhage resulted. This is a clinical indication of the severity of the inflammatory reaction in this case of periodontitis ("gingivitis").

Left: Stained supragingival plaque. Plaque accumulation on the mesial surface of tooth 14 is minimal, and does not correlate with the copious hemorrhage in this region. The etiology is likely a strong reaction to the subgingival periodontopathic bacteria.

After the Hygiene Phase

616 Buccal View

Two weeks after supragingival plaque and calculus removal, initial motivation and OHI, the gingivae are already less erythematous and swollen. The enamel defect on the distoincisal of tooth 13 was attributed to bruxism.

Right: *Sub*gingival concrements and plaque persist.

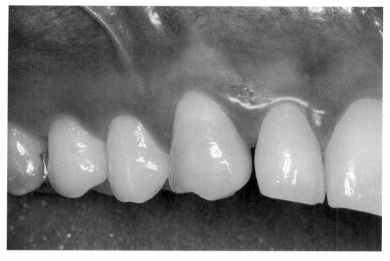
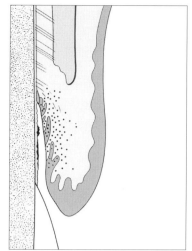

617 Palatal View

Following the first phase of initial therapy—oral hygiene and professional supragingival debridement—the gingivae are still slightly edematous.

Of note in this photograph is the pronounced wear facet on tooth 13. The patient must be made aware of the stress-elicited bruxing habit, and be encouraged to reduce this parafunction.

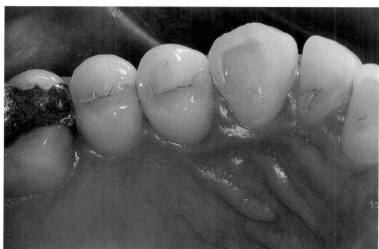

Subgingival Debridement

618 Anesthesia

Subgingival debridement is performed using hand instruments, generally with infiltration or nerve block anesthesia.

With the use of slim ultrasonic instruments ("Slimline," Cavitron) it is often possible to treat shallow pockets without any need for infiltration anesthesia.

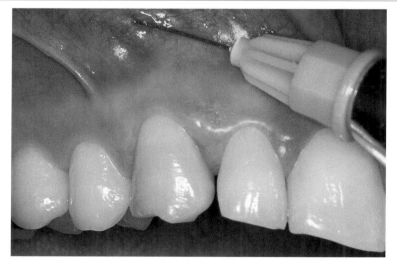

619 Probing the Depth of the Pocket

Before any mechanical treatment of the root surface, the depth of the pocket is ascertained circumferentially under anesthesia. The floor of the pocket is usually irregular. Usually only isolated sites on the root surface exhibit pronounced attachment loss.

Right: The radiograph reveals that the periodontal probe, using a force of 0.25 N, almost reaches the interseptal bone.

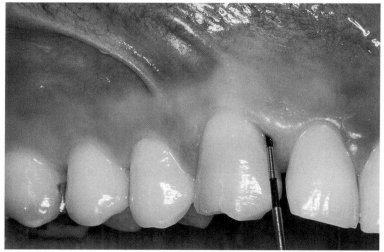
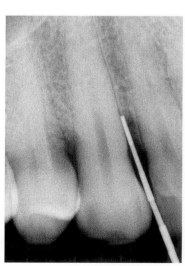

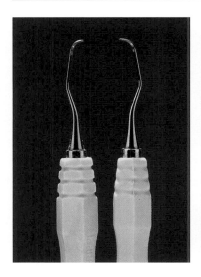

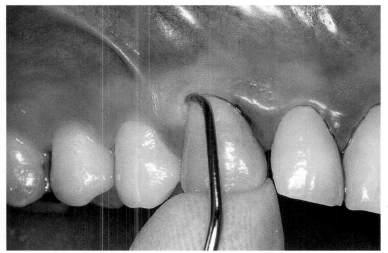

Double-ended Curette (Gracey 5–6, yellow) Used in the Anterior Segment

In the anterior and canine regions, the double-ended curette is applied to treat root surfaces on two adjacent surfaces.

620 Gracey 5—Distobuccal
Using this end of the curette, with overlapping and primarily vertical strokes, plaque and calculus are removed.

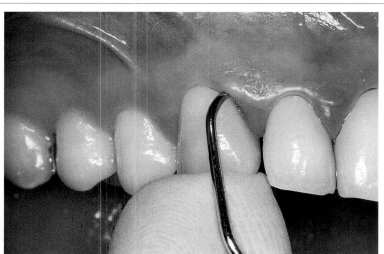

621 Gracey 5—Mesiopalatal
The same working end of the curette that treated the distobuccal surface, can also clean the diagonally opposed mesiopalatal root surface.

Note: Photographic limitations do not permit depiction of the fulcrum.

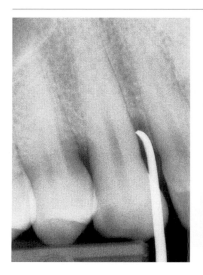

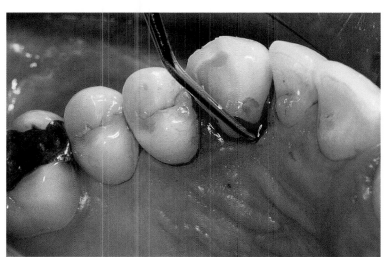

622 Gracey 6—Mesiobuccal
This end of the curette functions mesiobuccally and distopalatally. If the first "long" shaft of the curette is parallel to the root surface, the effective angle of the "face" is the desired value of ca. 80°.

Left: The Gracey curette does not achieve the fundus of the pocket, in contrast to the more elegant curettes (e. g., "minifive") with their shorter and narrower working ends.

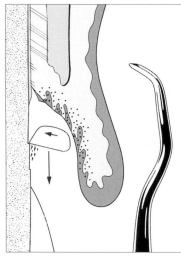

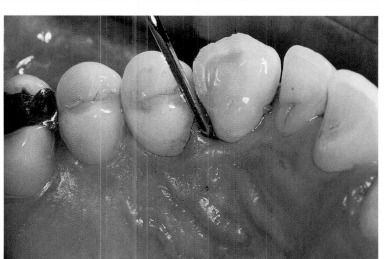

623 Gracey 6—Distopalatal
The same working end of the curette (above, Fig. 622) also serves for treatment of the distopalatal root surface.

Left: The angle of the curette blade to the root surface should be ca. 80°.

The working end of all Gracey curettes is sharpened on only one surface!

Scaling with Gracey Curettes in the Posterior Area
Double-ended Curette, GRA 11/12 (red), for Use on Mesial Surfaces

624 Gracey 12—Mesiobuccal
The mesial root surfaces of premolars and molars are best approached with the two paired working ends of the double-angled Gracey 11/12 curettes; shown here in the maxillary right quadrant, with GR 12 from the buccal, and GR 11 from the palatal.

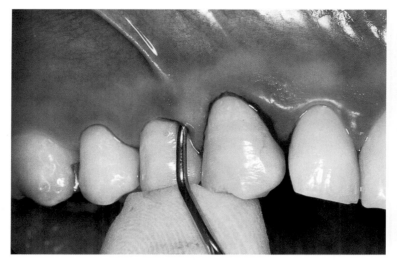
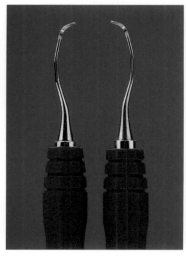

625 Gracey 11—Mesiopalatal
This blade of the double-ended 11/12 cleans the mesial surfaces of the premolar from the palatal aspect.
The mesial surfaces treated with the double-ended 11/12 curette must also be treated in the interdental area with overlapping strokes.

(In the maxillary left quadrant, the Gracey 11 is applied buccally and the Gracey 12 from the palatal approach.)

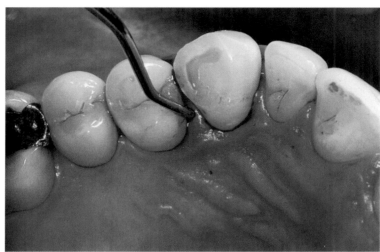

Double-ended Curettes, Gracey 13/14 (blue), for Treating Distal Surfaces

626 Gracey 13—Distobuccal
The distal aspect of the premolar (tooth 14) is treated from the buccal approach.

(On the left side of the maxilla, Gracey 14 would be used.)

Right: The working ends of the double-ended Gracey curette 13/14.

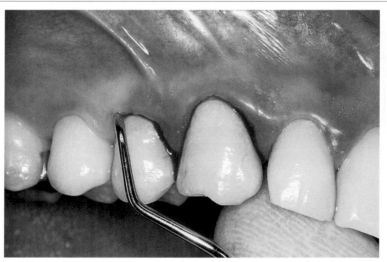
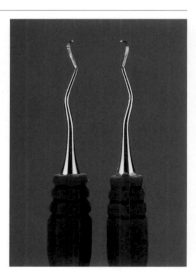
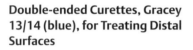

627 Gracey 14—Distopalatal
Note that the terminal shank of the instrument is parallel to the root surface.

Right: Remarkable is the "hourglass" profile of the root surface, exhibiting furcation entrances that must be probed and as far as possible effectively cleaned.

The morphology of the roots and use of the wrong instruments establish the limits of subgingival scaling even more than the absolute pocket depth.

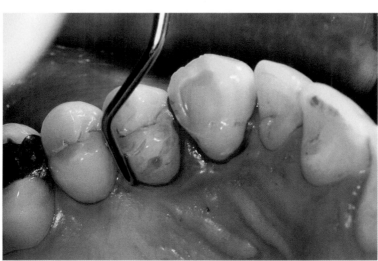
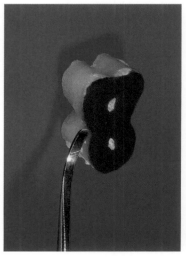

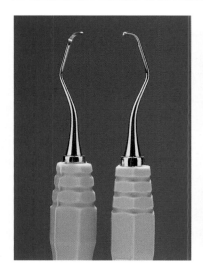

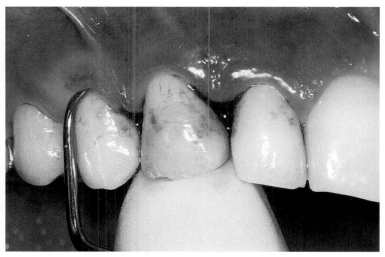

Double-ended Curette, Gracey 7/8 (Gray), Indicated for Root Planing on Buccal and Oral Surfaces in Posterior Segments

628 Gracey 7—Facial
Usually, subgingival debridement is performed from the *buccal* and *oral* aspects; depicted here in the maxillary right quadrant, Gracey curette 7 is used from the buccal approach up to the line angle and into the mesial interdental space.

Left: Working ends of the double-ended Gracey 7/8 curette.

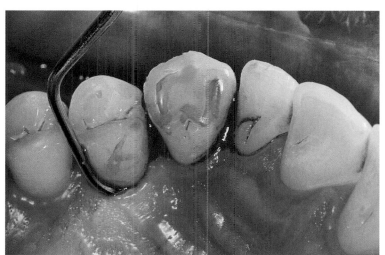

629 Gracey 8—Oral
In most cases, during the scaling of mesial (Gracey 11/12) and distal (Gracey 13/14) root surfaces (p. 274), the usually shallower buccal and oral pockets and the corresponding line angles are also effectively treated. Thus, using the Gracey 8, the palatal treatment of tooth 14 can be quickely completed.

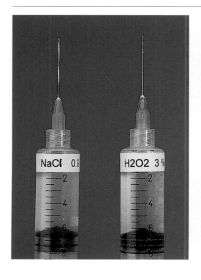

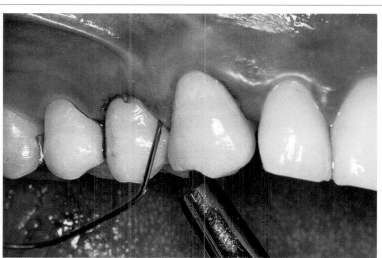

630 Pocket Rinsing
Following mechanical/instrumental treatment, the pocket should be thoroughly rinsed with NaCl 0.9 % and/or H_2O_2 3 % in order to remove from the pocket any remaining microbial plaque, calculus or cementum. This final phase of closed therapy will enhance the anti-infectious component of treatment.

Left: NaCl (0.9 %) and H_2O_2 (3 %) solutions. The canula must be blunt (e. g. Max-I-Probe, Hawe Co.)

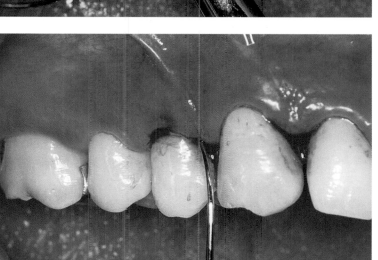

631 Root Surface Evaluation
Using a fine, pointed probe (depicted: EXS3A; Hu-Friedy) the surface of the root is evaluated with regard to its smoothness. This simple clinical test reveals whether the treatment procedure using curettes has effectively reached all segments of the root and removed all deposits.

But the most important aspect is not the planing and smoothing of the root surface, rather the removal or the destruction of the subgingival bacterial biofilm.

Closed Therapy in Quadrant 1 ...

Summary

Initially, the 29-year-old patient with aggressive periodontitis exhibited only moderate compliance with oral hygiene instructions. Following initial supragingival prophylaxis and repeated OHI, the patient's compliance improved. The visible gingival inflammation was reduced; however, BOP persisted.

Closed root planing was performed in the entire dentition, as depicted for the maxillary right quadrant. Teeth 17 through 11 did *not* require surgical intervention following the closed scaling therapy (cf. probing depths, lack of furcation involvement), but in several other quadrants, especially in the molar regions, flap surgery was indicated.

This case illustrates again that periodontitis is seldom generalized. It is the rule that each tooth, even each surface of each tooth, will exhibit differing severities of periodontal defects (single-tooth diagnosis, p. 196).

Initial Findings Before Initiation of Treatment

632 Clinical View
Gingivitis and generalized mild, but localized severe periodontitis. The gingiva bled copiously upon probing. The patient had never been adequately informed about oral hygiene.

Right: Pocket "filled" with plaque and calculus (red bar = pocket depth), pocket epithelium and infiltrated subepithelial connective tissue.

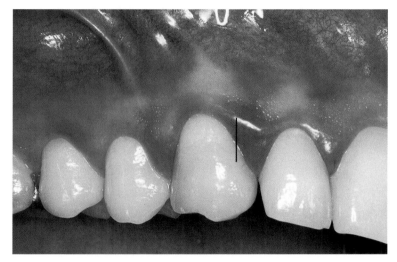
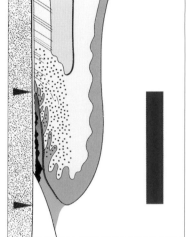

633 Probing Depths—Initial Findings (Quadrant 1)
Because of the gingival swelling, the *attachment loss* must be somewhat less valued than the measured probing depths (p. 169).

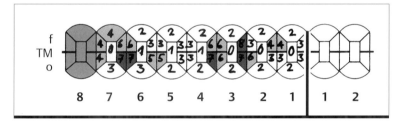

Before

Three Years after Subgingival Debridement
Physiologic probing depths are in evidence, resulting from the gingival shrinkage and connective tissue repair. Only one site shows a probing depth beyond 3 mm.

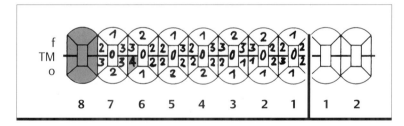

After

634 Clinical View, Three Years after Treatment
Professional treatment and the patient's oral hygiene endeavors led to mild recession yet fully healthy gingiva, but without pronounced stippling.

Right: An active pocket responded to the treatment and the result is a shallow, inactive "residual pocket" (red bar).

1 Shrinkage
2 Attachment gain (repair)

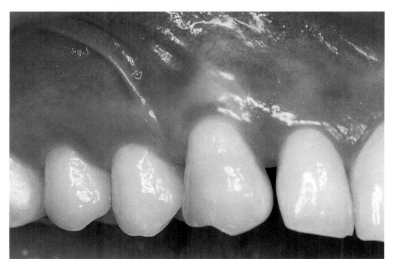
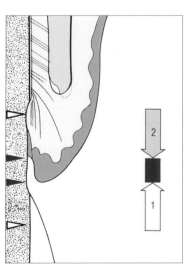

... and in the Rest of the Dentition?

Summary of the Entire Case

Following closed subgingival root planing in the entire dentition, not unexpectedly some sites exhibited persistent deep and active pockets in quadrants 2, 3 and 4.

Therefore, on teeth 25 (distal), 26 (distal), 36 (mesial) and 46 (mesial) paper points were used to harvest microbiologic samples for the preparation of *cultures* (Fig. 636, left). The presence of *Aa* was, at that time (1991), only qualitative ("yes/no"). On the other hand, the black-pigmenting Bacteroides types (BPB) and the sum of all anaerobic flora were quantitatively determined ("colony forming units," CFU).

Flap surgical procedures were performed on all of the remaining deep pockets, combined with systemic administration of amoxicillin and metronidazol (van Winkelhoff et al. 1989). The patient remained on a 3-month recall schedule. Two years later, physiologic probing depths were in evidence, with only a few exceptions.

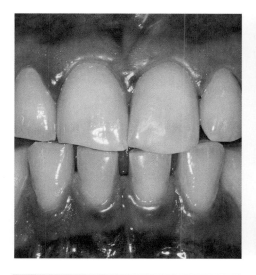

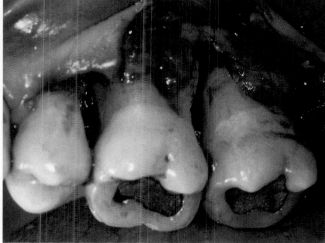

635 Intra-Operation View of Teeth 25, 26, 27
Deep bony pockets, but the furcations are closed. Even with direct vision, root planing was difficult and time-consuming.

Left: Initial anterior view. The gingiva, especially in the maxilla, is erythematous, swollen and not stippled. But this clinical view does not provide any clues as to the severity of periodontitis.

Microorganisms	Tooth sites			
	16d	26d	36m	46m
Aa	–	–	+	+
BPB	10^5	10^7	10^5	10^7
Σ Anaerobes	10^7	$>10^8$	10^7	10^8

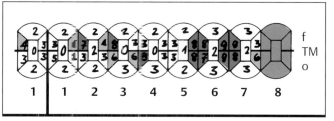

636 Probing Depths and Tooth Mobility—Initial Findings
Periodontal pockets up to 9 mm.

Left: Bacterial culture—findings from active residual pockets following Phase 1 therapy.

Microorganisms	Tooth sites			
	16d	26d	36m	46m
Aa	–	–	–	–
BPB	$>10^2$	10^5	10^3	10^4
Σ Anaerobes	10^4	10^5	10^4	10^5

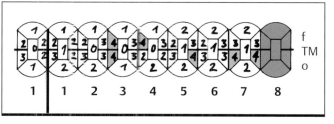

Probing Depths and Tooth Mobility—Two Years Later

Left: Bacterial culture—significantly reduced findings six months after completion of treatment.

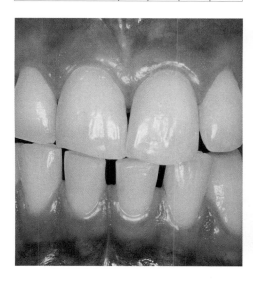

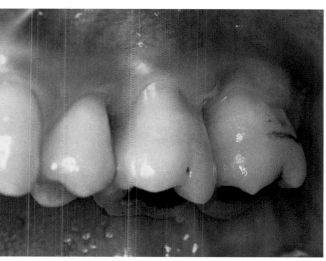

637 Teeth 25, 26, 27— Findings after Two Years
Irregular course of the gingival margin (shrinkage, cf. bony configuration in Fig. 635).
Reduction of probing depths: 2–4 mm.

Left: Final view, anterior segment. The gingiva is inflammation-free and very thin, and therefore does not exhibit stippling.

Limitations of Closed Therapy

The boundaries between closed and open (surgical) root treatment are dependent upon a myriad of criteria, and therefore not always easy to clearly define:

- Closed *and* open treatment may be necessary, and the latter always follows the former. Frequently, following optimum debridement, a few areas will require surgical therapy, e.g., in poorly accessible regions (molars and furcations) and with expansively progressive diseases.

- *Wound healing* occurs more rapidly following closed procedures, and often with fewer pain complications.

- The treatment procedures are also dependent upon the *philosophy* of the individual practice: In almost all cases the dental hygienist will initially perform the closed therapy. In mild/slight cases, this may be the only therapy required, but in more severe situations, surgical treatment may be necessary subsequently.

**638 Initial View—
Occlusal, Maxilla**
Periodontitis accompanied by severe gingivitis. The gingivae are severely erythematous and hyperplastic. BOP is ubiquitous. The patient practiced *no* oral hygiene. The teeth were severely stained. The initial supragingival debridement and OHI had to be careful and supportive.

Right: Pre-treatment view of teeth 13, 12; 21.

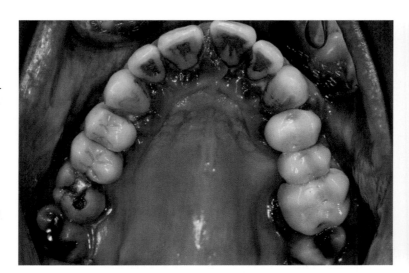
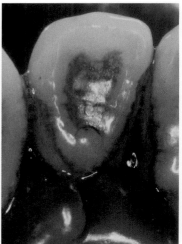

**639 Initial Findings,
Anterior Segment**
Initial ulcerations were obvious on several papillae. The diastema between teeth 11 and 12 had remained unchanged over the past two years. Note gingival recession on teeth 34, 33 and 43, 44.

Right: Initial probing depths and tooth mobility.
The severity of this case made it difficult to believe that treatment consisting solely of closed debridement would bring a successful result.

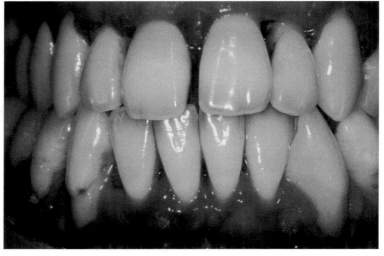
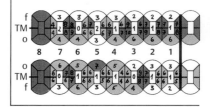

Before

After

640 Radiographic Findings
The radiographs confirmed the clinical diagnosis of severe, aggressive periodontitis. The mandibular molars also exhibit furcation involvement (F1), confirming the clinical findings. Tooth 16 was extracted.

Right: Probing depths and tooth mobility *after* treatment. At almost all sites, physiologic probing depths are in evidence. *How to explain such success?*

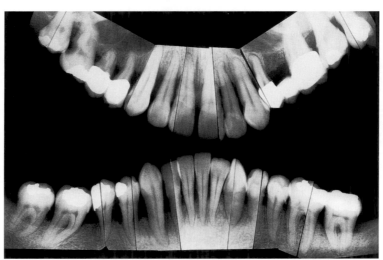
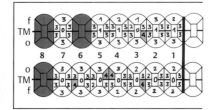

- The *philosophy* of the hygienist and the dentist also plays a role:
  Some prefer an optimum, precise and relatively hemorrhage-free conservative approach; others prefer a surgical approach and are quicker to move to the scalpel. Worthy of note, also, is that even surgical interventions may vary from extremely conservative toward relatively radical (see Surgery, p. 301).

- Last but not least, the patient's own wishes must be considered. The patient may also have an opinion regarding conservative treatment versus surgical intervention. In the case depicted here, advanced periodontitis was treated using closed therapy, with a successful result.

The 34-year-old patient suffered from generalized, aggressive periodontitis with simultaneously pronounced gingivitis, and exhibited ulcerations in some areas. Until recently, he had been a heavy smoker.

Initial findings:

PI: 70%	BOP: 78%	TM: 0–2

The figures below depict the clinical situation, probing depths and radiographic findings.

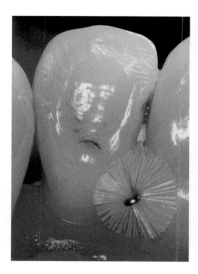

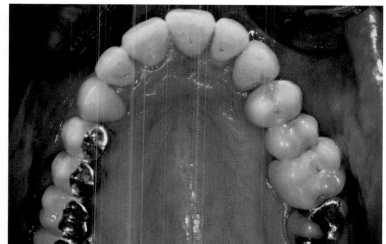

641 Clinical Findings Two Years after Closed Treatment—Occlusal View

Healthy gingival and periodontal conditions. Note the spontaneous closure of the diastema between teeth 11 and 21. In quadrant 1, a bridge was fabricated from teeth 14, 15 to 17. The old, overcontoured bridge in quadrant 2 was left in place because of financial considerations.

Left: Clinical view of teeth 13, 12 and 11 after therapy and optimum oral hygiene.

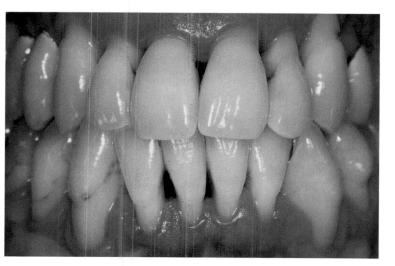

642 Final Result, Two Years after Closed Therapy—Anterior View

As depicted in this clinical photograph, purely closed treatment led to relatively favorable results, including some shrinkage of the gingival tissues; however, the degree of gingival recession had increased. The clinical, esthetic result necessitated free gingival grafting procedures above the canines.

Left: Initial probing depths (left side).

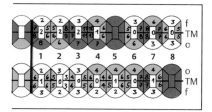

Before

After

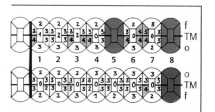

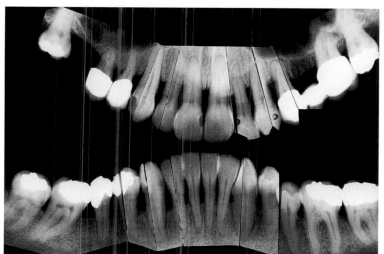

643 Radiographic Findings Two Years after Treatment

The intraoral conditions have "stabilized." Several teeth exhibit new bone apposition, e. g., mesial of tooth 43 and in the mandibular furcations.

Left: Probing depths and tooth mobility two years after therapy (cf. Fig. 640, right).

Courtesy L. Ritz

Possibilities and Limitations of Closed Therapy ...

Phase 1 therapy (I: plaque control, *supragingival* debridement; II: *subgingival* scaling, root planing and eventual curettage) is certainly the most important and fundamental measure for comprehensive treatment of periodontal disease. Phase 1 therapy is truly causal therapy, the *gold standard*.

The often necessary adjunct to Phase 1 therapy is periodontal surgery. This permits treatment of the root surfaces with direct vision, and is therefore also "causal" therapy. In addition, surgical approaches can eliminate or correct symptoms or consequences (defects) of the disease process.

... in Gingivitis

In most cases of gingivitis, initial therapy (Phase I) is the only treatment necessary. One exception is fibrous gingival hyperplasia, which may persist even after elimination of the inflammation. This is often the case following severe gingivitis, with mouth breathing, as well as chronic ingestion of certain medications that have gingival overgrowth as a side effect (phenytoin, dihydropyridine, cyclosporine-A; p. 121). In such cases, Phase 1 therapy must be followed by surgery (gingivectomy/gingivoplasty).

644 Pocket Depth Reduction and Gain of Attachment after Various Treatment Methods in 4–6 mm Pockets (Knowles et al. 1979)

——————— Root planing and curettage
——————— Modified Widman procedure
– – – – – – Surgical pocket elimination

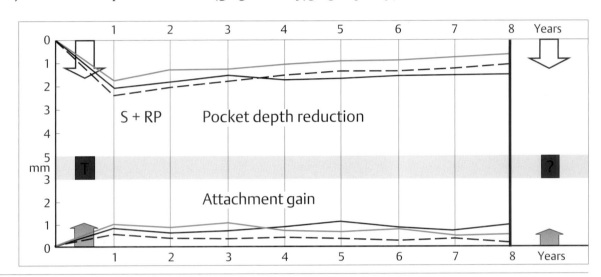

645 Changes in Pocket Depths Following Closed, Non-surgical Therapy
Badersten et al. (1984) demonstrated early on the advantages and shortcomings of closed treatment. Ideal areas are those with probing depths (PD) up to ca. 6 mm (blue region). Attachment loss is present with PD of 3 mm and less, to deep "residual pockets" with PD greater than 7 mm. In such cases, other techniques (surgery) or the use of medications is more promising (p. 287).

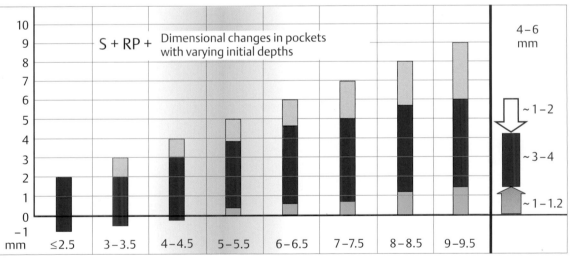

... in Mild Periodontitis

In such cases, especially on single-rooted teeth, Phase 1 therapy alone usually leads to good results (Badersten 1984; Badersten et al. 1984a, b; cf. Fig. 644).

... in Moderate and Advanced Periodontitis

In such cases, success after only Phase 1 therapy is rare. As already noted, subgingival plaque and calculus removal becomes more difficult as pocket depth increases (Waerhaug 1978).

Root irregularities, grooves, furcations and fusions cannot be perfectly cleaned; scaling and planing of the root surface can be performed only incompletely at best. The consequences include a total lack of new attachment (regeneration) and re-infection of the residual pockets.

It is therefore absolutely necessary to re-evaluate the patient's periodontal condition ca. 8 weeks after completion of Phase 1 therapy ("Phase 1 evaluation"). At this time, a decision can be made regarding the necessity for surgical intervention.

FMT—"Full Mouth Therapy"

- **Non-surgical Therapy, plus ...**
- **FMD—"Full Mouth Disinfection"**

"Full Mouth Disinfection"—FMD

It is becoming more and more clear that purely mechanical, non-surgical periodontitis therapy can be greatly improved if all of the currently available pharmacologic possibilities are utilized. Such possibilities improve the success rates for pocket reduction and clinical attachment gain to the levels achieved by surgical methods (Drisko 2002; Quirynen et al. 2002).

The therapeutic terms *antimicrobial* and *anti-infectious* do not imply only that the root surfaces in the area of pockets are scraped clean; rather, that the microbial colonizers of the pocket must be reduced, and those microbes with pathogenic potential must be eliminated. This principle also holds true for the entire oral cavity with all of its plaque retentive niches, and the recolonization of residual pockets; the oral cavity must therefore also be thoroughly disinfected (FMD). And finally, the oral cavity of the patient's *partner* must be examined and treated as necessary.

The principal procedure for "full mouth therapy" including "full mouth disinfection" is portrayed in the figure below (Fig. 646).

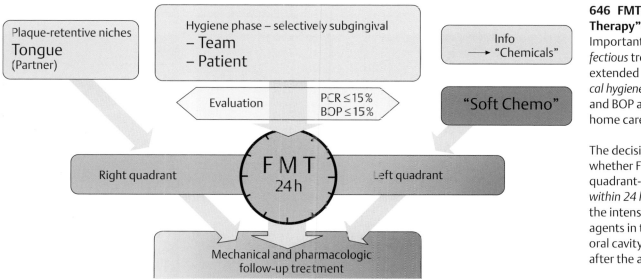

646 FMT—"Full Mouth Therapy"—Schematic
Important: The *intensive anti-infectious* treatment begins with an extended *phase of purely mechanical hygiene*, until the patient's PI and BOP are reduced to 15 % by home care procedures.

The decision is then made whether FMT will be performed quadrant-by-quadrant or (better) *within 24 hours*. Now also begins the intensive use of antiseptic agents in the pockets and in the oral cavity, before, during and after the active FM therapy.

Practical Procedure for FMT

The procedure is simple and includes the following steps (Quirynen et al. 2001; Saxer 2001):
- An extended hygiene phase; goal: PI and BOP ≤ 15 %
- Actual closed pocket therapy—FMT, pharmacomechanical, within a short period of time
- Supervised follow-up care (mouth, tongue, teeth)

During the *hygiene phase* the patient is motivated in toothbrushing technique, tongue cleansing with a brush or scraper, and the periodontal pockets are *purely mechanically* debrided, deeper and deeper at each appointment.

After achieving the established hygiene goals, the actual "full mouth therapy," now *pharmacomechanical*, is instituted within a 24-hour period of time (p. 210):

- Oral rinses (CHX 0.1–0.2 %) 1–2 days before initiating therapy (reduction of the "bacterial load" in the oral cavity)
- *Mechanical pocket therapy*, including: Use of antiseptics during the FMT; repeated pocket rinsing (CHX 0.2 %; H_2O_2 3 % plus betadine 0.5 %), and "filling" the pocket with CHX gel after treatment
- Supervised follow-up care (tongue cleansing with CHX).

FMT—Instrumental/Mechanical and ...

Is "full mouth therapy" the *wonder concept* of the future? Here remains the controversy! Where praise is heard, criticism is not far behind. The loudest outcry against FMT: The "brutal" hours-long *stress situation* for the patients during the 24-hour treatment, and the occasionally occurring *bout of fever* following therapy!

It has long been known that fever, even septic shock, may be the reaction after massive antibiotic administration and the subsequent massive death of bacteria; this also leads to an equally large release of bacterial metabolic by-products,

e.g., LPS (also PGE2, IL-1, IL-6 etc.). The host response may be overcome.

The proper use of FMT prevents this type of stress and fever: During the *extended hygiene phase*, the bacterial mass in the oral cavity and within pockets is reduced successively from appointment to appointment using careful mechanical instrumentation and without local anesthesia. Thus, at the end of the hygiene phase, most shallow pockets are already "healed" and only a few deep and active pockets remain to be treated by the FMT method.

647 Fine Tips for the Ultrasonic Device—Cavitron
The use of thin, fine tips with internal cooling (pictured, the paired Slimline tips) permits effective subgingival debridement in areas where curettes are difficult to maneuver, and usually without anesthesia (caution: contaminated spray aerosol!).

Right: Using the thin, curved ultrasonic tips, even the narrowest furcations can be debrided with a "closed" approach.

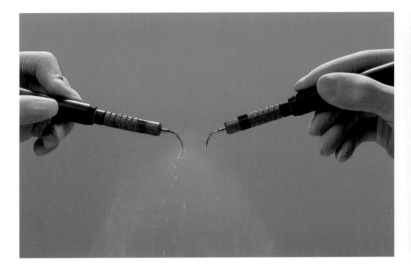 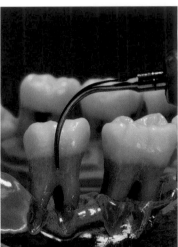

648 Linear Vibrations of the Vector Ultrasonic Device without Spray Aerosol
The Vector device is only mildly abrasive and therefore not indicated for the removal of hard calculus. However, for the destruction and removal of *subgingival biofilm* it is ideal and also gentle on exposed root surfaces. It is therefore well indicated for follow-up care postoperatively and during recall.

Right: Unusual characteristic—the Vector without any spray aerosol.

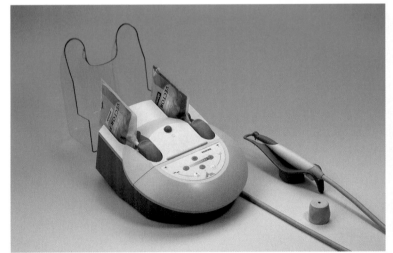 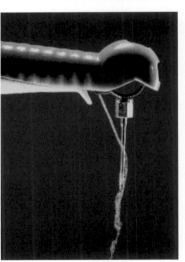

649 The Vector in Use—Delicate!
Two powder suspensions provide the mild abrasiveness for polishing capability of the device. The purely linear vibrations reduce pain sensation. Only very few patients require local anesthesia.

Right: **EMS—Handy 2**
This powder-water spray device, with its special fine tip, can also be used subgingivally, thanks to the minimally abrasive powder (amino acid glycine; Petersilka et al. 2003).

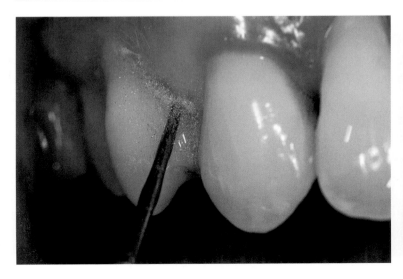 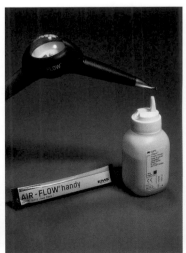

... Pharmacologic Therapy

If this more "patient" procedure is employed, neither fever nor particular stress will occur. And, 9 out of 10 patients questioned reported that they would decide on this form of therapy again. The overriding question is, what does the patient consider to be less burdensome: Long-term results and financial concerns? The choice of "getting it all over with" (FMT in 24 hours), or the more traditional approach to periodontal surgery, sextant by sextant? These questions must be answered by a thoroughly informed patient.

The authors who have enthusiastically endorsed closed, anti-infectious treatment methods (FMT) hope that their efforts will bring us closer to the goal stated by Dr. Jörgen Slots (2002): *"Effective, safe and affordable periodontal therapy"* (Bollen & Quirynen 1996; Vandekerckhove et al. 1996; Bollen et al. 1998; Quirynen et al. 1998; Mongardini et al. 1999; DeSoete et al. 2001, and others).

The antiseptic agents described below, and the various possibilities for their uses represent cost-effective pharmacologic agents for FMT.

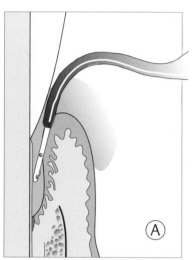

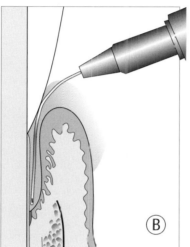

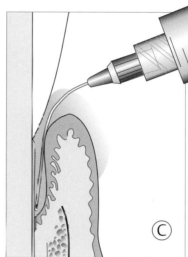

650 Pocket Rinsing with Antiseptics—Subgingival
Using the depicted blunt and therefore non-traumatic cannulae, the fundus of the pocket can be achieved in most cases.

A Perioflex (Oral-B)
B Periodontal Pik (WaterPik)
C Max-I-Probe (HaWe)
on a 10 ml syringe

A single rinsing has only a short-term effect. Prolonged effects can only be achieved with *repeated* irrigation using relatively high concentration disinfectants.

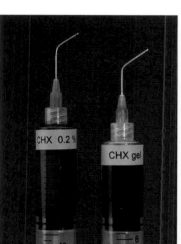

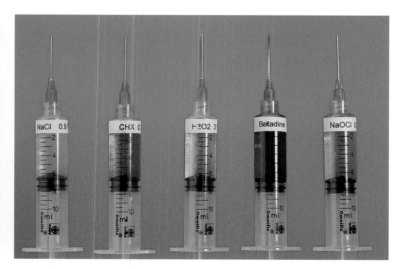

651 Rinsing and Disinfection Agents for Subgingival Application
The depicted agents can be used alone or in combination, together with the mechanical treatment:

- **NaCl** 0.9 %
- **CHX** 0.2 %
- **H₂O₂** 3 %
- **Betadine** 0.5 %
- **NaOCl** 0.5 %

Left: Two CHX modalities

- **CHX Rinsing Solution 0.2 %**
- **CHX Gel 2 %** (larger cannula)

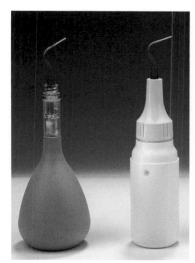

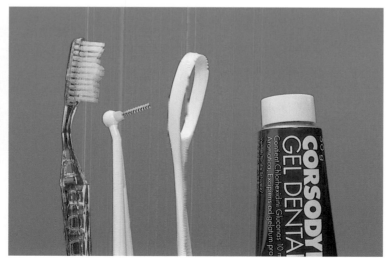

652 At-home Oral Hygiene, Brought to the Highest Level
In addition to toothbrushing and interdental cleaning, the "FMT patient" optimizes oral hygiene by regular use of a tongue cleansing device (cf. halitosis, p. 237). The regular brushing of the dorsum of the tongue with chlorhexidine gel helps to decimate the enormous bacterial reservoir.

Left: **Syrette** (Oral-B).
Using this device, the dextrous and instructed patient can rinse residual active pockets.

FMT—Radiographic Results

The biggest practical difficulties in any type of periodontitis therapy include, of course, deep pockets, roots with unusual morphology, limited physical access, poor visibility or none whatever, etc.

The most frequently encountered and most difficult problems, especially with closed treatment, include:

- Deep and *narrow* bony pockets
- Furcation involvement in multirooted teeth
- The distal pocket following third molar extraction.

The potential of "full mouth therapy" was tested in precisely these difficult situations. In the radiographs below, "bone fill" is demonstrated that is seldom achieved with conventional closed therapy, or even with "access surgery" (p. 300).

Bone fill does not, of course, reveal anything about true, effective *histologic* healing. On the other hand, bone fill never occurs in the vicinity of an active pocket! It is a testament to the dental hygiene profession that the cases depicted below were treated by students in a dental hygiene school!

---

653 Single-Rooted, Vital Premolar with Large Vertical Osseous Defects— Initial Situation (left)

Right: Five months after initiation of treatment (hygiene phase) and subsequent FMT with "full mouth disinfection" the osseous defect has regenerated almost completely.

Antiseptics used during the active FMT: Combined irrigations with H₂O₂ mixed 1:1 with betadine.

FMT / FMD—Single-Rooted Tooth

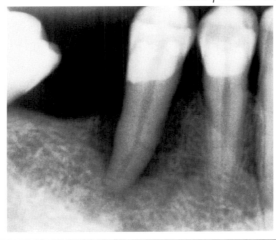
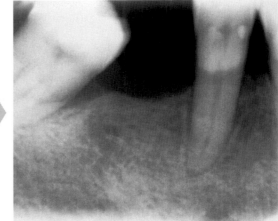

---

654 Molar 36 with a Distal Bony Defect and Severe Furcation Involvement— Initial Situation (left)

Right: Radiographic view two years later. The hygiene phase included removal of restoration overhangs, polishing as well as closed mechanical therapy/FMT. Note the almost complete osseous regeneration in the furcation.

FMT / FMD—Severe Furcation Involvement (F2)

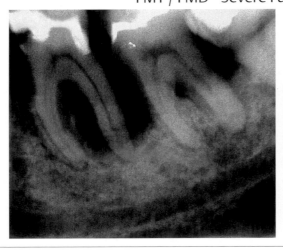
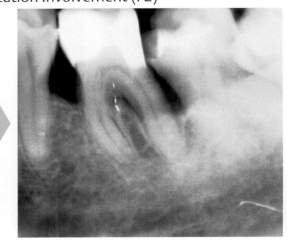

---

655 Distal Pocket Following Third Molar Extraction— Initial Situation (left)
Massive bone loss and an unfavorable open area (anatomic defects) for any future bone regeneration.

Right: Radiographic view two years later. The bone has regenerated, leaving only a small residual defect. The probing depth at this site was 4 mm.

FMT / FMD—Distal Pocket after Third Molar Extraction

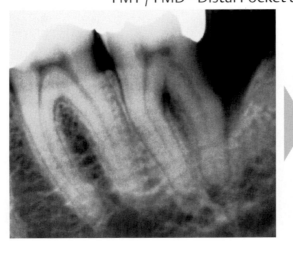
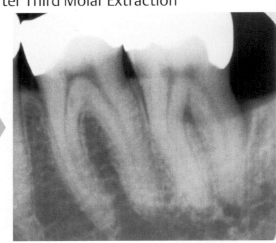

Courtesy *U. Saxer*

FMT—Statistical/Numerical Results

During the 1980's the Loma Linda group (Badersten et al. 1981, Badersten 1984, Badersten et al. 1984, Nordland et al. 1987) reported their imposing results using closed, mechanical, non-surgical therapy, and described the successful results and the presumed limitations of that gold standard.

New knowledge acquired during the 1990s—the characteristics of plaque "biofilm," the colonization of niches as well as epithelial cells throughout the entire oral cavity, even by periodontopathic microorganisms, their transfer from site to site and even from person to person—led to a true *paradigm shift* and to re-thinking of the then-contemporary treatment strategies.

The results of this re-thinking about periodontitis was a combined *pharmacologic-mechanical* treatment concept that also included niches outside the actual periodontal pocket: The "full mouth therapy" (FMT) including its important component "full mouth disinfection" (FMD). The results of FMT are, indeed, promising. Figures 656 and 657 (below) summarize a clinical study by the Leuwen group (Quirynen et al. 2000).

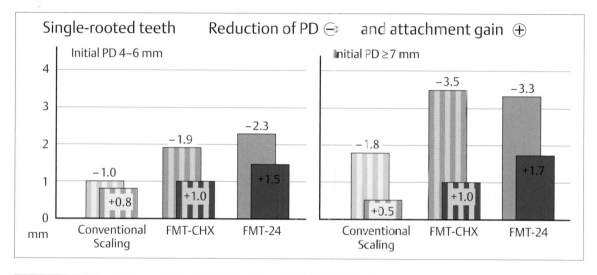

Comparison of Three Types of Closed Therapy

656 Treatment of Single-rooted Teeth

Legends, see Fig. 657

Negative values: Reduction of PD
Positive values: Attachment gain

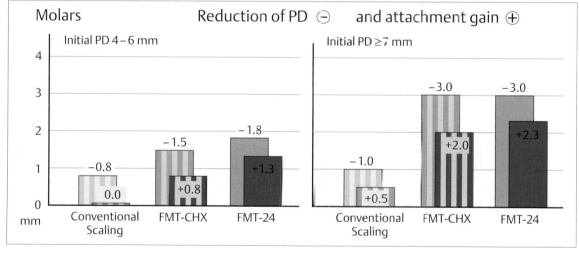

657 Treatment of Molars
- Left:
  Initial probing depths 4–6 mm
- Right:
  Initial probing depths ≥ 7 mm

Columns: Type of treatment
Left: Conventional scaling, 1 quadrant/1–2 weeks
Middle: FMT—scaling as above, with addition of FMD using CHX
Right: FMT 24—as with FMT, but treatment of all four quadrants within 24 hours

Results: Possibilities and Limitations

Using the FMT treatment concept, clinical healing rates are possible that far exceed results obtained using conventional closed therapy, and even those of surgical access therapy (pp. 299, 300). The successes of FMT are causing major changes in the philosophy of periodontal practice:
- Periodontitis is an infection that must be treated strictly anti-microbially ("pharmacomechanical").
- Any re-infection of a treated pocket must be prevented by optimum oral hygiene and rapid integration of subgingival treatment procedures (debridement, supported by antiseptics).

- Oral niches must be thoroughly and regularly cleaned both before and subsequent to treatment.

Some of the disadvantages of traditional therapy (scaling and root planing) also limit FMT, e. g., lack of direct vision in the field of operation and the still insufficient effect of antiseptic agents in the pocket.

New agents are being sought for "vision control," e. g., the pocket television (DV-TV). More highly concentrated antiseptics, eventually even topical antibiotics (p. 292) and root conditioning agents such as Emdogain are even today being developed and clinically evaluated.

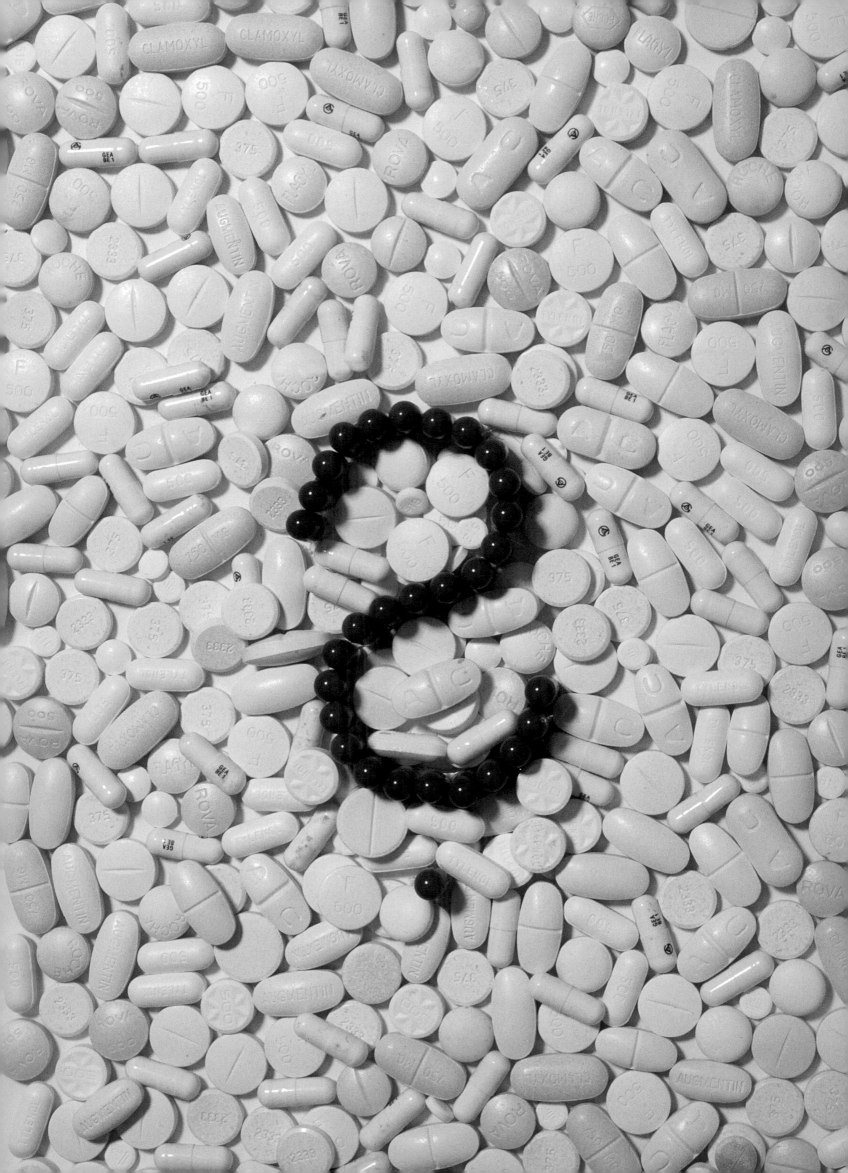

Medications

- Anti-microbial, Antibiotic, Anti-infective: Pharmacological Co-Treatment
- Host Factor Modulating Substances

Anti-infectious Supportive Therapy—Antibiotics in Periodontitis Therapy

The accumulation of bacteria upon the teeth represents the primary cause of gingivitis and periodontitis. The regular mechanical removal of plaque biofilm from all non-desquamating surfaces is therefore essential, and it is also the primary measure for prevention or inhibition of the progression of periodontitis (Mombelli 2003).

Through systematic, careful debridement of teeth and affected root surfaces, periodontitis can in many cases be successfully treated. Two disadvantages of this *non-specific mechanical* treatment, which is repeated regularly at recalls, are the irreversible and ever-increasing damage to tooth hard structure, especially roots within periodontal pockets, as well as gingival recession. In addition, it is virtually impossible to mechanically remove dental plaque from narrow grooves and scratches, narrow furcations and other bacterial reservoirs within the pocket area (p. 255).

Thus it is appropriate to combine mechanical plaque suppression with a medicinal, anti-infectious parallel therapy. Since only a few bacterial species are potentially periodontopathic, it is reasonable to eliminate these groups *specifically* (Mombelli, Slots, van Winkelhoff). These groups contain bacteria that can colonize cells of the pocket epithelium and thus escape both the host response and mechanical cleaning efforts (*A. actinomycetemcomitans, P. gingivalis, S. constellatus*; Herrera et al. 2002). This situation can be effectively combated using systemic antibiotics or topically-applied medicaments.

In addition to antimicrobial agents, mainly antibiotics with their well-known side effects and the ever-increasing emergence of resistant microbial stains, more and more new substances are being offered for use in periodontal therapy, especially agents that modulate the host response.

This chapter on "Medications" is arranged as follows:

- Decision-making criteria—When to use antibiotics?
- Systemic antibiotics for periodontitis therapy
- Antibiotics—Bacterial sensitivity and resistance
- Systemic versus topical antimicrobial treatment
- Topical antimicrobial treatment—Controlled release drugs
- Host response—modulating substances

p. 286
Which Pill is the Correct One?

Decision-Making Criteria—When to Use Antibiotics?

Remember: Periodontitis is an *infectious disease*, caused by periodontopathic, usually opportunistic microorganisms that are organized within a protective biofilm.

Both non-pathogenic and pathogenic species live everywhere in the oral cavity, above all in niches of every sort. They construct a biofilm characterized by close community interrelationships, and exchange metabolic by-products, virulence factors, resistance factors etc. The biofilm protects against the host response as well as against antimicrobial pharmacologic agents (Haffajee et al. 2003).

Even though purely mechanical/instrumental treatment—surgical or non-surgical—will usually very much improve the clinical parameters in most cases, in certain situations an *antimicrobial supportive therapy*, applied systemically or topically, can improve the treatment outcome (Hung & Douglass 2002, Mombelli 2003).

Antibiotics help to subdue the infection; they do not affect healing. Only the host organism can do this. The sensitivity and the nature of the colonization will determine the choice of an antibiotic.

658 Medicinal Supportive Therapy—Yes or No?
Severely progressive cases of chronic periodontitis/Type II, particularly periodontitis cases associated with compromised host response (aggressive periodontitis/Type III, and periodontitis with systemic diseases/Type IV etc.) require systemic supportive therapy in addition to mechanical/instrumental treatment. It is imperative that treatment failure not be caused by the patient's own poor oral hygiene!

The flow-chart depicted here shows a reasonable "decision tree."

The question always arises, whether and when are microbiologic tests indicated. Such tests provide better information about the necessity to employ systemic antibiotics against specific microbial pathogens. Additional tests after therapy can reveal whether or not the targeted microbial species have been eliminated.

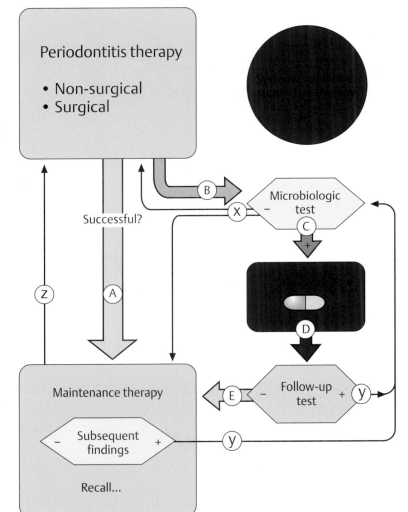

A Successful therapy
→ maintenance therapy
B Failure
→ microbial test
C Positive test result (+):
→ antibiotic targeted toward *pathogenic flora*
D Follow-up, four weeks after antibiotic regimen
E Normal healing
→ maintenance therapy/recall
x Negative test is "positive" for the patient
→ maintenance therapy
y Check-up result with a positive test: → pharmacomechanical treatment repeated
z* Recurrence/recolonization: → repeated instrumental/mechanical therapy
***** For remaining active sites, possible topical medication using a "controlled release drug" (CRD)

Modified from *van Winkelhoff et al. 1996*

659 Test Results— Example of the IAI PadoTest 4.5
On the basis of its affinity for pathogenic species *Aa, Tf, Pg,* and *Td*, this test (p. 185) defines five pocket types (clusters), and provides decision-making information about the use of antibiotics. Beyond the reduction of probing depths that can be achieved by improved oral hygiene alone, better clinical results usually follow scaling and root planing (S + RP), especially S + RP combined with a systemic antibiotic in types 4 and 5.

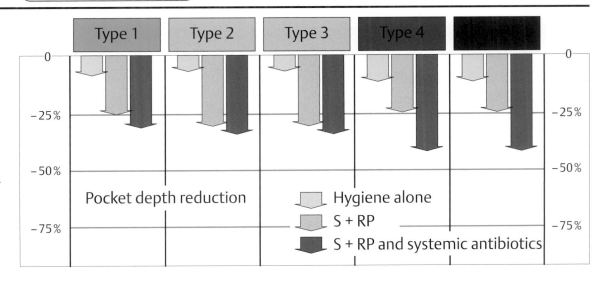

Microbiologic Testing

- Tests *before* treatment define the pathogenic species, above all the presence of *Aa* and/or *Pg*, and provide a basis for selecting an antibiotic.
- Tests *after* treatment show whether or not the maker bacteria have been eliminated.

Pooled Findings or Individual Findings?

With the use of systemic antibiotics, pooled findings are sufficient. However, if individual active residual pockets remain after treatment, the pooled findings provide no information about the initial status.

When Indicated: Which Antibiotic to Prescribe?

The spectrum of efficacy of antibiotics, their important side effects and the compliance of the patient must be understood in advance: Oral ingestion (tablets) over an extended period of time demands discipline from an informed patient (Newman & van Winkelhoff 2001).

In general, broad spectrum antibiotics (e.g., tetracyclines) are used only for special indications. While the commensal flora consists primarily of gram-positive aerobes, the periodontopathic organisms are mainly gram-negative and anaerobic.

Systemic antibiotics – adjunctive periodontal therapy (choices)

Class	Antibiotic	Adult dose (mg/day)	Duration Days
Tetrazykline* bacteriostatic (-stat)	• **Tetracyclin-HCl** • **Doxycyclin-HCl** • **Minocyclon-HCl**	4 x 250 1 x 100 (1 per day x 100) 1 x 200	14 – 21 14 – 21 14 – 21
Penizilline* bakterizid (-cidal)	• **Amoxicillin** plus 125 mg **Clavulonic acid:** →**Augmentin****	3 x 500	7 – 10
Nitroimidazole (-cidal)	• **Metronidazol** • **Ornidazol**	3 x 500 2 x 500	7 – 10 7 – 10
Makrolide (-cidal)	• **Azithromycin** • **Spiramycin** combined with **Metronizadol:** →**Rodogyl****	2 x 250 3 x 33 M.I.E	3 >4
Lincosamide (-static/cidal)	• **Clindamycin**	4 x 300	7 – 10
Chinolone (-cidal)	• **Ciprofloxacin** • **Ofloxacin**	2 x 500 2 x 200	7 – 10 5
Combinations: (-cidal)	„*parallel*" • **Augmentin**** see above • **Rodogyl**** see above • **Amoxicillin 375 + Metronidazol 250** • **Metronidazol 500 + Ciprofloxacin 500**	3 x 625 2 x 2 3 x tid 1 2 x tid 1	7 – 10 7 – 10 7 – 10 7 – 10
Combinations	"*Serial*" use */* • Bacteriocidal, then bacteriostatic		

660 Established and Frequently Employed Systemic Antibiotics for Supportive Periodontitis Therapy

Medication class, average dosage and duration of medication are shown.

In order to prevent the emergence of resistant bacterial strains, medication should never be prescribed with excessively low doses or short regimens!

Bacteriocidal antibiotics (AB; "-cidal") exert their effects much quicker than bacteriostatic ("-static") agents. Bacteriocidal agents should *never* be given simultaneously with bacteriostatic antibiotics.

On the other hand, the serial use of antibiotics (one-after-the-other, see combinations) may provide optimal effects (cf. varying treatment of HIV, p. 149):

*   Successive drug use: Penicillin → tetracycline

**   Augmentin: Combination of amoxicillin (AB) and the penicillinase inhibitor clavulanic acid

*** Rodogyl: Combination of metronidazole and spiramycin

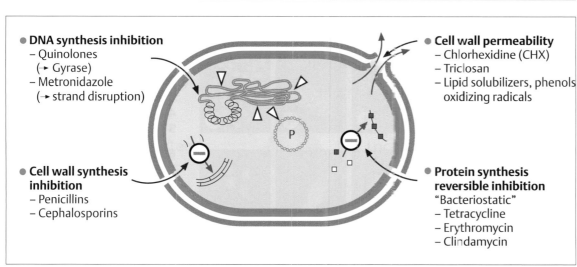

- **DNA synthesis inhibition**
  - Quinolones
    (→ Gyrase)
  - Metronidazole
    (→ strand disruption)

- **Cell wall permeability**
  - Chlorhexidine (CHX)
  - Triclosan
  - Lipid solubilizers, phenols oxidizing radicals

- **Cell wall synthesis inhibition**
  - Penicillins
  - Cephalosporins

- **Protein synthesis reversible inhibition**
  "Bacteriostatic"
  - Tetracycline
  - Erythromycin
  - Clindamycin

661 Effect of Various Antibiotics and Antiseptics on the Target Organisms

Bacteriocidal agents effect the ...

- Cell wall integrity
- Cell wall synthesis
- DNA synthesis and packaging

Bacteriostatic agents inhibit ...

- Protein synthesis

Modified from *J. Goodson 1994*

Local (Topical) Antimicrobial Therapy—"Controlled Release Drugs" (CRD)

It has been routine in dentistry for decades that local, acute processes such as abscesses or NUG lesions are treated with topical medicaments for so long a time as necessary to stop the acute symptoms. Oral rinsing and irrigation have only limited effects if subgingival debridement of the bacterial colonization is not performed simultaneously. All of these types of applications are associated with the disadvantage that the medicament applied is effective for only a very short period of time because it is rapidly rinsed out of the pocket by sulcus fluid secretions.

Only with the development of targeted carrier systems did

it become possible to apply topical medicaments with effective, high doses and controlled release at the appropriate site.

The problem, however, was the same as with systemic antibiotics, namely, what are the *indications* for use of topically applied antimicrobials? Research studies have not yet provided adequate information concerning how long mechanical therapy should be continued and at what point the use of "controlled release drugs" should begin. To date, this decision remains in the hands and mind of each clinician.

667 Effective Subgingival Concentration Following Four Methods of Application
With all systems, the initial concentration far exceeds the minimal inhibitory concentration (**MIC**), but these concentrations decrease quite variably.

A **Irrigation** (cf. p. 283)
B **SRD**
  "sustained release drug"
C **PCH** CHX — PerioChip
D **CRD** "controlled release drug"

Modified from *M. Tonetti 1997*

Subgingival Medicament Concentration

(A) Irrigation
(B) SRD
(C) PCH
(D) CRD

0   ▲   1   3   5   10 Days

MIC*

668 PerioChip
Active ingredient: 2.5 mg
chlorhexidine digluconate
Vehicle: Resorbable gelatin

The vehicle was temperature sensitive and for this reason the sterile packaging had to be maintained in a refrigerator.
This problem is now solved.

Right: Close view of the PerioChip, ca. 3 x 4 mm in size.

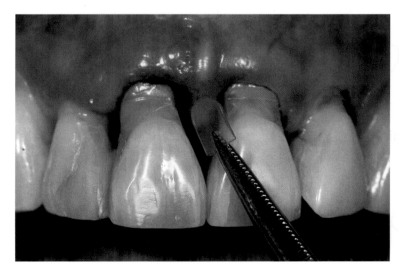
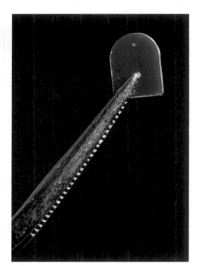

669 Inserting the PerioChip into a Periodontal Pocket
The chip is removed from the refrigerator immediately before its insertion into the periodontal pocket; this is necessary to insure that the chip retains the necessary stiffness. Using a forceps, the PerioChip is slowly inserted, at least 5 mm into the periodontal pocket ...

Right: ... and forced to the depth of the pocket, using the forceps. The chip should be completely subgingival.

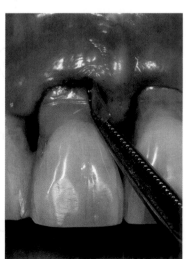

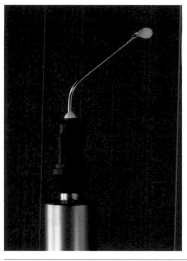

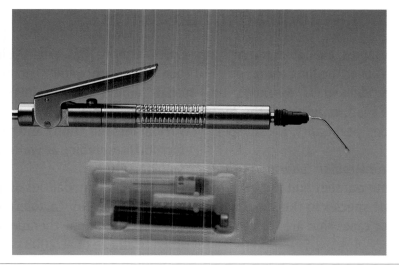

670 Elyzol (Colgate)
Active agent: 25 % Metronidazole benzoate
Vehicle: Mixture of glycerol-monooleate/sesame oil.
Effective time: 24–36 hours.
Application of the prepared contents of the carpule, via the special cannula, directly into the pocket. The gel solidifies upon contact with fluid. Application should be repeated seven days later.

Left: Detailed view of the cannula and the gel.

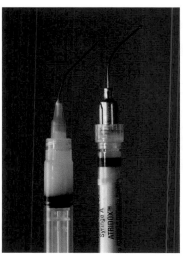

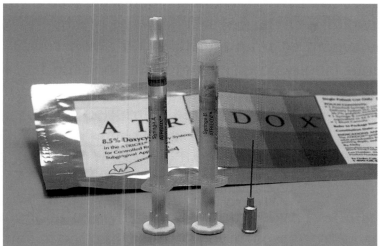

Atridox (Block Drug)

671 The Product . . .
Active ingredient: 8.5 % doxycycline hyclate
Vehicle: Atrigel technology; must be refrigerated.
The active ingredient and vehicle are provided separately as a two-syringe mixing system (ready for use after coupling of the two syringes and 50 back-and-forth movements).

Left: Atridox in comparison to a 2 ml ointment syringe.

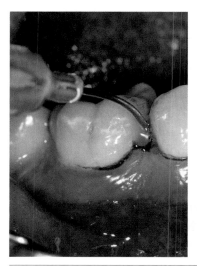

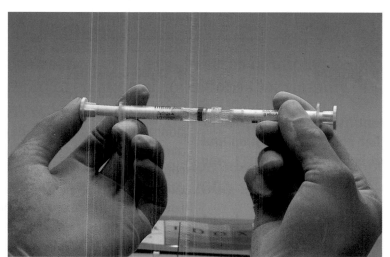

672 ... and the Final Mixing and Application
After final mixing, the syringes are separated and the cannula is affixed.

Left: The cannula is inserted into the 6 mm pocket. The pocket is filled from its apical aspect, rapidly, because the gel quickly begins to solidify.
Following deposition, the cannula is quickly removed from the pocket.

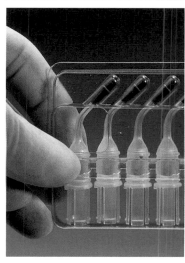

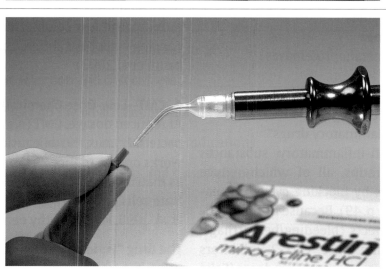

673 Arestin (Ora Pharma)
Active ingredient: 1 mg minocycline-HCl per dose
Vehicle: Microcapsules, powder-form

Arestin is the newest development on the market (2001). Pre-prepared Arestin portions are provided within a disposable tip. The powder is "blown" via air pressure within the metal tip into the pocket.

Left: Arestin portions. Each pocket receives an individual portion.

Factors that Influence the Treatment Result

On the previous pages, we discussed factors about patient selection and periodontal defect morphology, which are of importance for the selection of an effective surgical procedure. The term *success* (a *positive treatment result*) must be defined, and especially must differentiate between *short-term* and *long-term* success.

In the *short-term*, these goals could be achieved by means of the classical—decades-long acknowledged—methods of open or closed root scaling and planing, if adequate plaque control is subsequently insured.

The goal must, however, include *long-term* measures after active therapy, over years and decades, to insure a healthy periodontium and therewith the patient's oral integrity. The most important criteria of success include:
- Regeneration of the alveolar bone
- Attachment gain or at least maintenance of the attachment level, reduction of pocket depth and/or pocket elimination
- Elimination of symptoms of disease activity (bleeding)
- Stabilization of tooth mobility
- Maintenance therapy!

676 Factors that Influence the Treatment "Outcome"
An optimum, *long-term* treatment result depends not only on precise local treatment, but is also "steered" by a myriad of influences and factors.

Purely mechanical plaque control remains the cornerstone of treatment, supported in cases of aggressive periodontitis by medicinal adjunctive therapies.
In addition, however, efforts should also be targeted toward influencing co-factors within the overall etiology. Systemic diseases can usually be successfully treated; tooth position, tooth and alveolar defective morphologies as well as occlusal disharmonies can be corrected; endo-perio problems can usually be solved. On the other hand, correction of the genetic constellation of a patient is not possible, the aging process cannot be halted, and a patient addicted to smoking is extremely difficult to manage.

Modified from *K. Kornman & P. Robertson 2000*

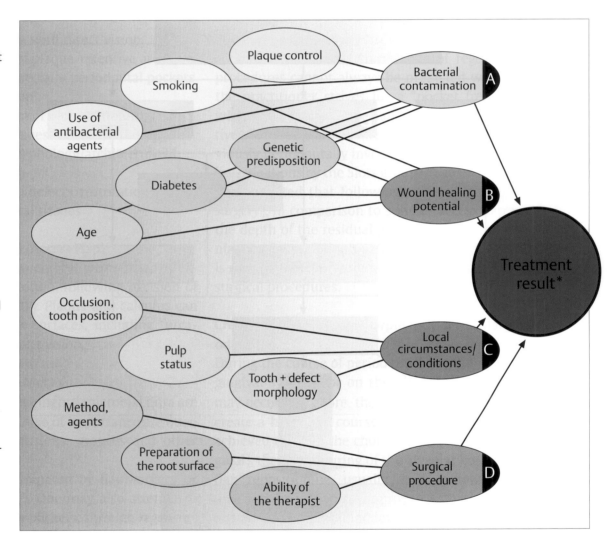

The long-term success is dependent upon many factors:

A Without question, the "bacterial load" plays a determining role, but in addition to the microbiologic load, the pathogenicity and specificity of the microorganisms are critical (Etiology and Pathogenesis, p. 21; Diagnosis, p. 165).
B In addition, the wound healing potential plays an important role, and this can vary considerably from patient to patient through genetic determination, systemic disorders or even heavy tobacco use.

C Oral, local and morphologic situations may be of significance.
D In addition, the type of therapy, i.e., the surgical procedure itself, plays an important role in determining the long-term success.

These four primary parameters are based upon a myriad of other influences (Fig. 676). In the final analysis, long-term success is determined not only by the proper choice of a treatment methodology and its flawless performance, but also by the expertise of the surgeon. But the most important variable remains optimum plaque control (Hygienist! Recall!).

Methods of Periodontal Surgery and their Indications

Which periodontal surgical procedure to select? The choice depends primarily upon the disease *type* (AAP classification, 1999, p. 327), as well as the *severity* and the *expanse* of the disease.

If the patient presents with *aggressive periodontitis* (AAP Type III), and if the etiology includes not only periodontopathic bacteria but also significant co-factors (see p. 298), a more radical surgical procedure should be considered, also possibly incorporating systemic or topical medicaments, and perhaps even extraction of severely involved teeth. On the other hand, if the patient's cooperation and compliance (as assessed during Phase 1 therapy) are not optimum, one must consider whether simple palliative treatment (debridement) should be performed, because the long-term results of extensive surgical procedures would be compromised from the onset.

The *degree of severity* of the disease, i.e., the present state of progression, Class III (severe form) demands pharmacologic support following radical or intensive surgical procedures, much more than the therapy of less severe cases (Class I or Class II).

In addition to the type and severity of disease, the *pathomorphology* of the diseased periodontium will also determine the nature of surgical intervention. Are the gingiva and/or the alveolar bone thin, or thick? Is the periodontal bone loss horizontal in nature, or are vertical (angular) osseous defects present? Does the patient present with a complete dentition, or are teeth missing? Even the morphology of the individual teeth and their position in the arch can influence the choice of a surgical procedure.

This myriad of factors will determine, in an individual patient, or even in a given segment of the dentition, which of the various surgical methods must be employed adjacent to each other or combined in a surgical procedure.

Periodontal Surgical Procedures

- *"Access flap surgery,"* open flap debridement (OFD), e.g., modified Widman flap (MWF), p. 300
- *Wedge excisions* on lone-standing or individual teeth
- *Regenerative methods*, pocket implantation with bone or bone replacement materials, "guided tissue regeneration" (GTR), use of matrix proteins or growth factors (p. 301)
- *Resective procedures* (osseous surgery, pocket elimination, crown lengthening; p. 301)
- *Gingivectomy (GV)/gingivoplasty (GP)*: These procedures are included in the resective or modeling methods
- *Surgical furcation therapy*
- *Mucogingival plastic surgery*

"Access flap" (p. 300) connotes the creation of visual access to periodontally involved root surfaces. The methods comprise for the most part the techniques formerly referred to as "modified Widman procedures." In principle, even in the more complicated flap procedures the goal is to create access. The guiding principles of the modified Widman flap procedure—incisions, creation of the flap, tight adaptation during flap repositioning—must also be adhered to.

Wedge excisions may be indicated when, distally, an end-standing or a lone-standing tooth exhibits bony pockets.

Regenerative methods are becoming more and more popular in periodontitis therapy. In contrast to the more traditional resective methods, these attempt to rebuild lost tissues, and the regeneration of periodontal defects is surely a desirable goal. Unfortunately, today, the long-term results cannot yet be predicted with certainty. Regenerative treatment techniques are indicated primarily in cases of vertical osseous defects, in furcation involvement (F1 or F2; p. 306), and for covering areas of gingival recession (Class I and Class II).

Resective procedures retain, even today, their position as the most predictable of success, even long-term. Resective procedures are indicated with irregular alveolar bone loss, and when the osseous morphology requires osteoplasty or ostectomy. There are significant disadvantages to resective therapy, which temper their indication.

Gingivectomy (GV) and *gingivoplasty (GP)* represent surgical techniques within the rubric of resective soft tissue treatment methods. As a treatment modality for periodontitis, GV is only rarely employed today. On the other hand, GP remains the treatment of choice for contouring hyperplastic gingiva.

Surgical furcation therapy is indicated in Class F3 furcation involvement, and often also F2 involvement. Such treatment may be resective or maintenance. Amputation of individual tooth roots, hemi- and tri-section with maintenance of individual or all roots can be recommended for maintenance of the masticatory efficiency of a dental quadrant or if a tooth must be maintained as a component of a total arch reconstruction. The alternative may involve the use of osseointegrated, root-form dental implants.

Mucoplastic Procedures

Mucogingival surgery is not truly a method for the treatment of periodontitis. It is indicated primarily for the treatment of progressive gingival recession and its consequences, as well as in the treatment of alveolar ridge defects. It is truly a form of plastic surgery, which helps to eliminate esthetic problems.

Furcation Involvement—Classifications

The varying degrees of severity of furcation involvement in multi-rooted teeth have already been discussed in the chapters "Forms" (p. 102) and "Data Collection—Diagnosis—Prognosis" (p. 165).

On the basis of horizontal probing, in this *Atlas* we will differentiate degrees of severity F1 to F3, as described by Hamp et al. (1975). It is also important for both diagnosis and treatment planning whether the root trunk between the crown and the divergence of the roots is long or short. Furthermore, the vertical interradicular dimension of the de-

fect between the roof of the furcation and the alveolar bone niveau is important. Tarnow & Fletcher (1994) have categorized this vertical dimension in three subclasses: A = 1–3 mm, B = 4–6 mm and C > 6 mm. This classification can only be precisely verified during surgery.

Also important for treatment planning is the angle between/among the roots and their proximity to each other. With a long root trunk or with close root proximity, hemisection is seldom possible, and totally impossible if the roots are fused.

Score – Horizontal measurement	
Measured from (an imaginary) tangent (Hemp et al. 1975)	
F0	No horizontal probing depth
F1	1–3 mm
F2	> 3 mm, but not through-and-through
F3	Through-and-through

Score – Vertical measurement	
Measured interradicularly from the furcation roof (Tarnow and Fletcher 1984)	
A	1–3 mm
B	4–6 mm
C	> 6 mm

692 Classifications
– Horizontal Severity
Left: Horizontal probing depth/severity (F0-F3), measured from the tangent of the three roots, along the roof of the furcation (red tangents in Fig. 919, left).

– Vertical Severity
Right: Probing severities (A, B, C) in the vertical direction measured from the roof of the furcation to the niveau of the alveolar bone of the adjacent two roots (cf. Fig. 693, right).

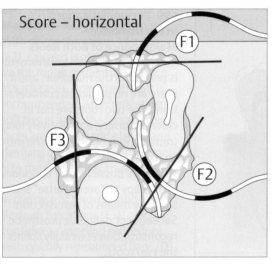

Score – horizontal

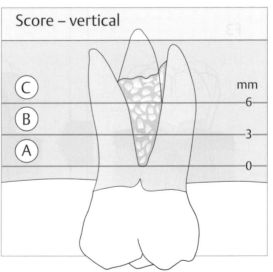

Score – vertical

693 Maxillary Molar—"F-Degree"—Horizontal and Vertical
Left: The furcation probe (Nabers; Hu-Friedy) reveals a complex situation: Between the two buccal roots, **F1**, between the mesiobuccal and palatal root, **F2,** and a class **F3** furcation around the palatal root.

Right: Determining the *vertical* bone loss emanating from the roof of the furcation.
A precise measurement, with direct vision, is only possible during surgery.

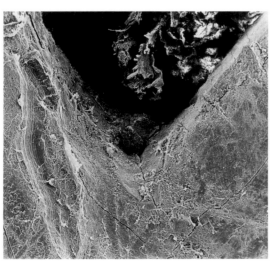

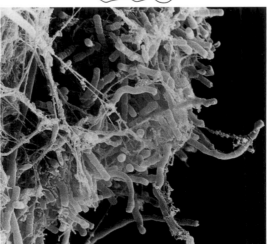

694 Roof of the Furcation, SEM—Details
Left: Tooth 16 exhibits class F3 furcation involvement. After curetting the furcation, the tooth was extracted and prepared for SEM examination. Between the palatal (left) and the distobuccal root (right) the furcation is less than 1 mm wide (the width of a curette is 0.95–1.2 mm!).

Right: Plaque bacteria in the furcation region that were *not* eliminated by mechanical therapy.

Furcation Involvement, F2, in the Maxilla—Furcationplasty

Several therapeutic options are available for the treatment of F2 furcation involvement in both maxilla and mandible, depending upon the morphologic situation. One may employ purely *conservative* methods as with F1 cases and simply open the plaque-retentive areas (Fig. 696), or one may intervene *surgically*, e.g., using GTR techniques in an effort to induce tissue regeneration in the furcation. If the F2 involvement is on a maxillary molar between/among all three roots, some authors suggest hemisection or trisection (Carnevale et al. 1995).

It is common in F2 involvement that the roots join the root trunk forming narrow interradicular areas. In such circumstances, root planing is impossible even with the narrowest curettes. If the overall treatment plan calls for the maintenance of the tooth, the problem can often be solved by odontoplasty (furcationplasty). Initially using course diamonds (75–40 µm), the furcation entrance is widened such that it can be effectively treated with a slender curette. The area is then polished with the 15 µm diamond.

It is best to perform grade 2 furcationplasty carefully and with direct vision, i.e., after careful reflection of the gingiva.

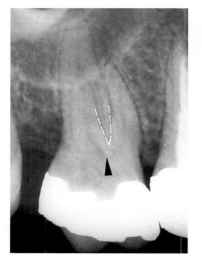
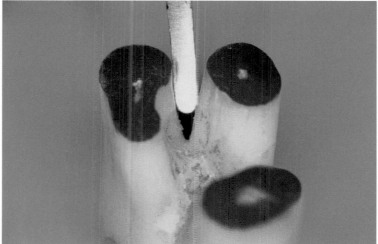

695 Narrow Buccal Furcation
Even the extremely slender (only 0.9 mm wide) curette cannot reach the roof of the affected furcation.

Left: The radiograph reveals the closely spaced buccal roots (arrow). However, the severity of the furcation involvement (periodontal pocket, plaque, calculus) cannot be ascertained radiographically especially in three-rooted maxillary molars.

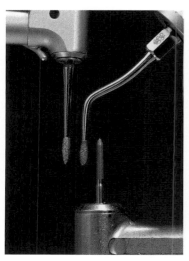
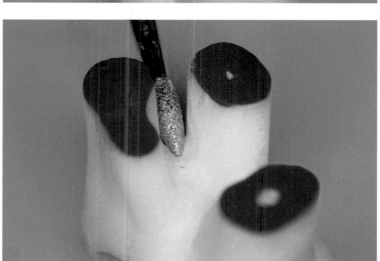

696 Furcationplasty
If clinical access is good, the procedure can be performed "closed," but it is easier to do after reflecting a small flap. Various instruments can be used to open such an involved furcation so curettes can be used for cleaning.
Left:

- **PerioSet Diamonds**
- **KaVo Sonic Scaler**
- **Polishing Diamonds**

Furcations that have undergone odontoplasty are particularly susceptible to caries!

697 Hygiene made Possible
Debridement and root planing with fine curettes can now be performed during the course of periodontal therapy as well as at each recall appointment.

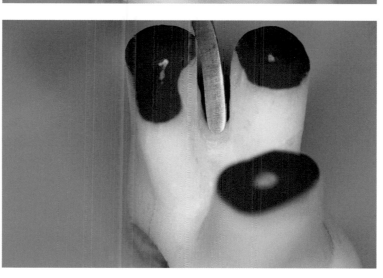

In such cases, cervical sensitivity may be particularly troublesome and persistent. The treated furcation must be polished and fluoridated. This will enhance surface remineralization, reduce plaque formation and lessen cervical sensitivity.

Phase 3 Therapy
Periodontal Maintenance Therapy—Recall

Dental Hygienists *Rule*!

The long-term success of periodontal therapy depends less on the manner in which the case was actively treated (Phase 1 and 2) than on rigorous follow-up of the wound healing process immediately after therapy and on how well the case is maintained in subsequent recall (Rosling et al. 1976, Nyman et al. 1977, Knowles et al. 1979. Ramfjord et al. 1982, Wilson 1996; Axelsson 2002, AAP 2003).

Clinical research by Axelsson & Lindhe (1981, Axelsson et al. 1991) demonstrated dramatically the effects of preventive measures during recall (Fig. 698). This truly classic clinical study, which is ongoing even today (!), continues to demonstrate that regular and short-interval (2–3 months) prophylaxis by the dental hygienist (!) results in virtually no new *caries* and not the slightest periodontal *attachment loss*. This landmark clinical study, originally planned for 6 years duration, casts some serious doubts about "classical" reparative dentistry!

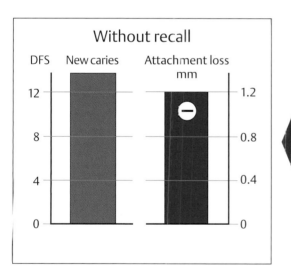

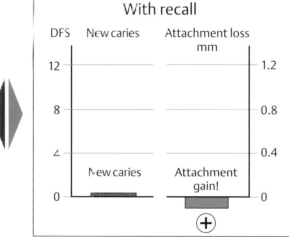

698 Axelsson Study: Caries and Attachment Loss with and without Recall

Left: Patients who received neither homecare motivation nor preventive measures during one dental visit per year had 14 new caries and progressive attachment loss over the 6-year period.

Right: Similar patients who received intensive professional prophylaxis every 2–3 months developed essentially no new carious lesions and actually exhibited some attachment gain!

The primary goals of maintenance therapy include:

- Maintenance of oral health (including cancer screening)
- Maintenance of chewing function, phonetics and esthetics
- Prevention of new infection (gingivitis, periodontitis)
- Prevention of re-infection of inactive residual pockets (periodontitis)
- Prevention of dental caries

These goals can be achieved through:

- Re-examination and re-evaluation
- Re-motivation and new information for the patient
- Re-instruction in oral hygiene and update of oral hygiene informative materials
- Supragingival plaque and calculus removal
- Subgingival debridement of pockets and root surfaces in areas exhibiting disease activity
- Topical fluoride application

The "Recall Hour"—Practical Periodontal Maintenance Therapy

Clinical Findings
- *At every recall appointment*:
  - Gingival condition (BOP or PBI)
  - Plaque accumulation (PI/PCR or API; disclosing solution)
  - Activity of residual pockets
- *Additionally, every 6–24 months*:
  - Pocket probing depths, radiographs (?)
  - Occlusion, reconstructions (tooth vitality), caries
- *Additionally, every 3–4 years*:
  - Panoramic radiograph and individual PA films, p.r.n.

Clinical Procedures
Depending upon the findings, the following procedures should be performed:
- *At every recall appointment (e.g., every 2–6 months)*:
  - Medical history up-date
  - OHI and re-instruction
  - Re-motivation of patient compliance
  - Plaque and calculus removal *where indicated*!
  - Treatment of disease recurrence, p.r.n: debridement, topical meds (p. 291); additional appointments.

See also the *10-point program plus X*, below.

702 The "Recall Hour"
The diagram portrays a rough approximation of a typical 1-hour recall visit. Rationalization of the instrumentarium (ultrasonic instruments) may compensate for the "lost time" required today for the thorough disinfection of the operatory. The fact is that the dental hygienist really has only about 50 minutes per patient.

The division of the "prophy hour" is in four most important segments, depicted on page 313:

1 Patient history, clinical data collection (ca. 15 minutes*)
2 Patient instruction, *instrumentation* (ca. 25 minutes*)
3 Treatment of active sites (ca. 5 minutes *)
4 Polishing, fluoride application (ca. 5 minutes*)

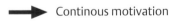 Continous motivation

* The times required will vary from case to case.

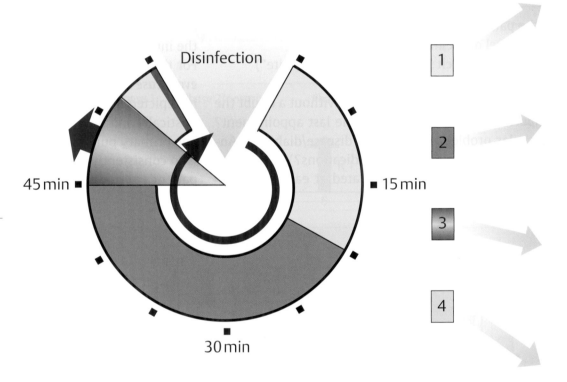

Checklist: 10-Point Program Plus X
1 Medical history update . . . . . new systemic risks
2 Mucosal examination . . . . oral cancer prevention
3 Evaluation of inflammation . motivation
4 Pocket probing depths . . . . . . activity?
5 OHI. . . . . compliance
6 Oral hygiene . . . . re-instruction
7 Calculus removal . . . . targeted!
8 Biofilm removal . . . . mild instrumentation
9 Polishing restorations. . . . . . . minimal abrasiveness
10 Fluoridation of the teeth . . . . information about its effectiveness
X Extra measures. . . . . radiographs, vitality, sensitivity, surgery etc.

Recall—"As Fine as Possible"
Of top priority at recall appointment is the instrumentation of *root surfaces* and *any exposed dentin surfaces*. Just as we advise patients to not use any abrasive dentifrice when cleaning interdental areas, the dental hygienist is also well advised to use only the *gentlest* machines and hand instruments as well as the least abrasive prophy pastes as she/he cleans and polishes tooth surfaces.

Goal: Clean, but not abrasive/destructive! Even after 100 recall appointments (20–40 years), there should be no gross evidence of excessive "scraping" on the teeth (cf. Fig. 713)!

Examination

Re-Evaluation

Diagnosis

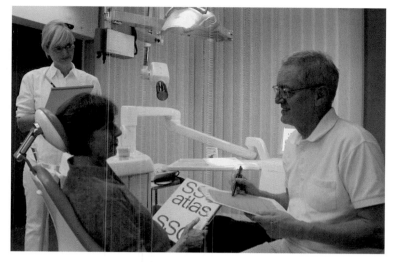

703 Data Collection, Re-Evaluation, Diagnosis
The current status of the patient is evaluated.
The patient's personal and even family difficulties are discussed as well as a follow-up of the general systemic health. Changes in medications are particularly important with older patients (stress?). Have any other risk factors changed (smoking)?
Note: Five minutes of attentive listening is much more important than dental instrumentation, even when time is of the essence.

Motivation

Re-Instruction

Instrumentation

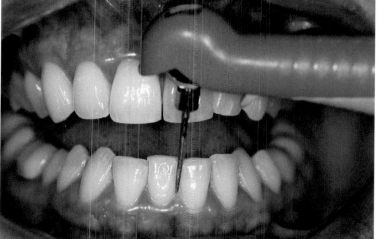
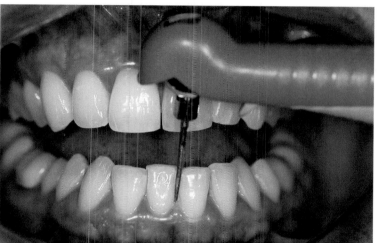

704 Motivation, Re-Instruction, Instrumentation
The latest scientific findings show us the way: Perform scaling only where calculus is present, and remove microbial biofilm using the most gentle of instruments. Evaluate new developments! For example, the Vector ultrasonic device (pictured here); water-powder spray devices with minimally abrasive powder (EMS-Handy 2; p. 282) etc.

Re-Treatment
of Active Sites

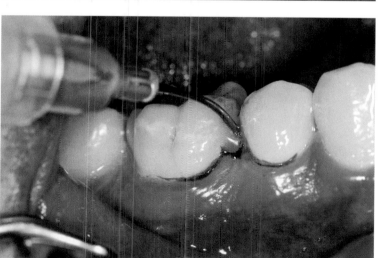

705 Treatment of Active Sites (Re-infected or Newly Infected)
Individual active pockets can often be treated during the recall appointment (scaling; topical irrigation, e. g., betadine or controlled-release drugs). Pictured is an Atridox application into a "refractory pocket" (cf. p. 293).

Multiple active sites or true recurrence of periodontitis will require separate appointments for treatment (scaling or surgery, supported by medicaments, p.r.n).

Polishing

Fluoride Application

Re-scheduling

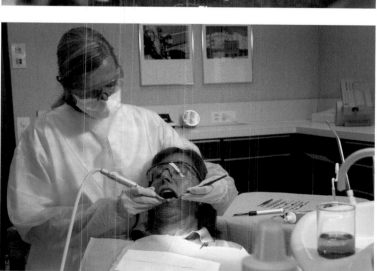
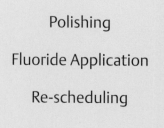

706 Polishing, Fluoridation, Scheduling the Next Appointment ... Recall Interval
Before applying fluoride, all teeth are polished with the rubber cup and a fluoride-containing prophy paste.

Determination of the recall interval is made on the basis of risk assessment (type and severity of periodontitis, systemic and local risk factors, plaque control and patient compliance etc).

Dental Hygienist and Dentist—The "Preventive Team"

Cost-effective and modern preventive measures—true "pro-phylaxis"—would be impossible today without the *highly qualified, highly skilled and highly educated* dental hygienist. The dental hygienist can actually *replace* the dentist in many procedures such as data gathering, prophylaxis, initial ther-apy and maintenance therapy (recall). A full time dental hy-gienist can provide care and maintenance for over 500 pa-tients per year, based upon 3–4 one-hour appointments per year. In most states, clinical care by the dental hygienist

must be performed unter the direct aegis of a dentist: how-ever, many states are pushing for "independent" dental hy-giene practice, and one (Colorado) has so far succeeded. The dental hygienist and other auxiliary personnel can also be of significant assistance to the dentist in the care and maintenance of all other dental patients, e.g., patients with all types of dental replacements (denture care, preventive measures on abutment teeth, dental implants and fixed bridgework etc.).

707 Relief of the Dentist (Gray) by the Dental Hygienist (Laven-der)
The dental hygienist (DH) is re-sponsible for over 90 % of each re-call appointment (**D**), but the DH can also augment the dentist in other areas.
For example during data gathe-ring (**A**) and especially during *ini-tial therapy* (**B**) the DH assumes more than 80 % of the work.
Even during the surgical phase of therapy (**C**) the DH plays a signifi-cant role in post-surgical wound management.

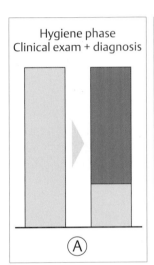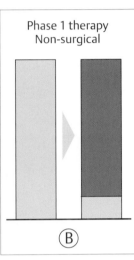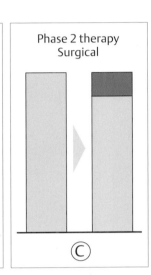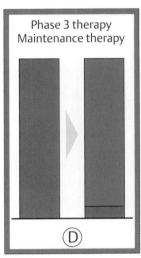

Auxiliary Personnel and Treatment Needs

Hamburg Clinical Study, 1987—CPITN

Ninety-seven percent of individuals examined in the Ham-burg study required some type of periodontal care (TN = "treatment need" of the CPITN; p.72; Ahrens & Bublitz 1987). The type of treatment indicated varied dramatically:

- A total of 12 % (3 % of the healthy and 9 % of patients with plaque-induced bleeding on probing)—required repeated OHI.

- 72 % of those exhibiting calculus, and patients with pro-bing depths to 5.5 mm required subgingival scaling.
- "Only" 16 % of patients exhibiting deeper pockets required more complex periodontal therapy (surgery).

Based on the study, 84 % of the population—the relatively healthy and those exhibiting gingivitis/periodontitis—could be treated prophylactically *and* therapeutically by auxiliary personnel: 12 % by trained dental assistants alone and fully 72 % by *highly qualified and educated dental hygienists*.

708 "Treatment Need/TN" in the Hamburg Study (1987)
TN I Oral hygiene instruction and *supragingival* plaque and calculus removal
TN II As above, plus *subgingival* debridement/scaling
TN III As above plus more com-plex therapy
A 100 % of prophylaxis (TN I) is performed by the skilled hy-gienist.
B 84 % of TN II can be performed by the dental hygienist
C For TN III, 16 % of cases require a dentist or a specialist.

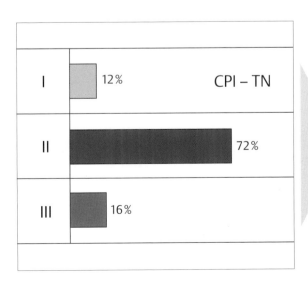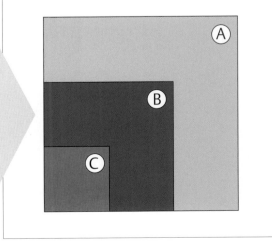

Failures—Lack of Periodontal Maintenance Therapy

Success in Periodontal Therapy

- Inflammation (gingival bleeding) eliminated
- Pocket activity eliminated
- Probing depths reduced
- Attachment loss halted
- Tooth mobility stabilized or reduced

Failures of Periodontal Therapy

- Persistent bleeding
- Persistent pocket activity
- Increasing probing depths
- Advancing attachment loss
- Increasing tooth mobility

Most failures in the treatment of periodontitis can be explained. The most common causes of failure include: Incorrect dental and systemic medical history, incorrect diagnosis and/or prognosis, inappropriate treatment plan, inadequate therapy, *insufficient patient compliance* and *lack of maintenance* (Becker et al. 1984, Rateitschak 1985).

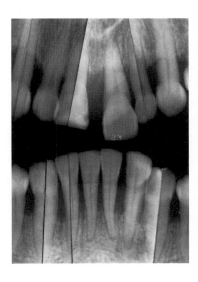

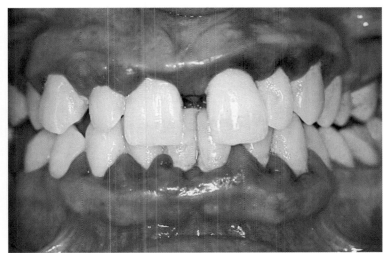

709 Advanced, Rapidly Progressing Periodontitis
When this 38-year-old female presented, she had never been instructed in oral hygiene. She only wanted a dental check-up; she had no complaints!
Clinical findings:

PCR	100%
PBI	3.8
PD	up to 8 mm, many active pockets
TM	very elevated, with tooth migration

Left: Radiographic appearance

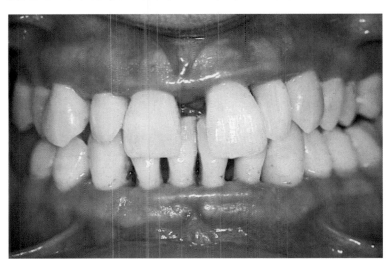

710 Following Initial Therapy
The clinical picture is significantly improved following thorough scaling and root planing. The patient's compliance with homecare instructions was inadequate from the beginning, and therefore no surgical procedures were performed. Shortly after initial therapy, plaque and calculus accumulation occurred (mandibular anterior area).
The patient refused to enter a regular maintenance recall schedule or to undergo orthodontic treatment.

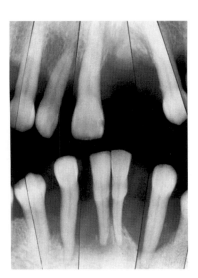

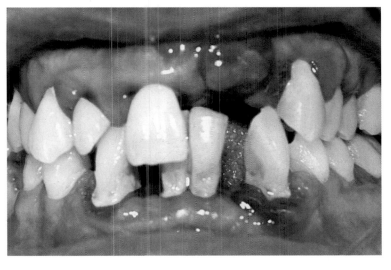

711 Five Years Later, without Recall
The patient presented again, after teeth 22, 23, 32 and 42 had spontaneously exfoliated. The treating clinician elected not to attempt extensive periodontal therapy.

Therapy:
Maxilla: Complete denture
Mandible: Retain four premolars via periodontal therapy; removable partial denture.

Left: Radiographic findings five years later, without recall.

Negative Results of Therapy

- Long teeth—exposed dentin
- Tooth mobility
- Phonetic problems
- Compromised esthetics (maxillary anterior region)

Depending upon the severity of the initial periodontitis, therapeutic measures (closed as well as surgical therapy) will lead to more or less pronounced gingival shrinkage and therefore to "lengthening" of the teeth. The patient must be warned of such possible consequences *before* any therapy is initiated!

Long teeth with their typically attendant dark interdental spaces represent the greatest problem, especially in patients with a high smile line (short upper lip). This situation not only compromises phonetics, but also esthetics, which has become ever more important today. These problems can be dealt with by means of very expensive prosthetics measures, but can also be solved using simple and inexpensive treatments which, unfortunately, usually become "permanent temporary" solutions (p. 317).
(The problems of tooth neck hypersensitivity are discussed on page 318.)

Successful (?) Periodontal Therapy

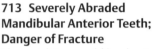

712 "Long Teeth"—Excessive "Compliance" by the Patient?
This 32-year-old female exhibited gingival recession even prior to surgery, and her esthetic appearance worsened after periodontal surgery, when her chief complaints included poor esthetics, phonetics, and tooth neck sensitivity.
She had not yet noticed the wedge-shaped defects on the posterior teeth.

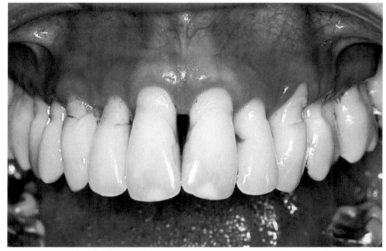

Results of therapy:

- Gingival recession
- Hypersensitive dentin
- Dark-appearing interdental spaces

713 Severely Abraded Mandibular Anterior Teeth; Danger of Fracture
The condition could be due to overzealous homecare by the patient or to overaggressive scaling/root planing during recall appointments.
The patient must be instructed to use *no abrasive dentifrice* on the interdental brushes, rather only fluoride- or CHX-containing gel. At recall appointments, the dental hygienist should use minimally aggressive instruments and prophy paste in the interdental region.

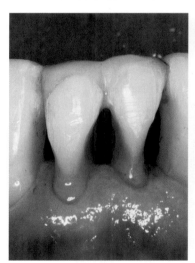
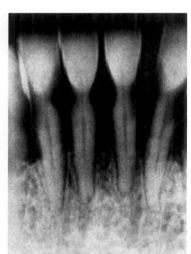

Oral hygiene "too good":

- Wedge-shaped defects
- Narrowing of the interdental tooth substance

714 Cervical Caries
Note the deep wedge-shaped cervical defect with also a small but very deep carious lesion (*left*); removal of the caries led to pulp exposure: Root canal treatment was performed (*right*) without a rubber dam!
Note: The question remains how to perform gentle *yet thorough* treatment?
The regimen included once per day perfect plaque removal using a soft toothbrush, very little force, a gentle technique and a non-abrasive dentifrice.

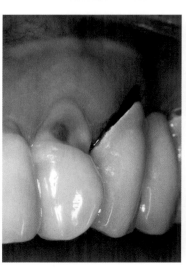
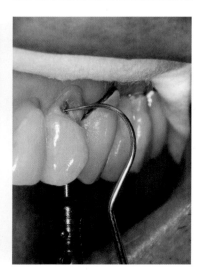

"Inadequate oral hygiene":

- Cervical caries!
- Gingivitis
- Recurrence of periodontitis?

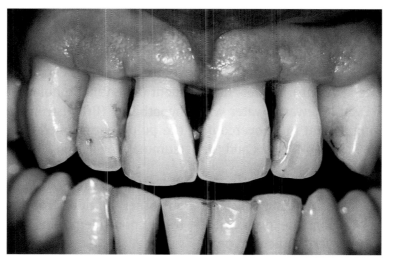

Esthetic Improvement for Negative Therapeutic Results

715 Clinical Appearance after Periodontal Therapy

The maxillary anterior teeth are unesthetically proportioned. The interdental spaces are large, appearing as "black triangles," which disturbed this young female patient. Dental reconstruction by means of veneers or crowns exceeded the patient's financial situation.
Planning: Restorations and a gingival mask.

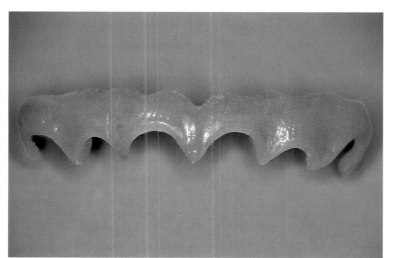

716 Gingival Mask Fabricated from Denture Base Acrylic Resin

Initially, interdental composite resin restorations were placed (acid etch technique). These were over-contoured to reduce the expanse of the interdental space. Using a rubber-elastic material, an impression was made for use in fabricating the color-matched gingival mask.

Left: Denture base acrylic resin in various shades, to blend perfectly with the patient's tissues.

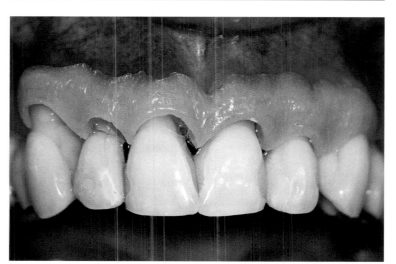

717 Inserting the Gingival Mask

The wedge-shaped interdental portions of the mask snap into place with minimum pressure, into the interdental areas.

In this case, the patient first seats the left side of the gingival mask, distal to tooth 23 and then with a rolling motion of the finger seats the gingival mask into the remaining interdental spaces.

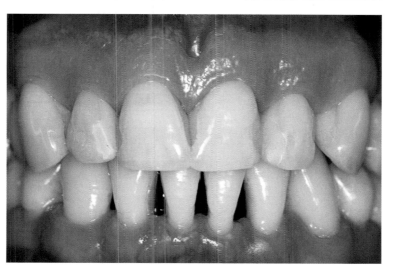

718 Much-improved Esthetics

The margin of the gingival mask at the mucogingival junction is scarcely visible. This patient had a "low smile line" which led to an excellent esthetic (invisible) result.

Note: Because damage of such acrylic gingival masks is not uncommon, it is wise to prepare several masks for the patient.
Soft masks—on the other hand—become quickly discolored.

Determinative Diagnostic Criteria

Tooth Maintenance or Dental Implant?

This question can only be answered on a case-by-case basis. In healthy patients, implant success rates of 99% after 15 years have been reported (Lindquist et al. 1996). In patients suffering systemic disease, as well as those manifesting aggressive periodontitis, the success rate is much lower. Thus the predictability of success is also reduced, and there can be no "guaranteed" prognosis. Local risk factors (oral hygiene, compliance etc.), and above all general systemic risks (smoking, diabetes, osteoporosis, hematologic disorders) must be definitively characterized and diagnosed before making the decision about whether a tooth should be maintained "at all costs" (van Steenberghe 2003).

These decisions demand careful examination of the general medical history and all specific clinical data. It remains within the competency of the dentist to interpret the numerous aspects of each case in order to determine the appropriate and long-term functional treatment plan.

Maintenance of natural teeth
Not only in dental implantology, but also in regenerative periodontal therapy, enormous advances have been made. If periodontal therapy—alone—can lead to success, implant therapy is not indicated; this is especially true for teeth in the "risk areas" such as the maxillary posterior segment (maxillary sinus) or mandibular molars (mandibular canal/mental foramen).

If a prospective abutment tooth requires initial endodontic treatment, post build-up etc., it is important to consider and compare the length of treatment, the costs and the prognosis in comparison to dental implant therapy. Especially in such cases, the well-informed patient must participate in the decision.

Replacement via dental implants
In many partially edentulous patients, such decisions are not even necessary; the decision is simply between fixed bridgework including dental implants, or a removable partial denture.
Teeth that exhibit severe periodontal compromise and which are in danger of progressive disease are better extracted early on in order to preclude extensive loss of the osseous fundament that will be necessary for subsequent dental implant therapy.

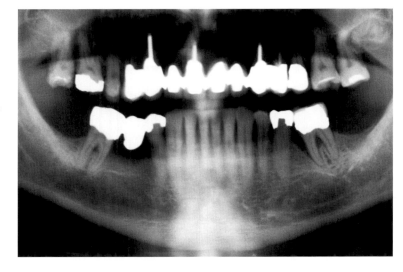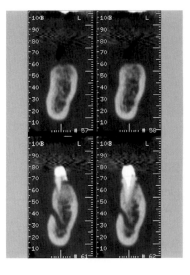

723 Panoramic Radiograph of an "At-Risk" Patient with Periodontally Involved Mandibular Molars Bilaterally
Questions: In this advanced case (risk factors: smoking, oral hygiene), should regenerative periodontal surgical therapy be undertaken or should dental implants be placed following extraction?
Right: More complex diagnostic measures provide information about anatomic structures (jaw dimension, alveolar ridge width, mandibular canal etc.). CT (jaw cross section in a Dentascan).

Diagnosis before Dental Implant Therapy

Before making a definitive decision in favor of dental implants, the identical clinical examinations and findings must be collated as for all periodontitis patients (p. 165). Additional radiographic examinations (CT scans) provide information in complex or risk-rich cases concerning shape, structure, and thickness of the alveolar ridge, as well as concerning special structures such as the maxillary sinus, mandibular canal, persistent areas of ostitis, thickness of the compact bone layers and therefore indirectly concerning the bone *quality* (Lekholm & Zarb 1985).
Simultaneously, the prosthetically relevant parameters as they relate to the set-up plan and positions of the fixtures can be depicted in the radiographs (templates with marker points). This permits the observation of the implant sites before the surgical procedure.
In cases in which the alveolar process is significantly deformed, the implants may have to be positioned in unconventional areas of the alveolar ridge. Today, implants are not necessarily placed where bone remains, rather in locations where the prosthodontist needs them for her/his crown and/or bridge constructions ("backward planning"); additional surgical procedures may be necessary.

Therapeutic Concepts—Therapeutic Results

Treatment Planning—Planning Problems

The prosthodontic concept of modern dental implant therapy is associated with the fact that implants must often be placed in areas where alveolar bone is minimal. Today there are numerous ridge-augmentation procedures that can be performed before placement of dental implants or, under certain conditions, simultaneously.

All of these surgical procedures can only be attempted with great care in *periodontitis-prone patients*. Above all the risk factor "heavy smoking," in combination with poor oral hygiene and compliance, as well as other risks—diabetes, IL-1 and other gene polymorphisms that lessen host response—must be considered when planning such surgical procedures.

Patients today demand not only masticatory function, but also esthetically satisfying treatment, and this makes treatment planning all the more difficult. The dentist must sometimes reduce a patient's utopic thoughts by providing appropriate information and whenever possible using a written treatment plan, including costs and time considerations.

Augmentation Techniques

These surgical procedures are identical for the most part to those of periodontal and mucogingival surgery (p. 295). *Soft tissue augmentation* should usually be performed before hard tissue procedures. Using connective tissue grafts (CTG), tissue augmentation and esthetics can be achieved. This can provide thickening of thin alveolar ridge mucosa so that the surgical site after flap reflection and GBR ("guided bone regeneration") can be closed tightly, without tension. Even reconstruction of papillae can be accomplished using thick mucosa; the "emergence profile" of an ovate pontic can provide the appearance of a natural tooth.

Osseous Alveolar augmentation for stabilization of the implant bed can, depending on the anatomic situation, be performed *simultaneously* during the seating of the fixture, or as a *second* procedure.

Examples of these procedures include:
- Guided bone regeneration (GBR)
- Osseous block transplants
- Sinus lift procedures
- Distraction osteogenesis

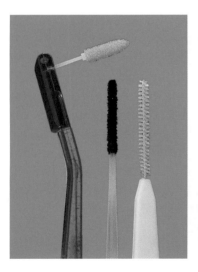
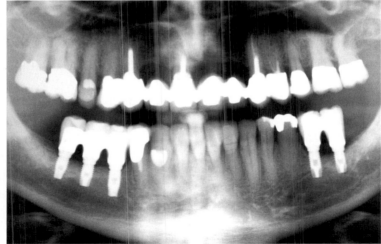

724 Panoramic Radiograph of the "At-Risk" Patient 3 Years after Implant Placement
Following bilateral extraction of the periodontally involved mandibular molars and a six-month waiting period for healing—without ridge augmentation—5 screw-type implants with micro-etched surfaces were placed.
Left: The oral hygiene compliance was significantly improved, permitting the patient to be placed on a 3–4 month recall schedule. Unfortunately, the patient did not stop smoking!

Long-Term Results—Oral Hygiene

The "chances for maintenance" of natural teeth and dental implants in a partially dentulous periodontitis patient are similar, but are clearly poorer than in a "periodontally healthy" patient. The chances of success depend upon the reaction of the patient (oral hygiene, compliance), her, his risk profile (smoking, clenching and bruxism), and above all the microbiologic colonization of the marginal soft tissues, and the "interface" between the tooth/implant and its surrounding soft tissue. A highly susceptible patient reacts to even a small colonization of shallow pockets with pathogenic microorganisms in a manner that is much less "con-

trolled" than in a healthy patient. In the gingival sulcus and in pockets around dental implants, one finds virtually the same microbiologic flora as around natural teeth. Predominating are *Tannerella forsythensis*, *Peptostreptococcus micros* etc.

Fact: In a partially edentulous periodontitis patient with dental implants, the most important requirement for a favorable long-term prognosis is conscientious and careful plaque control and professional maintenance therapy (recall), *by the dental hygienist!*

Recall—Management of Implant Problems

Early failures of dental implants often result for purely biologic reasons. Overheating the bone during preparation of the implant bed may lead to necrosis and contamination of the wound bed, and to subsequent infection. Qualitatively or quantitatively insufficient bone, critical primary stability or premature loading can prevent successful osseointegration. *Late failures*, on the other hand, in healthy patients are usually of a mechanical (overloading, parafunctions) or technical nature (fracture of implant components). It is different in treated periodontitis patients, where peri-implant inflammatory processes more often occur.

Peri-implant problems must be diagnosed as early as possible, depending upon the recall interval and the type of disease, in order to institute the simplest possible measures to halt the disease process (see CIST classes).

For this reason, at *every* recall appointment, the following biological parameters must be evaluated:
- Plaque accumulation on the implant structures
- BOP of the peri-implant tissues
- Suppuration, initial pocket formation
- Probing pocket depths (PPD)
- Peri-implant bone loss (radiograph)

725 "Therapy Cascade"— CIST
   C Cumulative
   I Interceptive
   S Supportive
   T Therapy

The check-list (right) can be a big help to the dental hygienist; she is, after all, responsible for the recall organization and for early recognition of therapeutic problems. Treatment "package" **A** is initiated in all cases where the disease is *progressing*.

Note: **E** stands for *hopeless*, a virtual synonym for *implant loss*.

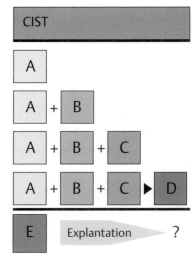

PPD mm	PI Plaque	BOP Bleeding	Bone Loss	CIST
≤3	–/+	–/+	–	A
4–5	+	+	–	A + B
>5	+	+	≤2 mm ↓	A + B + C
	+	+	>2 mm ↓	A + B + C ▶ D
Mobility / pain		Clinical and radiographic findings		E Explantation ?

Cumulative Management—Treatment Classes

A-E in the table (above) represent aspects of treatment that must be enhanced according to the "CIST" classes (Mombelli et al. 2003):

Procedure A—Mechanical Debridement
With inflammation (mucositis and probing depths to 3 mm): Mechanical cleaning of the implant using rubber cup and paste, calculus removal using plastic instruments.

Procedures A+B—Antiseptic Therapy
With suppuration, an early symptom of the destruction of peri-implant tissues, and 4–5 mm deep pockets: Treatment A plus pocket rinsing with CHX 0.2%; the patient should also use CHX spray or at-home pocket irrigation.

Procedures A+B+C—Antibiotic Therapy
With probing depths above 5 mm and bone loss (radiography → peri-implantitis): Microbiologic tests may be indicated (Mombelli et al. 1987, Mombelli & Lang 1992, Luterbacher et al. 2000): Procedures A+B with additional antibiotic therapy against anaerobic microorganisms (systemic metronidazole, 1 g for 10 days, or topical application of "controlled released drugs," e. g., Atridox etc.).

Procedures A+B+C+D—Regenerative or Resective
With significant bone loss it may be necessary to intervene surgically (D) following antibiotic administration, in order to avoid osseo-disintegration of the implant. The surgical procedure may be resective, or one may attempt a regenerative-augmentive procedure in order to fill the osseous defect, following detoxification of the exposed implant surface (acids, mechanical removal of rough implant layers, "sandblasting" with biocompatible abrasive powders etc.); in extreme cases, re-osseointegration can be tried and may occur (Wetzel et al. 1999). Such more radical procedures may prevent loss of the dental implant.

Procedure E—Extraction, Explantation
Explantation. Pain and mobility indicate loss of osseointegration, a "failed implant." The implant should be quickly removed in order to give the "alveolus" the best possibility for regeneration. Thus, later, at the same site, a new implant can be placed.

Note: Oral hygiene and the absolutely necessary and regular implant follow-up professional care must always be performed using instruments that do not scratch the implant surface. With such routine care, implants can be maintained into old age.

Geriatric Periodontology?—The Periodontium in the Elderly

Different Circumstances—Modified Concepts of Treatment

The percentage of elderly individuals within the entire population continues to increase, but differences exist between the "Third World" and the industrialized nations (Fig. 726).

Problem 1 for dentistry and dental hygiene is the increasingly wide chasm between that which is *absolutely necessary* and that which is *possible*. This intriguing development brings with it socioeconomic considerations, technical health insurance matters and medical-ethical dilemmas, the magnitude of which has only been recognized in recent years.

The World Health Organization categorizes our aging population in four classes:

- Aging individuals   45–60 years old
- Older individuals   61–75 years old
- Old individuals   76–90 years old
- Very old individuals   91–100 years old

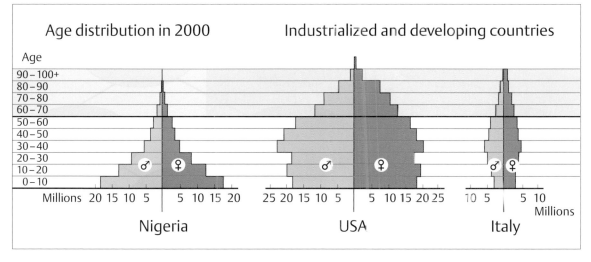

726 Age Distribution in a Developing Country and in Industrialized Nations
In the "Third World" (example, Nigeria), one observes a high birth rate resulting in a broad and youthful population pyramid. The USA exhibits a "belly-like" age pyramid, which has resulted from a certain reduction in birth rate and a much higher life expectancy. The Italian curve exhibits the same shape as that of the USA, but is dramatically slimmer because of the significantly lower total population.

It is clear, of course, that the overall state of health of individual persons cannot be considered solely on the basis of age. Much more than age, each individual's physical, psychic and spectral conditions are most meaningful for individual quality of life. Diseases and the medications used to treat them may therefore prejudge dental treatment planning (ASA classification, medical history; p. 212).

Despite the increasing number of elderly persons, fewer complete dentures are fabricated today compared to earlier decades. This is likely due to enhanced knowledge of the etiology and pathogenesis of dental and periodontal structures in the second half of the twentieth century, which has

increased enormously. This knowledge has led to comprehensive and intensive prophylaxis, which continues its effectiveness even into old age.

In addition, dental treatment techniques and preventive strategies have continued to develop and to be refined, so that a significantly extended maintenance of the natural teeth is virtually guaranteed.

Age-related Changes—Influence Upon Treatment Planning

In this *Atlas*, we have repeatedly stated that certain prerequisites must be fulfilled before initiation of comprehensive periodontitis treatment:

- Time, understanding and resiliency of the patient
- Persistent and appropriate compliance with regard to oral hygiene
- Good general systemic health
- Reduction of risk factors

Even in elderly individuals, these prerequisites can surely also remain, if the patient is psychologically and physically healthy. Particularly, the elderly today often *demand* optimum treatment, similar to that offered to younger patients. These older patients seek no compromises in their treatment, simply because they are old! They often do not even want to compromise when it comes to oral esthetics.

On the other hand, some elderly patients will not fulfill the above-listed criteria for periodontal therapy, or fulfill them only partially. Their reduced capacities ("it is no longer worth it"!) must often lead to therapeutic compromises. In many cases, the mental capacity/understanding for systematic treatment is lacking. Only the "most necessary" or pain-alleviating treatment should be performed: The patient, in

her/his age-related inflexibility, often knows better what to do—or what not to do—than the dental team itself.

Also severe systemic diseases such as diabetes, Alzheimer's, tumors, autoimmune disease, Parkinson's, hematologic disorders, and medication side effects must influence the oral/dental treatment plan significantly.

In general, manual dexterity decreases with age. Elderly patients with diseases such as those listed above may often not understand the importance of oral hygiene, or may be incapable of performing it. It is not always possible to replace the manual toothbrush with an electric device or by medicinal oral rinsing (CHX; cf. p. 235). The result is often greater plaque accumulation, and as a result, gingivitis and even periodontitis. Statistical studies have demonstrated that periodontal diseases develop more rapidly and more severely in the elderly as compared to young persons (Imfeld 1985). *Nevertheless*, periodontitis can no longer be categorized as a "disease of aging."

In addition to the previously discussed systemic health problems and oral hygiene difficulties of elderly patients, the dentition will also exhibit manifestations of age such as attrition, abrasion, gingival recession and tooth discoloration.

729 80-Year-Old Male
This mentally alert patient suffered from mild Parkinson's disease. He had major difficulties with mechanical oral hygiene, but wanted to have "clean" teeth. Following professional tooth cleaning and periodontal therapy, an electric toothbrush was demonstrated, and a case-specific rinsing regimen with CHX (with the help of the patient's family), and the patient was scheduled for short-interval recall.

Right: CHX rinsing program.

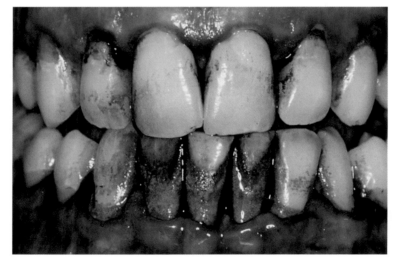

**CHX Rinsing Program—
Two Possible Regimens**

A

1 month long, daily 2 x CHX,
  0.1–0.2 %
3 months *no* CHX
1 month CHX
3 months *no* CHX

B

Daily low dose CHX rinsing
(0.06 %) as a permanent replacement for the patient's insufficient home care
(e. g., retirement home!)

Modified Treatment Planning

Old but still mentally and physically healthy patients usually do not require any changes in dental treatment planning. However, in patients who are mentally and/or physically handicapped, the treatment plan must be adapted to the actual situation. Teeth with a questionable prognosis should probably be extracted. A perhaps somewhat extreme approach would be to treat periodontally only those teeth that can be expected to be maintained until life's end.

Missing teeth in non-visible jaw segments beg the question of whether replacement is necessary. If replacement is un-

avoidable for functional reasons, a removable partial denture is often preferable to a fixed reconstruction.
It is better to incorporate a dental prosthesis at an age at which the patient can become accustomed to it, instead of persisting with years-long (decades-long) periodontal therapy, leading finally only to a complete denture that the patient can no longer successfully accept.

Teeth need not be maintained "at all costs" in elderly patients; rather it is the sense of oral well-being (health, function, phonetics, esthetics) and therewith the patient's own feeling of self worth.

Classification of Periodontal Diseases

Most Recent Re-Classification of Periodontal Diseases (1999)

As demonstrated in the chapter "Forms of Plaque-associated Diseases" (p. 79), new scientific and clinical findings, accumulating long-term experiences as well as the rapid exchange of this knowledge (internet) resulted in the necessity to freshly define the classifications and nomenclature of diseases and clinical "conditions."

Toward the end of 1999, a workshop in Oak Brook, Illinois, was convened with members of the American Academy of Periodontology (AAP) and the European Federation of Periodontology (EFP), and the result of this meeting is presented on the following two pages as the original and unabridged illustration of the new classification (Types I-VIII), as published by Armitage (1999) in *Annals of Periodontology*.

Type	1999 Classification of periodontal disorders
I	**Gingival diseases**
II	**Chronic periodontitis**
III	**Aggressive periodontitis**
IV	**Periodontitis as a manifestation of systemic disease**
V	**Necrotizing periodontal diseases**
VI	**Periodontal abscess**
VII	**Periodontitis in combination with endodontic lesions**
VIII	**Developmental or inherited conditions**

730 Periodontal Disease Types—Classification, 1999
The new classification of periodontal disease in eight primary groups/types will be depicted on the following two pages, including all subclassifications.

Classification 1999—For and Against

The "old classification" (AAP 1989) described five disease classes. This classification too heavily weighted the *patient age at disease onset*—e.g., "early onset periodontitis," EOP and "adult periodontitis," AP, as well as the course of the disease, e.g., rapidly-progressing (EOP/RPP). It was necessary to change this type of classification because "rapidly progressive periodontitis" (RPP) does not occur only in young patients, and also a chronic periodontitis (AP) in elderly patients with reduced immune function can unexpectedly and quickly evolve into an acute status.

But even the new 1999 classification will only last for a limited period of time: It is too all-inclusive and *combines* the disease entities that are *practice-relevant* and most common with those disease entities that are rather quite rare. The 1999 classification is similar in many ways to the extensive catalog provided by the WHO list of diseases, but does not consider the multifactorial character of periodontal diseases (risks!).

This problem has been described thematically in numerous subsequent publications (Van der Velden 2000, Burgermeister & Schlagenhauf 2002, Brunner et al. 2002, DGP 2002, Bengel 2003, Lang 2003).

Classification 1999—Gingiva

731 Classification—Original Version (AAP 1999)
This classification of periodontal diseases has been universally accepted world-wide, and is presented here in its original and unabridged English text version (abbreviated classification, p. 78).

Gingival Diseases
These occur in the periodontal tissues *without* simultaneous periodontal attachment or bone loss.

(Even with periodontitis, one of the primary symptoms is gingival disease.)

Plaque-induced Gingival Diseases (A)
Above all, plaque-induced gingivitis (type I A) is a ubiquitous disease. It occurs more or less in all oral, periodontal diseases and is easy to treat. Deeper periodontal structures are not affected within this definition.

Non Plaque-induced Gingival Lesions (B)
Also with these disease processes, an "additional" plaque-induced gingivitis may be present.
This is a group of diseases/lesions that are relatively seldom observed. Exceptions: Viral lesions that affect the periodontal tissues as well as the oral mucosa. Treatment may be difficult, with varying success results. In many cases, medical specialists must be called upon, especially in life-threatening forms (e. g., *Pemphigus vulgaris*; I B 5a 3).

Type I—Gingival Diseases
- **A.** Dental plaque-induced gingival diseases
  1. Gingivitis associated with dental plaque only
     a. without other local contributing factors
     b. with local contributing factors (see VIII A)
  2. Gingival diseases modified by systemic factors
     a. associated with the endocrine system
        1) puberty-associated gingivitis
        2) menstrual cycle-associated gingivitis
        3) pregnancy-associated
           a) gingivitis
           b) pyogenic granuloma
        4) diabetes mellitus-associated gingivitis
     b. associated with blood dyscrasias
        1) leukemia-associated gingivitis
        2) other
  3. Gingival diseases modified by medications
     a. drug-influenced gingival diseases
        1) drug-influenced gingival enlargements
        2) drug-influenced gingivitis
           a) oral contraceptive-associated gingivitis
           b) other
  4. Gingival diseases modified by malnutrition
     a. ascorbid acid-deficiency gingivitis
     b. other

- **B.** Non-plaque-induced gingival lesions
  1. Gingival diseases of specific bacterial origin
     a. *Neisseria gonorrhea*-associated lesions
     b. *Treponema pallidum*-associated lesions
     c. streptococcal species-associated lesions
     d. other
  2. Gingival diseases of viral origin
     a. herpes virus infections
        1) primary herpetic gingivostomatitis
        2) recurrent oral herpes
        3) varicella-zoster infections
     b. other
  3. Gingival diseases of fungal origin
     a. *Candida*-species infections
        1) generalized gingival candidosis
     b. linear gingival erythema
     c. histoplasmosis
     d. other
  4. Gingival lesions of genetic origin
     a. hereditary gingival fibromatosis
     b. other
  5. Gingival manifestations of systemic conditions
     a. mucocutaneous disorders
        1) lichen planus
        2) pemphigoid
        3) pemphigus vulgaris
        4) erythema multiforme
        5) lupus erythematosus
        6) drug-induced
        7) other
     b. allergic reactions
        1) dental restorative materials
           a) mercury
           b) nickel
           c) acrylic
           d) other
        2) reactions attributable to
           a) toothpaste/dentifrices
           b) mouthrinses/mouthwashes
           c) chewing gum additives
           d) other
  6. Traumatic lesions (factitious, iatrogenic, accidental)
     a. chemical injury
     b. physical injury
     c. thermal injury
  7. Foreign body reactions
  8. Not otherwise specified (NOS)

Type I—Gingival Diseases
- **Plaque-induced Gingival Diseases**
  - gingivitis caused solely by plaque
  - gingivitis modified by systemic factors

  - Gingival diseases modified by medications

  - Gingival diseases modified by malnutrition

- **Non Plaque-induced Gingival Lesions**
  - specific bacterial lesions

  - viral lesions

  - fungal lesions

  - genetically-elicited lesions

  - systemically-related lesions

  - traumatic lesions

  - foreign body reactions
  - others

**Type II—
Chronic Periodontitis, CP**

**Type III—
Aggressive Periodontitis, AP**

**Type IV—Periodontitis
with Systemic Diseases**

- blood dyscrasia
- genetic factors

- non-specified

Type V—Necrotizing Gingivitis (NUG) and Periodontitis (NUP)

Type VI—Abscesses

Type VII—Periodontitis in Combination with Endodontic Lesions

Type VIII—Developmental and Inherited Deformities and Conditions

- localized dental factors, which enhance plaque retention
- mucogingival problems within the dental arch
- mucogingival problems within the edentulous alveolar ridge
- occlusal trauma

Classification 1999—Periodontium

Type II **Chronic Periodontitis (CP)** * *
- **A.** Localized
- **B.** Generalized

Type III **Aggressive Periodontitis (AP)** * *
- **A.** Localized
- **B.** Generalized

Type IV **Periodontitis as a Manifestation of Systemic Diseases**
- **A.** Associated with hematologic disorders
  1. Acquired neutropenia
  2. Leukemia
  3. Other
- **B.** Associated with genetic disorders
  1. Familial and cyclic neutropenia
  2. Down syndrome
  3. Leukocyte adhesion deficiency syndromes
  4. Papillon-Lefèvre syndrome
  5. Chediak-Higashi syndrome
  6. Histiocytosis syndromes
  7. Glycogen storage disease
  8. Infantile genetic agranulocytosis
  9. Cohen syndrome
  10. Ehlers-Danlos syndrome (Types IV and VIII)
  11. Hypophosphatasia
  12. Other
- **C.** Not otherwise specified (NOS)

Type V **Necrotizing Periodontal Diseases**
- **A.** Necrotizing ulcerative gingivitis (NUG)
- **B.** Necrotizing ulcerative periodontitis (NUP)

Type VI **Abscesses of the Periodontium**
- **A.** Gingival abscess
- **B.** Periodontal abscess
- **C.** Pericoronal abscess

Type VII **Periodontitis Associated with Endodontic Lesions**
- **A.** Combined periodontal-endodontic lesions

Type VIII **Developmental or Acquired Deformities and Conditions**
- **A.** Localized tooth-related factors that modify or predispose to plaque-induced gingival diseases/periodontitis
  1. Tooth anatomic factors
  2. Dental anatomic factors
  3. Root fractures
  4. Cervical root resorption and cemental tears
- **B.** Mucogingival deformities and conditions around teeth
  1. Gingival/soft tissue recession
     a. facial or lingual surfaces
     b. interproximal (papillary)
  2. Lack of keratinized gingiva
  3. Decreased vestibular depth
  4. Aberrant frenum/muscle position
  5. Gingival excess
     a. pseudopocket
     b. inconsistent gingival margin
     c. excessive gingival display
     d. gingival enlargement (see I A3 and I B4)
  6. Abnormal color
- **C.** Mucogingival deformities and conditions on edentulous ridges
  1. Vertical and/or horizontal ridge deficiency
  2. Lack of gingiva/keratinized tissue
  3. Gingival/soft tissue enlargement
  4. Aberrant frenum/muscle position
  5. Decreased vestibular depth
  6. Abnormal color
- **D.** Occlusal trauma
  1. Primary occlusal trauma
  2. Secondary occlusal trauma

732 Periodontitis—Types II to VIII

Chronic (II) and Aggressive (III) Periodontitis

Chronic periodontitis (previously AP) is the most common form of the disease (> 80 % of all cases).

More aggressive forms (formerly EOP, as PP, LJP, RPP are rare).

In addition to the *pathobiologic* form (p. 96), the *pathomorphologic* expanse (p. 98) and the localization of the attachment loss must be considered:

*** * Localized/Generalized**
In a case with less than 30 % involvement of all sites, the case is categorized as *localized*.
More serious and expansive involvement is categorized as *generalized*.

*** * Degree of Severity**
Clinical attachment loss (CAL) is described as follows:

- "slight" up to 2 mm
- "moderate" 3–4 mm
- "severe" 5+ mm

* *In addition to the globally accepted AAP-Classification (1999), one must also consider the degree of severity (CAL) alone and with the corresponding prospective therapeutic involvement, as described in the ADA/AAP classification of "*case patterns*" or "*case types*" (American Dental Association):

ADA—"Case Types"

• Grade	Severity Evaluation
I	Gingivitis – 3 degrees of severity
II	Early periodontitis
III	Moderate periodontitis
IV	Advanced periodontitis

Changes—Comparing the 1989 and 1999 Classifications

Any classification of a complicated disease process can only be an attempt to describe the *overall* disease process in a short format, hopefully leading to better understanding of the complex nature over the long-term.

Therefore, it is not possible to assess/address alongside the name of the disease, also the etiologies, the initiation, the clinical condition and its severity and course, and ultimately the causes of the specific disease types in simple terms, or to distinguish the individual disease process from other diseases.

On the other hand, a classification may elicit and describe the relevance and the prevalence of the disease process, and therefore target the therapeutic energies of each dental practitioner!

The authors of this *Atlas* have attempted to use the new classification, while also noting the previous system. Above all, it was our goal to describe and portray the *most important periodontal disease forms* in our text and illustrations for the dental hygienist, dentist and periodontist.

733 Changes and Alterations within the 1999 AAP Classification
These are depicted in the table (right).

The term "apical" is retained for the more rare forms of periodontitis.

Note: Reasonable abbreviations for the new classifications are for the most part lacking!

Modified from *Meyle et al. 2002; DGP/QV*

1989/99	Changes in the classification	1989 5 classes	1999 8 types
⊕	• Enhancement of the classification "gingival disorders"	—	I
	• Enhancement of the classification "periodontal abscess"	—	VI
	• Enhancement of the classification "periodontitis in conjunction with endodontic lesions"	—	VII
	• Enhancement of the classification "developmental or genetic conditions"	—	VIII
△	• Differentiation among the term "periodontitis as a manifestation of systemic disease"	III	IV
▶○▶	• Replacement of the term "adult periodontitis" with the term "chronic periodontitis"	I AP	II CP
	• Replacement of the term "early onset periodontitis" with the term "aggressive periodontitis"	II EOP $\begin{smallmatrix}PPP\\LJP\\RPP\end{smallmatrix}$	III AP
	• Replacement of the term "necrotizing ulcerative periodontitis" with the term " necrotizing periodontal disease"	IV ANUG/P	V NUG/P
⊖	• Elimination of the terms "refractory and recurrent periodontitis" as individual categories	V RP	✕

Limitations—Examples of Criticism

The new classification (1999) has too many sub-classifications (hierarchy); for example, pregnancy gingivitis is found in I A 2a 3a/b! In addition, it would appear to be totally impractical that the most commonly occurring disease entities are not identified with simple abbreviations, except for CP, AP, NUG/NUP.
Possibly the most important chapter in this *Atlas*, "Oral manifestations of HIV-infection and AIDS " (p. 142) is not even *listed* in the new classification, even though this severe immunodeficiency not only manifests as necrotizing ulcerative gingivitis/periodontitis (NUG/NUP), but also as a specific "linear gingival erythema," and a long list of opportunistic secondary infections in the oral mucosa and periodontium (bacterial, viral and fungal infections, as well as tumors such as the Kaposi sarcoma, p. 146).

"Classical gingival recession," which has become more and more common in industrialized nations in recent years (p. 155), is classified under VIIIB1a, "mucogingival deformations and conditions." Any "soft tissue recession" usually oc-

curs only after some form of osseous dehiscence. Whether this "condition" should be classified as a disease or only as a morphologic variation of the healthy periodontium is really irrelevant for a dental hygienist (improper oral hygiene, functional dysfunction).

Each dental hygienist and dentist must come to grips with the fact that the patient is not interested only in oral health but also, more and more, esthetic problems (gingival recession, "long teeth"), which can only be addressed through mucogingival/plastic surgery.

In the most recent classification, entire disease entities are not represented (infectious diseases—HIV/AIDS), or are inadequately represented (gingival recession), and some "conditions" such as pericoronal abscess (VI C) find themselves on the highest level.

Acknowledgments for Figures

The individuals listed below provided us with illustrative materials for this publication.
All other illustrations and figures derived from the archives of the authors, and Drs. K.H. & E.M. Rateitschak (University of Basle), their departments or private practices.

Photographs of objects were made exclusively by author Herbert F. Wolf.

All of the *histologic illustrations*—with exception of special illustrations—were provided to us by Dr. Alice Kallenberger (emeritus, Basle).

All of the *schematic and graphic illustrations* were prepared and provided, according to detailed illustrations by H.F. Wolf, by the scientific illustration company B. Struchen & Partner (Zurich), and by J. Hormann, Graphic Design (Stuttgart).

Because many of the figures contain more than one photograph, each acknowledgement contains an exact description of the donor's contribution (e. g., L, M or R for left, middle or right; A, B, C etc.).

University of Basle, Switzerland

B. Maeglin	261L, 262, 265, 266–268, 271, 271R, 272, 272L, 273, 275, 275R, 276, 276R
B. Daiker	285, 285L, 286, 286L
R. Guggenheim	255L
J. Meyer	71, 71L
H. Müller	290
L. Ritz	638–643
B. Widmer	247

University of Berne, Switzerland

D. Bosshardt	S. 6, 26R, 28L, 30L
N. Lang	21R, 23, 25L, 278
M. Grassi	320R

University of California, San Francisco, USA

G. Armitage	377
J. Winkler	310

University of Geneva, Switzerland

G. Cimasoni	47, 360
A. Mombelli	410–412, 662, 663

Loma Linda University, USA

J. Egelberg	37R, 155R, 158R

University of Pennsylvania, Philadelphia, USA

M A. Listgarten	45, 46, 46L, 54, 563

University of Zurich, Switzerland

B. Guggenheim	56, 56R, 57, 58, 58L, 59, 73R, 75R
F. Lutz	51L
W. Mörmann	38
H. R. Mühlemann	13R, 269R
P. Schüpbach	S. 200
H. Schroeder	18, 18L, 19, 23L, 26R–28L, 31R, 32, 48R, 455, 446

Dental Hygiene School, PSZN Zurich-North, Switzerland

U. Saxer	270, 299, 301, 653–655

Private practitioners

U. Hersberger (Frenkendorf, BL)	239–241, 244
F. Wolgensinger (Kilchberg, ZH)	11

Periodontology—Related specialties

- Dental Hygiene
- Basics
- Types
- Findings, diagnosis
- Prevention
- Initial treatment—Phase 1 therapy
- Medicaments
- Surgical treatment—Phase 2 therapy
- Phase 3 therapy—Maintenance therapy (see Dental Hygiene) Recall
- Esthetic integration
- Varia

Dental Hygiene

Allen DL, McFall WT, Jenzano JW. Periodontics for the Dental Hygienist, 4th Ed. Philadelphia: Lea & Fibeger; 1987.

Botticelli AT. Manual of Dental Hygiene. London: Quintessence; 2002.

Daniel ST, Harfst SA 9th Eds, Mosby's Dental Hygiene Concepts, Cases, and Competencies. St. Louis: Mosby; 2002

Darby ML (ed.). Mosby's Comprehensive Review of Dental Hygiene, 5th Ed. St. Louis: Mosby; 2002.

Haring JI, Jansen L. Dental Radiography, Principles and Techniques, 2nd Ed. Philadelphia: WB Saunders; 2000.

Nathe CN. Dental Public Health: Contemporary Practice for the Dental Hygienist, 2nd Ed. Upper Saddle River, NJ: Pearson-Prentice Hall; 2005

Neild-Gehrig JS, Fundamentals of Periodontal Instrumentation, 5th edition, Lippincott, Williams and Wilkins 2000, ISBN 0-7807-2860-6.

Phagan-Schostok PA, Maloney KL. Contemporary Dental Hygiene Practice. Chicago: Quintessence; 1988.

Walsh TF, Figures KH, Lamb DJ. Clinical Dental Hygiene: A Handbook for the Dental Team. Oxford: Wright; 1992.

Wilkins EM, Clinical Practice of the Dental Hygienist, 8th edition, Lippincott, Williams and Wilkins 1999, ISBN 0-683-30362-7.

Wilkins EM, Clinical Practice of the Dental Hygienist, 9th Ed. Philadelphia: Lippincott Williams & Wilkins; 2005.

Woodall IR. Comprehensive Dental Hygiene Care, 4th Ed. St. Louis: Mosby; 1993.

Wyche C, Wilkins EM. Student Workbook for Clinical Practice of the Dental Hygienist. Philadelphia: Lippincott Williams & Wilkins; 2005.

Basics

Abbas AK, Lichtman AH, Prober JS. Immunologie. Bern: Huber; 1996.

Avery JK, Steele PF. Essentials of Oral Histology and Embryology: A Clinical Approach. St. Louis: Mosby; 1992.

Bartold PM, Narayanan AS. Biology of the Periodontal Connective Tissues. Chicago: Quintessence Books; 1998.

Bergquist LM, Pogosian B. Microbiology: Principles and Health Science Applications. Philadelphia: WB Saunders; 2000.

Cohen S, Burns RC (eds.). Pathways of the Pulp, 7th Ed. St. Louis: Mosby; 1998.

Fejerskov O, Ekstrand J, Burt BA (eds.). Fluoride in Dentistry, 2nd Ed. Copenhagen: Munksgaard; 1996.

Gemsa D, Kalden JR, Resch K, eds. Immunologie. 4. Aufl. Stuttgart: Thieme; 1997.

Genco R, Goldman HM, Cohen DW. Periodontics Contemporary Standards. St. Louis: Mosby; 1990.

Genco R, Hamada S, Lehner T, McGhee J, Mergenhagen S. Molecular Pathogenesis of Periodontal Disease. Washington D.C.: ASM Press; 1994.

Genetics in Dentistry: Focus Group Research with Dental Health Professionals Rockville, MD: US Department of Health and Human Services, National Institutes of Health, National Institute of Dental and Craniofacial Research, March 2003.

Hamada S, Holt SC, McGhee JR, eds. Periodontal Disease. Pathogens and Host Immune Responses. Tokyo: Quintessence; 1991.

Ibsen OAC, Phelan JA. Oral Pathology for the Dental Hygienist, 3rd Ed. Philadelphia: WB Saunders; 2000.

Jansen van Rensburg BG. Oral Biology. Chicago: Quintessence; 1995.

Karlson P, Doenecke D, Koolman J. Kurzes Lehrbuch der Biochemie. 14. Aufl. Stuttgart: Thieme; 1994.

Marsh P, Martin MV. Oral Microbiology, 4th Ed. Oxford: Wright; 1999.

Page RC, Schroeder HE. Periodontitis in Man and Other Animals. A Comparative Review. Basel: Karger; 1982.

Roitt I, Brostoff J, Male D. Immunology. London: Gower; 1985.

Roitt IM, Brostoff J, Male DK. Kurzes Lehrbuch der Immunologie. 3. Aufl. Stuttgart: Thieme; 1995.

Samaranayake LP. Essential Microbiology for Dentistry. New York: Chuchill Livingstone; 1996.

Sanderink RBA, Bernhardt H, Knoke M, Meyer J, Weber C, Weiger R. Orale Mikrobiologie und Immunologie. Berlin 2004.

Schroeder HE. Formation and Inhibition of Dental Calculus. Vienna: Hans Huber Publishers: 1969.

Schroeder HE, Listgarten MA. Fine Structure of the Developing Epithelial Attachment of Human Teeth. 2nd ed. Basel: Karger; 1977.

Schroeder HE. The Periodontium. Berlin: Springer; 1986.

Ten Cate AR. Oral Histology, Development, Structure and Function, 5th Ed. St. Louis: Mosby; 1998.

Zinkernagl RM. In: Kayser FH, Bienz KA, Eckert J, Zinkernagl RM. Medizinische Mikrobiologie. Stuttgart: Thieme; 1998, S. 76–78.

Disease manifestations including HIV/AIDS

DeVita VT, Hellman S, Rosenberg SA (eds.). AIDS: Etiology, Diagnosis, Treatment and Prevention, 4th Ed. Philadelphia: Lippincott-Raven; 1997.

Greenspan D, Greenspan JS, Schidt M, Pindborg JJ. AIDS and the Mounth: Diagnosis and Management of Oral Lesions. Copenhagen: Munksgaard; 1990.

Hassell TM. Epilepsy and the Oral Manifestations of Phenytoin Therapy. Basel: Karger; 1981.

Keyes GG, Waithe ME. HIV Infection in Dentistry: Ethical and Legal Issues. In, Weinstein BD. Dental Ethics. Philadelphia: Lea & Febiger; 1993.

Little JW, Falace DA, Miller CS, Thodus NL. Dental Management of the Medically Compromised Patient, 5th Ed. St. Louis: Mosby; 1997.

Pindborg JJ. Atlas of Diseases of the Oral Mucosa. Copenhagen: Munksgaard; 1985.

Reichert PA, Philipsen HP. Color Atlas of Dental Medicine—Oral Pathology. New York and Stuttgart: Thieme Medical Publishers; 2000.

Clinical findings, Diagnosis

Armitage GC. Development of a Classification System for Periodontal Diseases and Conditions. Annals of Periodontology 1999; 4: 1–6.

Axelsson P. Periodontal Diseases. Diagnosis and Risk Prediction. Vol. 3. Chicago: Quintessence; 2002.

Egelberg J, Claffey N. Periodontal Re-Evaluation—The Scientific Way. Copenhagen: Munksgaard; 1994.

Egelberg J. Periodontics—The Scientific Way. 2nd ed. Malmö: Odonto Science; 1995.

Mueller-Joseph L, Petersen M. Dental Hygiene Process: Diagnosis and Care Planning. Albany: Delmar; 1995.

Prevention

Axelsson P. An Introduction to Risk Prediction and Preventive Dentistry. Preventive Dentistry. Chicago: Quintessence; 1999.

Benenson AS (ed.) Control of Communicable Diseases in Man 16th Ed. Washington, DC: American Public Health Association; 1995.

Cuttone JA, Terezhalmy GT, Molinari JA. Practical Infection Control in Dentistry, 2nd Ed. Philadelphia: William & Wilkins; 1996.

Harris NO, Christien AG. Primary Preventive Dentistry, 4th Ed. Norwalk, CT: Appleton &Lange; 1995.

Malamed SF. Handbook of Medical Emergencies in the Dental Office, 5th Ed. St. Louis: Mosby; 2000.

Phase 1 therapy—Initial treatment

Dionne RA, Phero JC, Becker DE. Management of Pain and Anxiety in the Dental Office. Philadelphia: WB Saunders; 2002.

Hodges KO. Concepts in Non-Surgical Periodontal Therapy. New York: Delmar; 1997.

Hodges KO (ed.). Concepts in Non-Surgical Periodontal Therapy. Albany, NY: Delmar; 1998.

Lang NP, Attström R, Löe H. Proceedings of the European Workshop on Mechanical Plaque Control. Chicago: Quintessence; 1998.

Nield-Gehrig JS, Houseman GA. Fundamentals of Periodontal Instrumentation, 3rd Ed. Baltimore: Williams & Wilkins; 1996.

Pattison G, Pattison AM. Periodontal Instrumentation. Restor Reston Publ.; 1979.

Pattison AM, Pattison G. Periodontal Instrumentation, 2nd Ed. Norwalk, CT: Appleton & Lange; 1992.

Schoen DH, Dean M-C. Contemporary Periodontal Instrumentation. Philadelphia: WB Saunders; 1996.

Medicaments

American Dental Association, Council on Scientific Affairs: ADA Guide to Dental Therapeutics, 2nd Ed. Chicago: ADA Publishing Co.; 2000.

Lang NP, Karring T, Lindhe J. Proceedings of the 2nd European Workshop on Periodontology, Chemicals in Periodontics. London: Quintessenz; 1996.

Lowinson JH, Ruiz P, Millman RB, Langrod JG (eds.). Substance Abuse: A Comprehensive Textbook, 3rd Ed. Baltimore: Williams&Wilkins; 1997.

Mandel ID. Chemical Agents for Control of Plaque and Gingivitis; Committee on Research, Science and Therapy, American Academy of Periodontology—Position Paper. Chicago: April 1994. See www.perio.org.

Newman MG, van Winkelhoff AJ. Antibiotic and Antimicrobial Use in Dental Practice. Chicago: Quintessence; 2001.

Rose LF, Genco, RJ, Cohen, DW, Mealey BL (eds.) Periodontal Medicine. Hamilton, ONT: BC Decker; 2000.

Phase 2 therapy—Surgical treatment

Polson AM. Periodontal Regeneration. Chicago: Quintessence; 1994.

Wennström J, Heijl L, Lindhe J. Periodontal Surgery: Access Therapy. In: Lindhe J, Karring T, Lang NP. Clinical Periodontology and Implant Dentistry. 3rd ed. Copenhagen: Munksgaard; 1997, pp. 508–549.

Esthetic integration

Cohen ES. Atlas of Cosmetic and Reconstructive Periodontal Surgery. 2nd ed. Philadelphia: Lea & Febiger; 1994.

Magne P, Belser U. Bonded Porcelain Restorations. Chicago: Quintessence; 2002.

Varia

Beemsterboer PL. Ethics and Law in Dental Hygiene. Philadelphia: WB Saunders; 2001.

Bricker SL, Langlais RP, Miller CS. Oral Diagnosis, Oral Medicine, and Treatment Planning, 2nd Ed. Hamilton: BC Decker; 2002.

Carranza F, Shklar G. History of Periodontology. Chicago: Quintessence; 2003.

Dennis C, Gallagher R. The Human Genome. London: Palgrave/Nature; 2001.

Gladwin M, Bagby M. Clinical Aspects of Dental Materials. Philadelphia: Lippincott Williams & Wilkins; 2000.

Malamed SF. Sedation. 3rd ed. St. Louis: Mosby; 1995.

McDonald RE, Avery DR. Dentistry for Children and the Adolescent, 7th Ed. St. Louis: Mosby; 2000.

Palmer CA. Diet and Nutrition in Oral Health. New Jersey: Prentice Hall; 2003.

Reichel W (ed.). Care of the Elderly: Clinical Aspects of Aging, 4th Ed. Baltimore: Williams & Wilkins; 1995.

Schijatschky MM. Life-threatening Emergencies in Dental Practice. Berlin: Quintessenz; 1992.

Spallek H, Spallek G. The Global Village of Dentistry. Berlin: Quintessence; 1997.

Index